How Animals Heal Us

'Weaving humour, empathy, pathos and so much more, Griffiths shows that animals are braided throughout the human psyche. An absolute fountain of fact, culture and raw animal power!' Carl Safina, author of *Beyond Words: What Animals Think and Feel*

'A book of boundless passion and compassion. As she explores the worlds of animals, Jay Griffiths makes the case for a different way of living: a joyous, vital inclusivity. This is how a book should be – genuinely mind-expanding'
Tom Bullough, author of *Sarn Helen*

'Griffiths's genius is to reveal the familiar as wondrous, strange, miraculous. Incredible and heart-wrenching, this gift of a book will shift your relationship to animals'
Ben Rawlence, author of *The Treeline*

'Deeply researched and highly readable, this is a moving and exquisitely written exploration of how we are shaped by different creatures, from tigers to teddy bears'
Caroline Eden, author of *Samarkand*

'Griffiths weaves a poetic tapestry of wonders; a searing, soaring manifesto for reviving our vital communion with other creatures'
Natalie Lawrence, author of *Enchanted Creatures*

'A wise, deep, and tender account of animal healing, written in lyrical language that sings with compassion' Pascale Petit, author of *My Hummingbird Father*

'Jay Griffiths is an artist, and this book is poetry – buzzing with courage and honesty. *How Animals Heal Us* is wonder and grief combined, speaking passionately to vibrant ways of being, a true visionary work' Laura Coleman, author of *The Puma Years*

'Imagine meeting someone on a train who turns to you and starts telling you the most amazing stories about animals. Each one makes you go "Wow!" And she can talk for hours – eloquently, magically. This is Jay Griffiths. Then she puts it all in a wonderful book, and you can return to these tales again and again' David Rothenberg, author of *Why Birds Sing*

'An exhilarating epic journey that made me see our companions through Griffiths's fresh and compassionate eyes. What we owe our fellow animals is humbling' Gwyneth Lewis, author of *Nightshade Mother: A Disentangling*

'Revelatory and utterly fascinating, a moving, inspiring and joyous book' James Macdonald Lockhart, author of *Wild Air: In Search of Birdsong*

'A shrewd, funny, tender, downright clever mapping of the human soul; a celebration of the potency of relationship; a prescription that can heal and save, if we'll take it, and an astringent political antiseptic' Charles A. Foster, author of *Being a Beast*

'Beautiful and important . . . Griffiths provides a deeply personal and intelligent account of the vital importance of having animals in our lives, and in our world' Dr Hannah Burgon, author of *Equine-Assisted Therapy and Learning with At-Risk Young People*

'Essential reading . . . When we figure out how to live compassionately alongside animals, we will resolve our human problems . . . That is no easy task, but after reading Griffiths's wonderful book, it is at least an easy choice' Dr Alex Lockwood, author of *The Pig in Thin Air: An Identification*

'I am so grateful to Jay Griffiths for breathing fresh and poetic life into a subject that is not only dear to my heart but that I feel is so crucial to the very survival of the human animal . . . It is my deepest hope that this book reaches as many people as possible' Dr Dawn Prince-Hughes, author of *Songs of the Gorilla Nation: My Journey Through Autism*

BY THE SAME AUTHOR

NON-FICTION

Why Rebel

Nemesis, My Friend

Tristimania: A Diary of Manic Depression

Kith: The Riddle of the Childscape

Wild: An Elemental Journey

Pip Pip: A Sideways Look at Time

FICTION

A Love Letter from a Stray Moon

Anarchipelago

How Animals Heal Us

JAY GRIFFITHS

HAMISH HAMILTON
an imprint of
PENGUIN BOOKS

HAMISH HAMILTON

UK | USA | Canada | Ireland | Australia
India | New Zealand | South Africa

Hamish Hamilton is part of the Penguin Random House group of companies
whose addresses can be found at global.penguinrandomhouse.com

Penguin Random House UK,
One Embassy Gardens, 8 Viaduct Gardens, London SW11 7BW

penguin.co.uk

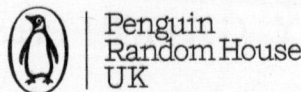

First published 2025

001

Copyright © Jay Griffiths, 2025

The moral right of the author has been asserted

Extract on page 5 from 'Four for Sir John Davies' by Theodore Roethke;
and extract on page 249 from 'The Thought-Fox' in *The Hawk in the Rain*
by Ted Hughes, reproduced by permission of Faber and Faber Ltd

The permissions on page 369 constitute an extension of this copyright page

No part of this book may be used or reproduced in any manner for the
purpose of training artificial intelligence technologies or systems. In accordance
with Article 4(3) of the DSM Directive 2019/790, Penguin Random House
expressly reserves this work from the text and data mining exception

Set in 12.5/16pt Fournier MT Pro
Typeset by Jouve (UK), Milton Keynes
Printed and bound in Great Britain by Clays Ltd, Elcograf S.p.A.

The authorized representative in the EEA is Penguin Random House Ireland,
Morrison Chambers, 32 Nassau Street, Dublin D02 YH68

A CIP catalogue record for this book is available from the British Library

ISBN: 978-0-241-61435-8

Penguin Random House is committed to a sustainable future
for our business, our readers and our planet. This book is made from
Forest Stewardship Council® certified paper

To Tom and Otter, who'll never know,
and to all who listen, with love

Contents

Introduction ... 1

PART ONE
How Animals Heal the Individual Psyche

1. Bouncing with Rude Health ... 5
2. A Remedy for the Lonely ... 26
3. Untangling the Psyche ... 45
4. Oh God, Get That Young Woman a Dog ... 63

PART TWO
How Animals Heal the Individual Body

5. Emergency Services ... 83
6. Dog Doctors ... 105
7. The Animal Apothecaries ... 124
8. Midwives for the Dying ... 142

PART THREE
How Animals Heal the Body Politic

9	Key Signatures for a Sound World	163
10	Wolves at the Core of Ethics	181
11	The Fair Play of Justice	198
12	Political Animals	219

PART FOUR
How Animals Heal the Soul Politic

13	Pink Pink Stink Nice Drink	241
14	Wild Alleluia	262
15	Spiderling, Chickadee, Finch and Friends	279
16	Shifting the Shape of the Mind	296

Coda	317
Notes	319
Select Bibliography	351
Index	361
In Thanks	369

Introduction

While I was working on this book, the research just bubbled out of me. 'Did you know,' I said to a stranger on a train, 'that baby jumping spiders dream?' 'Woodlice!' I said to a friend. '*Woodlice!*' They display emotional contagion, the first building block for empathy. Red deer make decisions by referendum, as do African buffaloes.

I kissed a whale in open waters. I fell in love with a wolf called Wolf 21 and a donkey called Leo. I read studies showing how fairness really matters to some animals. I was tested for Covid by a dog, and met other dogs who can detect diseases including some cancers. Knowing that ravens play King of the Castle, I wondered whether it was a game they taught us.

This book began by taking a thought for a walk. Everyone who's had a pet knows how psychologically healing they are, and may not be surprised that they are also physically medicinal, increasing the cuddle hormone oxytocin and decreasing stress. But I didn't know that lions have saved the life of a kidnapped girl, that the sound of a cat's purr is good for the body, or that a dog can be trained to phone the emergency services. I had no idea that dolphins could lead us to another person in danger, or that whales could guide a boat to safe harbour. I had no sense that animals might put their lives on the line for us, or accompany us in our dying, or that some police dogs have demonstrated a stronger sense of ethics than their handlers. I couldn't have guessed that there are chimpanzees who dance in response to waterfalls and that a particular part of the human brain lights up just for animals.

Writing this was a huge adventure, not only in what I discovered about animals, but also in considering the vastness of what constitutes health. I wanted to look at how animals heal the individual psychologically, which is the subject of Part One. In this, we see how many animals laugh and play, offering us an uninhibited sense of vitality. This part then explores how animals can be therapists for the hurt psyche, how pets are a remedy for loneliness and how when a person is suicidal, sometimes the most important thing may be to get a dog to them as fast as possible.

Part Two considers how animals are healing for the individual physically, how they can work as our first responders, including a pig who saved her owner's life, and a parrot who saved the life of a child. This part explores the work of disease-detection dogs, who can smell an incipient medical event including diabetes and some forms of epilepsy and alert their owners. It looks at how animals self-medicate and how humans have learned from them. It explores how animals may guide us to safety and help us when we're dying, giving us a hospice for the heart.

Part Three looks at how animals are healing for society, the body politic. Music has long been a part of healing traditions and I'll explore how animals are healers in the sound world, from birdsong to pond life. For a society to be healthy, it needs to have a sense of ethical behaviour, and it's likely we humans learned our ethics from the wolves. A healthy body politic also needs to have a sense of justice: some animals can have a strong sense of fairness. Society needs healthy politics, and we'll look at what we can learn from animals as political players, including the Athenian street dog, who always supports the underdog.

Part Four explores how true health includes that of the collective psyche, the soul politic. The collective mind needs animated energy in its art and its spirituality, and animals are vital medicine in these arenas. The collective mind dreams, through folk tales and medicine stories, and in them the animals are guides to healing the psyche of society. The world's earliest healers were the shamans, who everywhere in the world, now and at every time in history, have always said that it is the animals who heal. Are they right?

PART ONE

How Animals Heal the Individual Psyche

This section explores how animal spirits vitalize our minds. Many animals laugh and play. They light up a part of our brains and encourage liveliness and curiosity. In an epidemic of loneliness, pets communicate with us and heal the pain of isolation. This part considers animals used in therapy and how successful that is for the hurt psyche, and looks at how animals may even step in to rescue those who are suicidal when human efforts fall short.

I

Bouncing with Rude Health

'This joy outleaps the dog' – Theodore Roethke

If I consider my cat Otter, it is his exorbitant vitality that strikes me. Cat of character, happy-go-lucky and highly communicative, Otter has a capacity for bright happiness like no other animal I've known. Like many cats, he is curious, playful and affectionate, but he has a charge of sheer spirit that makes people remember him after just one meeting. He is a comedian, a show-off since kittenhood: he jumps at mirrors and bats them with his paws, interrupting himself only to look over his shoulder and check that humans are watching. He often sleeps on his back with his paws on his chest like an otter does; he sometimes walks through doorways sideways like a dressage pony and may stand on his hind legs like a tiny Prussian horse, giving a little chirrup and nose-nudging my hand. Every time he does it, I feel a leap of delight.

He radiates vibrancy even in his older years, providing good medicine for me and my friends. His life force strengthens mine and if the idea for this book came from anyone, it came from him.

This chapter explores how we are healed by the vitality of animals, in their happiness, their play, through their senses, awareness and uproarious animal spirits.

Laughter is perhaps one of the most beguiling ways in which any animal – including humans – demonstrates full-on vitality. Otter's ability to make people laugh is unlike anything I've ever seen in a cat. I think, in his cat-way, he can 'laugh'. Many animals do.

Bonobos, if tickled, make a choked *he-he-he* gasp of laughter, followed by a *peeeep* of pleasure. In fact they laugh until they fart. Their laughter sounds like a human who is laughing so hard they are clean out of breath but still can't stop laughing.[1] You know the sort: fits of laughter, in stitches, when your entire body convulses with vibrations as if all your organs are being massaged by the bubbles of a hundred and one jacuzzis and you are both the jacuzzi and the jacuzzed.

That one. That kind of laughter. Famously the best medicine.[2]

Laughter reduces stress hormones, anxiety and depression, boosting the mood and self-esteem. Laughter makes us not just happier but healthier as it reduces inflammation, improves circulation and enhances the immune system, while also stimulating the heart and lungs and aiding muscle relaxation. Laughter therapy is cheap, drug-free and fast-acting. It is publicly available, indeed ubiquitous. Tickle a child and they will laugh and likely so will you. Tickle a chimp and her mouth will widen into her playing face and she will wheeze with laughter.[3] Orangutans and gorillas may laugh in buzzy purrs of breath, and apes can laugh while inhaling as well as exhaling, like bagpipers. Gorilla laughter may be quick and rhythmic – *ho-ho he ha HA!* – as if the laughter has been fermenting within and a tickle pops the cork, unleashing all the effervescence.

Chortling, laughing like a drain, gurgling, giggling and guffawing, the laugher laughs with all of themselves in bodily and emotional exuberance and most of us can self-medicate with laughter.

When it comes to vitality, laughter is the dog's bollocks. Or the chimpanzee's clitoris. Female chimpanzees may laugh when they tickle their own fancy, using a stick to rub their genitals.[4]

Laughter is a signal that the laugher is not only happy but wishes to spend more time with the laughee, welcoming the interaction as a reciprocal exchange. Rocky Mountain elk squeal with laughter. Dogs laugh in that panting-coughing *huh-ha*, the breathy exhalation when they play. The sound of dog laughter can comfort other dogs, even those not playing,[5] which is also how we humans may experience it.

Some sixty-five creatures laugh while playing, including many primates, foxes, badgers, polecats, mongooses, cats, cows, kangaroos and elephants, as well as whales and seals, while among birds, the Australian magpie, the kea parrot and budgerigar all laugh.[6] Laughter signals play, subverts aggression, creates social bonds and just feels good.

Dolphins laugh in a short burst of pulses followed by a whistle in a series of sounds they never make except when play-fighting.[7] Most animals laugh just loudly enough for their playmate to hear and many may laugh too quietly or too high for our hearing to catch. Rats laugh when they play-fight and play-chase each other and, if tickled, chirp with laughter. At 50 kHz, the chirps are far above our hearing range, but ultrasound microphones can record and replay them in a lower register. I've listened, and it is the sweetest sound, lit with chirrups and tiny squeaks. Rats like listening to other rats giggling and, given a choice in an experiment, will push a bar to hear that sound rather than any other rat-sound.

Researchers tickle rats, finding that they love being tickled on their backs and bellies. They enjoy it so much that they chase the researcher's hand for more, their whole bodies, tipsy with delight, doing 'joy-jumps'. Jaak Panksepp spent decades investigating joy in rats and other animals, and confirmed that dopamine is implicated in both human and rat laughter. He demonstrated that rats chirp when brain areas associated with positive feelings are activated, something that takes place in the most ancient parts of the brain, and he believed that the ability to feel emotions of joy and sadness probably exists throughout the animal realm. His rat-tickling research was geared towards creating antidepressants which stimulate the ancient brain pathways associated with joy.[8]

We may not be able to hear rats laughing, but some birds laugh right into the heart of our hearing range. Kea parrots, mischievous birds from New Zealand, with olive and orange colouring, are known as the clowns of the mountains. When they laugh, the sound cascades happily down an octave and triggers an automatic play-reaction in other keas, launching them into spontaneous aerial acrobatics, play-pouncing and tussling with each other. It also elicits a helplessly happy play-state in my mind and I want to chirp along with them. So does David Rothenberg,

American musician and philosopher. Rothenberg has listened to, and played music with, birds and animals across the world for the joy of it. Playing with thrushes, he notes, the 'laughing thrush keeps laughing with the clarinet. It's a jazz of the underbrush.'[9] Author Mary Webb calls the woodpecker 'a good laugher' and translates the call of the chiffchaff as 'Live! Laugh!' The laughter of animals is, she says, like a herb that heals 'all inward hurts and outward wounds'.[10]

We live in a laughing world. There are almost certainly many more laughing creatures surrounding us than we know, laughter both audible and inaudible, enveloping us in a brightness of spirit, a susurration of soft chuckles, a myriad of giggles, a wellspring of vitality.

~

Vitality is zest, enthusiasm, fizzing like a vitamin in the psyche. Vitality is the inextinguishable life force, the sap-rising iridescence. Vitality is one of the five character strengths most highly correlated with happiness. (The others are curiosity – which is contagious – optimism, gratitude and the ability to love and be beloved.)[11] Vitality is not necessarily correlated with age, and an eighty-year-old can be elastic with vitality as a core inner strength. It is a key measure of psychological health, the mind's appetite for life and vigour, the vivid experience of being alive, playful and alert.

Animals are vivifying in their humour as well as their laughter. In *monkeyshines* and *horseplay*, *parroting*, *aping* or *playing copy-cat*, language suggests that animals can be a company of clowns. Primates enjoy monkey-tricks. There is footage online of a man performing a magic trick for a baby orangutan where the man first puts a chestnut into a cup and shows it to the infant. Then, in a sleight of hand unseen by the baby, the man tips out the chestnut before showing the orangutan the now-empty cup. For a moment, the baby looks disbelieving, then his mouth unrolls into a smile the size of half his face – more – so funny does he find it that he falls about laughing on the floor. (The humour palls when you see the baby is in a cage in a zoo.)

Many animals have a sense of humour and we may be the butt of their jokes. The chimpanzee Washoe, born in 1965 and the first non-human who could communicate in American Sign Language, lived at the Institute of Primate Studies in Oklahoma. Washoe, trained by Roger Fouts, had a notably naughty sense of humour. Once, when Fouts was giving her a piggyback, she signed 'FUNNY' and he didn't know why. Then, he writes, 'I felt something wet and warm flowing down my back and into my pants.'[12]

Koko, a gorilla, was born in San Francisco Zoo and in the 1970s learned a thousand American Sign Language signs and understood about two thousand spoken words. She would play pranks on people to make them jump. She was funny. Once, when she had wrenched a steel sink off a wall in frustration, and the people around her looked cross, she indicated her pet kitten and signed 'CAT DID IT'. She also liked physical comedy, tying her trainer's shoelaces together, then signing 'CHASE'.[13]

An African grey parrot called Throckmorton could mimic his human family's mobile phones, getting everyone running from different parts of the house, and when one of them answered the phone the parrot would imitate the flat tone of a caller hanging up.[14]

The human psyche finds happy animals to be medicine and their joy leaps the gap between species. The naturalist and photographer Geoffroy Delorme was unhappy as a teenager, and left human society to spend seven years living with roe deer in a forest in France. He was accepted into their lives and was struck by their *joie de vivre*: 'it's hard to find grumpy roe deer, because happiness seems to be their natural state.'[15]

Joy is widely associated with birds. For the Koyukon people of Alaska, the first migrating birds to appear in spring indicate summer, light and vitality.[16] We speak with glad gratitude of the bluebird of happiness. In Russian folk tales, the bluebird symbolizes hope, while in Navajo culture the mountain bluebird is linked to the rising of the sun. In the folklore of Lorraine in north-eastern France, the bluebird lives in the longed-for blue country of our dreams, the *pays bleu*, and in one tale, two children are sent in search of the Bluebird of Happiness. They cannot find the bird, and return home empty-handed and heavy-hearted.

Only then do they see her. She has in fact been living in their house (in a cage) all along. They give her away to a neighbour's child who is very ill, as the bird of happiness is medicine for the sick.

There'll be bluebirds over the white cliffs of Dover – a time of happiness in the future whose existence is a remedy for the difficult present. Oscar Wilde, caged in prison because he had a heart full of love, wrote of a better time coming when love could fly freely, when 'over our heads will float the Blue Bird singing of beautiful and impossible things, of things that are lovely and that never happened, of things that are not and that should be.'

The joy of animals is both medicinal and infectious. Canids express joy in explosions of tail-wagging, muzzle-licking and squealing. I am a godmother to many children and to an English shepherd dog, Fflos, my god-dog. One of the times in my life when I felt most viscerally alive was in the puppy pen with her puppies. The five of them loved being with humans, each one of them wriggling and squirming, and their bodies tingled every cell of mine. It was pure puppy medicine, the elixir of vitality.

The human face changes when a person greets their dog. Studies show that the smile becomes gentler and more genuine while the frown-creases and lines of tension around the eyes and mouth smooth out and soften, making people look younger, more relaxed, more attractive to others, less forbidding and more friendly.[17] People's voices change too, becoming gentler, higher and slower than usual.[18]

I've seen the way that an animal can work like a shot of joy-juice on a human, when an old man, fretted by bitterness, unexpectedly met a puppy. Ten years of resentment washed right off his face. Frown-lines rippled out into smile-lines. His eyes grew as moist as the nose of the puppy, whose tiny tail went helicopter, wagging so hard that the little barrel of his body tipped over. He was one thrumming battery of wriggling joy, in every part of him, ears, paws, eyes, mouth. Be happy *here*; be happy *now*. And the old man assented to the puppy-command.

~

Play is a sign of good health, showing a creature's vitality of spirit. Play is also a route to good health, improving cognitive, physical, social and emotional well-being. Play is spontaneous and beguiling, but only occurs when animals feel safe, so among infant primates, for example, play is fragmentary or infrequent when the infant is orphaned, injured or seriously ill.[19] Play is a medicine that reaches beyond the player, spreading among an animal's friends and relations, as research on mirror neurons suggests.[20] Their playfulness infects humans too, as being with animals at play untasks us from work, unzipping our spirits.

When I read about a donkey playing with a butterfly, whose whole body was oriented to delight so even his ears were joyful,[21] my own ears perked up in joy, mirror neurons having a little party even through the page. Kittens chase their own tails as if they kept the catnip there. Leverets leap with a levity that is gravity-defying. All mammals at play do joy-jumps, including goats, dogs, cats and horses.[22] The caper of a kid goat puts the capriccio in me. Lambs put springs under the toes of my springtime when they leap vertically. This is understood by some as an involuntary nerve response but, no matter the cause, it throws them up into the air and they find, presumably to their utter amazement, that they can fly.

Watching any animal playing, I slip the leash of being merely human and I slide into a baby elephant's wriggling trunk or a quivering lamb's tail. My human borders crumble and my responsibilities to seriousness dissolve like a biscuit in tea.

Using a well-respected set of criteria for classifying play as something that is unnecessary, voluntary, unique, repeated and safe,[23] researchers show that frogs wrestle each other and ride air bubbles.[24] Several species of fish play by pushing balls around and balancing sticks on their snouts.[25] Fish in one experiment were seen to play with red, green and blue laser lights, chasing and tracking them, and different species were drawn to different colours.[26] Marsupials including kangaroos, wallabies, Tasmanian devils and wombats are playful, as is the duck-billed platypus and the Komodo dragon, who has been seen playing with old shoes, shaking them like a dog does a slipper.[27]

Animals play many of the same games that we do, including tag, chase and catch, going sledging, play-wrestling and jumping on a sleeping friend. For elephant calves, a favourite game is to climb on to a sleeping elephant who then jiggles to unseat the calf. When the calves play in wallows they become one shoogling mass of glorious mud, and when they chase each other they often try to catch each other by the tail. For a baby elephant, their trunk is a fabulous toy, wiggly and sensitive. It is something to swing, something to nose out into the world, something to whizz around in a circle, and is also a source of comfort, for a baby elephant may suck their trunk as a young child sucks their thumb.[28]

Turtles play tug-of-war,[29] and so does a Komodo dragon, playing with a keeper she likes.[30] Wolf pups too play tug-of-war, perhaps with an antler they have found. Wolves like finding new toys, tossing pine cones or kicking cans around.[31] They play tag with each other and pounce on sleeping wolves for fun, and they lie in ambush and leap out at their friends, while on the tundra a wolf has been seen playing frisbee with a piece of caribou hide.[32] Wolves slide down mountains in the snow and smash ice for fun, standing on a new-frozen lake and jumping on to their front paws until the ice cracks. They skate. Sort of. At least they go dodgems on the ice, purely for the fun of it.[33] Marc Bekoff, effervescent professor emeritus, American biologist and animal behaviourist, describes buffaloes running on to ice and sliding on it, 'excitedly bellowing *gwaaa* as they did so'.[34]

In one viral video, a deer is on a football pitch, on his own, and begins playing with the ball, antlers down and pushing it into the goal. As it hits the net, the deer begins to prance in a kind of victory lap on the grass. Spotted dolphins of the Bahamas may play a game of seaweed-football with each other[35] where one dolphin has a strand of sargassum seaweed and moves it around its body (pectoral fin to fluke to rostrum) while the others give chase until the first dolphin drops the strand, at which point another dolphin takes it and swims off. Within the rules of the game, the chasers must not snatch the seaweed away, and dolphins sometimes invite humans to play this game with them.[36]

Right whales use their tails for sails for twenty minutes at a time in a strong breeze, doing it for play not locomotion.[37] Grey whales blow blasts of bubbles at and under each other, while mother greys and their calves can gather together in huge play groups of perhaps twenty or more pairs and play chase, splashing each other, rolling, rubbing and diving. Young greys have been seen playing with a ball of kelp, lifting it on to their heads, wearing it like a hat, submerging it and watching it pop up again when released.[38] They may surf the waves, kicking their tails to rise and sliding down the wave as it breaks.[39]

In the waters off Hawaii, bottlenose dolphins and humpback whales play together, with the dolphin approaching the whale and lying across the whale's head. The whale then lifts its head high, and the dolphin slides down its back.[40] Spinner dolphins are the whirling dervishes of the oceans, their minds turning like djinns in the play of the planets.

Ravens have been recorded sledging down snowy slopes, rolling, legs akimbo, and a crow in Russia was filmed snowboarding down a steep roof on a pan lid and as soon as the bird reached the bottom of the slope, he would pick up the lid in his beak, flap up to the top of the roof and do it again. Two ravens have been seen playing King of the Castle with an extra trophy: one raven would perch on the top of the mound with a prized piece of dung in his beak – the king is in his counting house – and the other would storm the castle to snatch the dung-treasure.[41] Lambs everywhere play King of the Castle. Cranes play catch with small pebbles.

So here's a question: since humans are so late to the party and the animals were here long before us, did we learn games from the animals? Was it the elephant calf who taught us to play-pounce and mock-ambush? Did a whale's tail give us the idea of sailing? Did Wolf invent the frisbee and show it to the little Mowgli-us? Did Raven, some nine times older than us, first play King of the Castle three million years ago, and then teach it to us dirty rascals who followed? Maybe all the health benefits of play that we experience so magnificently were bequeathed to us by the animals.

When ancient Greeks spoke of their pets, the most common term they used was *athurma*, meaning 'plaything', a toy that caused joy. Otter used to play catch with me if I took a toy mouse to a particular mat, delighting us both. French Renaissance thinker Michel de Montaigne noted: 'When I play with my cat, who knows whether I am playing with her, or she with me? We equally amuse each other with our monkey-tricks.' Our pets generally feel safe enough with us to play, but to earn the trust of a wild creature such that it will play with you moves into a place of grace. Vet and author Dr Sean Wensley writes of meeting a fox cub whom he fed and befriended in his back garden. They began to play and, growing in confidence, the cub began to chew his shoelaces, then played a hiding game around a tree. Wensley brought tennis balls and the cub tossed them into the air, following them with a leap, then pouncing and batting at them when they landed.[42]

Octopuses play with LEGO blocks and bounce balls around with their water jets.[43] In footage of a human scuba diver playing with an octopus, the octopus seems to adore the sensation of headbutting the human's palm, repeatedly returning for more. In the Amazon, river dolphins swim in synchronized leaps in the river and, in a game that has gone on for years, Pirahã men in canoes follow them, trying to touch the dolphins with their paddles. They always surface just out of reach, and the game draws a laughing crowd on the banks because the men never can touch the dolphins, who seem to love the game, coming back, never getting tagged and only disappearing with the sunset.[44]

Dogs are persistent in demanding the stick game but dog-owners often complain that when they throw a stick for a dog, the dog will fetch it but never bring it the whole way back. The dog will drop it just out of reach of the human, and people often find this irking: if the dog wants to play stick-fetch, they say, the dog should bring it all the way to them. Probably from the dog's perspective, the fun is when the stick is thrown, and is 'in play', and bringing it back is a chore. But I have wondered if the dog is trying to show the human how to play fetch properly. Is the dog trying to teach us the joy it knows is hidden in the stick?

Animals play in the mind as well as in the body. Koko, the signing gorilla, found humour in wordplay, so when asked what she could think of that was hard, she signed both 'ROCK' and 'WORK'. Lucy, a chimpanzee born in 1964 and kept at the Institute for Primate Studies in Oklahoma, was also taught sign language, and when she needed new words, she played her way to invention. She didn't have a sign for 'watermelon', so she called it 'DRINK FRUIT' in sign language. She tasted radish and called it 'CRY HURT FOOD'. She named a stick of celery a 'FOOD PIPE'.[45]

Play depends on 'let's pretend'. Let's pretend to be a predator and jump on you. Let's pretend to fight but actually just rumble around a bit. As a youngster, Austin, a chimpanzee born in 1974 and living at Georgia State University, often pretended to eat imaginary food, sometimes with an equally imaginary dish and spoon. He'd eat it in his imagination, rolling it around his mouth. With another chimpanzee, Sherman, he watched *King Kong* on TV and then they pretended King Kong was in a cage with them, as the chimps threw things, made threat barks and sprayed King Kong with a hose.[46]

~

'Be a good animal, true to your animal instinct,' wrote D. H. Lawrence. Animals model a healthy way to be fully present in the body, not as an appendage to our emotional and mental lives but as the very axis of vitality. They offer an almost irresistible invitation to be physical, to inhabit our skins and smells, to feel ourselves as pelt, paw and feather. Leave your scent-marking on the gatepost. Catch leaves in your snout. Know the belly-drum and the barrel-cock, the shanks and teats and horns. Like this, we can breathe in electric air, brimful, right to the very edge of our carnal selves, lips on the rim.

Animals don't wear clothes. They can't artificially dress to impress and as they don't cover their bits, they can't operate in the fig-leaf-and-shame categories. They serve as exemplars of a specific kind of psychological health because the never-dressed body doesn't lie. Of course, some animals pretend: frightened cats fluff up their tails like bog brushes to appear fiercer than they are. Butterflies 'deceive' predators with eyespots. The chameleon, whose body alters by the minute, is a Scheherazade among the animals, telling a thousand and one tales. But it is still the body which is speaking its physiological truth. It really is the cat's fur bristling. It really is the lattice of nanocrystals in the iridophores of the chameleon and the chitin in the butterfly wing.

The very presence of animals is vitalizing. Through hearing, smelling, seeing and touching animals, we are drawn out of ourselves, into a greater world beyond, whether listening to the low hums of giraffes in a savannah at evening when they caress each other, or watching puffins, clowns of the air, the most visually cheering of all birds. Hedgehogs snore, a rising, appreciative half-voiced *wheep* and an outbreath whiffle. When bees bump into each other, they make a *whoop!* sound which had been understood as a warning to deter the other bee but is now thought to be an indication of a bee surprised by a bee.[47] We live in a whooping world.

Animals vitalize the atmosphere even when we cannot see or hear them. Joyce Poole, researcher at Kenya's Amboseli National Park, could tell if elephants were nearby. If the elephants were absent, the landscape had 'a stillness, an emptiness', but when they were near, 'there seemed to be a vibrancy in the air, a certain warmth,' Poole writes.[48] Even when the sounds are in the deep infrasound range of elephants, lower than our hearing, we can still *feel*, right inside our bodies, the deep pulses that throb the air.[49]

Animals lead us to that electric and tender place where we feel fully alive. *Here! Look!* A raucous scarlet macaw flies past, carrying in their beak a seed-bomb of unfettered life to explode all that is anti-animate. When we are physically ill, we may well lose our sense of taste or smell – garlic tastes of cardboard. So does mint. Honey tastes of cardboard soup. Wellness includes sharpened senses, and animals help us with this. Animals bring us to our senses or, perhaps better, animals bring us to *their* senses.

Animals have different sense-abilities from us, including their perception of electric fields. Barn owls have a visual sensitivity which is at least thirty-five times that of humans.[50] We can take a guess at what that might feel like, with binoculars or cameras. We cannot, though, know what it is like to be the barn owl, or to be a bat experiencing batness. We can't know in ourselves what a mosquito senses as a mosquito. (Mosquitoes can taste things with their feet so if they land on skin treated with DEET they detest the taste and fly off.) We definitely can't experience how a catfish tastes the world through their entire body, or know how a bee feels having pollen baskets at their knees, but even taking a step towards their experiences can thrill every nerve and give us a hint of multiple worlds through the *Umwelt* of multiple creatures. *Umwelt* combines *Um*, 'what is around', and *Welt*, 'the world'. *Umwelt* (the concept was defined by zoologist Jakob von Uexküll in 1909) is the animal's experience of being: their perceptual world, how they sense things.

Every bird is, according to William Blake, 'an immense world of delight'. Each species is a realm, and Earth is a myriad of universes, spiralling into galaxies of vitality.

Reading Ed Yong's book *An Immense World: How Animal Senses Reveal the Hidden Realms Around Us* took me gladdened into worlds I never knew. If we could hear them aright, cicadas would sound like cows, and katydids like revving chainsaws, he tells us. Caterpillars have hairs that can feel the particular air-churn of flying honeybees, and when the caterpillars feel it they freeze or vomit or fall to the ground. It's good for the plant, reducing the damage the caterpillar could have done to it.[51]

But why is it *healing* for us that animals have such senses? Because they can enhance our world into something larger and fuller than our senses alone may detect, and we are more vitalized the more we partake of the enlivening world of the others.

I would like to offer you a tiny vial of vivacity, with the active ingredient of treehoppers. This is how two treehoppers (small insects) communicate. A treehopper squeezes its tummy to send vibrations down its legs, along a plant stem and up the legs of other treehoppers, giving them good vibes. Humans can't hear the vibrations unless they are passed through a vibrometer which can convert them into audible sounds. I've heard it – a rumbly, soft kind of noise with upstrokes of jazz clarinet in miniature. Treehopper the First, who happens to be male, purrs, punctuating it with a highly suggestive ticking sound. You can almost hear it in translation: *I like you. I really, really do. Shall we, eh? Shall we, eh?* Treehopper the Second, who happens to be female, replies with a warm, assentive hum. I hear it in translation: *yes I said yes I will Yes.*

Mice a-wooing sing like songbirds though it is in ultrasound, too high for us to hear. The blue-throated hummingbird sings at an ultrasonic pitch too high for *itself* to hear, singing, perhaps, for the insects and the angels. Plant hoppers, trying to detect signals from other plant hoppers, lean forward, their feet pressed down, and surely don't we too, at least in childhood, instinctively lean forward on tiptoes to hear better? So do elephants. An elephant may freeze mid-stride, leaning forward on her massive toenails, listening with her feet and able to feel other elephants through her toes before she sees them or hears them with her ears.[52]

For elephants, the world is full of message, including the mayhem of smells they create when they greet each other, pissing and shitting, with the glands on their faces streaming emotion. They raise their heads, flap their ears and rumble with delight, clicking their tusks, corkscrewing their trunks around one another's and trumpeting with joy.

The ocean too is full of scent-message, a realm opened to us by the senses of seabirds who can smell a substance (dimethyl sulphide) that plankton give off when they are eaten by krill. Smelling of oysters and seaweed, it is the scent of the sea at its most alive, Molly-Blooming with plankton.

I wish I had whiskers. If I did, I'd whisk the air like a mouse, a hyrax or a naked mole-rat. Or I'd whisk the water like the manatee and the seal, who with their whiskers can track the swirl of water in the wake of a fish. But even knowing that they do this enlivens me. Whiskers are properly called vibrissae, from the Latin word for *vibrate*, and whisking helps a creature to be more aware of its surroundings. The common seal has some shorter vibrissae that can pick up higher frequencies of sound while its longer vibrissae pick up lower frequencies.[53]

Dolphins experience the world in part by clicking it, and those who have swum with dolphins can feel as if the clicks live within them, unforgettably enlivening them. The more we know of animal senses, the more we become conscious of vitality everywhere, in a wonderful net of inter-senses, each linked through all to *all* the worlds.

Decreased alertness is a sign of ill health, from the exhaustion of sickness to coma and vegetative states when the animal spirits are gone. Conversely, increased alertness is an indicator of health. In medical terms, the major characteristics of consciousness are being alert and being oriented to time and place, knowing who you are, where you are and when you are. Animals are superbly oriented to time and place. They bring us into the vitality of now. Just one dog. Just one sock. And they're off: engrossed, riveted, extracting every bit of smell, their attention dealt out at full pelt so in that moment there is nothing in the whole world but The Sock. (Until they get a whiff from the bin.)

Dogs can inhabit an enlarged present, smelling what is about to happen, including perhaps a beloved dog-friend on her way, smelled before being seen; and they can smell the past too, so a disliked dog who has marked a lamp post is visually gone but present in the pissed-off nose of a dog at the post. For dogs, smells contain reports, histories and foretellings. Dogs 'see' in smells, and as Alexandra Horowitz, dog-olfactory expert, writes, 'those who see smells must remember in smells too: when we imagine dogs' dreaming and daydreaming, we should envisage dream images made of scents.'[54] Bearing in mind how smells move in currents of air, imagine how the world shimmers for a dog sensing smells.

~

Animals embody curiosity, which as we have seen is another key feature of vitality. Curiosity is good for you. Curious people are happier,[55] and curiosity is associated with higher levels of positive emotions, lower levels of anxiety and more life satisfaction. Curiosity means the mind is active, and the mind, like a muscle, gets stronger through being exercised. High scorers on the curiosity-measure show more playfulness, wit and ability to bond emotionally with a stranger of the opposite sex.[56] Maintaining curiosity in old age protects us against cognitive and physical decline.[57] Curiosity affects the well-being of others too. If you meet a person of rank incuriosity then your spirits droop and in their company time sickens, grows wan and dies. Meeting someone curious, though, has the opposite effect. The very *air* perks up. And the animals are there, in on the act, curious, engaged, interested, invigorating us. Animals offer us an unparalleled invitation to be curious. For many children, animals are the first object of their curiosity, pointing with both finger and brain at *doggie!*, the child's eyes lit with interest.

The combination of curiosity, interest and eagerness is known as the brain's 'seeking' circuit, a primal urge among all us animals to seek out what we need.[58] It's exciting, this digging, exploring, inquisitive attitude. Even small creatures such as scallops demonstrate curiosity, and in one adorable experiment called Scallop TV some scallops were strapped by tiny seat belts into miniature seats[59] and then shown images of drifting particles that would, to a scallop, look like food. Their shells opened up, ready to feed, then tightened back down, again and again opening and closing like castanets not because they could taste or smell anything but because, the researchers maintain, they were curious.

Dolphins are curious, and they purposely experiment with the psychoactive drug produced by pufferfish.[60] They hold the fish very carefully in their mouths, squeezing it gently for a tiny puff of neurotoxin (with caution, because the toxin is fatal in large doses) that the fish releases. Having taken a puff, the dolphins pass the puffer around to each other and they then begin to act strangely, noses at the water surface as if mesmerized by the play of light or their own reflections.

I find it very hard to be curious about some things: banking and the stock market, for instance. (I used to find it hard to be curious about footballers, or their feet, wives or balls, assuming they had more or less two of each, until Marcus Rashford led the opposition to the Tory government, Gareth Southgate embodied public goodness, Gary Lineker stood up for refugees, and Messi and Mbappé electrified the world in the Argentina v France 2022 World Cup Final.) But stock markets and banking, no. Give me an ant, though, and I want to know what it knows.

Show me your world! How do you talk to your friends? What does it feel like to have your brain overtaken by the cordyceps fungus, which sends you as obsessively insane as your average kleptocrat and then explodes out of your head from the top of a stem of grass?

~

Animals animate us. Living right at the quick, in a click or a whisk, animals vitalize the world. The octopus can shrink and enlarge or flatten and bloom because to the octopus nothing is impossible. The octopus is the shapeshifter's shapeshifter, metamorphosing and protean – the embodiment of mind at its best. The animal realm teems with movement: they waddle, strut, soar, flit and slither. Swooping, prowling, loping and frisking, they are candles lit from the very wick of life.

In lockdown, we delighted in seeing animals in 'human' spaces: mountain goats in the Welsh town of Llandudno, jackals in Tel Aviv and cougars in Santiago, Chile.[61] When a mouse scampers along the tracks of the London Underground, coming from a dark tunnel, appearing for a moment in the light before disappearing again, there is a collective gasp from the commuters on the platform. *Mouse!* a child cries out. All eyes are fixed on it. People may smile at each other, brought to a shared moment of micro-glee as something as mere as a mouse makes exclamation marks in the sentence of the daily commute.

Sport is one way we play. Animals entering sporting arenas add a vivace to the score. Their appearances are unschedulable, spontaneous and wild. A snapping turtle crawls across a golf course. A kangaroo hops on to a racetrack in Bathurst in Australia, in the middle of a race. A giant lizard crosses a car racetrack. A goose interrupts a game of golf. There have been hares and skunks on baseball pitches in the middle of a game and an awful lot of squirrels. One squirrel scored in a baseball game between Kent State and Louisville in Ohio on 23 September 2017, and the crowd roared for it. The squirrel had made a magnificent run on the pitch, and in the clip the commentator's voice is as excited as an eight-year-old's – 'Oh my goodness, buddy, do it, do it, do it!' – and as the squirrel makes the touchdown, the commentator thrills with pride: 'Man, he's my favourite squirrel.' Some two months later, a grey cat finds its way on to the field at Marlins Park in Florida, hightails it down the pitch, then climbs the vertical purple scoreboard wall. The crowd lights up with the sheer aliveness of the moment. Cats running on to football pitches are widely loved, greeted with chants of 'Sign 'em up!'

We modern humans are not among the animals enough, and their unexpected appearances release us from the leashes of the hours, stuck in our cages of routine. When they come among us, we perk up and take notice and in those instants we feel party to the life of a widened world.

Perhaps literature's most vitalic cat is Jeoffry, 'a mixture of gravity and waggery', life alive in all his moments, whether playing, washing or sleeping. His human companion was the eighteenth-century poet Christopher Smart, who was wildly alert to animal medicine but whose brilliance could buckle to madness. In his ode 'My Cat Jeoffry', Smart writes:

> For in his morning orisons he loves the sun and the sun loves him.
> For he is of the tribe of Tiger . . .
> For there is nothing sweeter than his peace when at rest.
> For there is nothing brisker than his life when in motion.

Jeoffry is complete. Nose, paws, eyes, tail. 'For the divine spirit comes about his body to sustain it in complete cat.' Let's pause on this word *complete*. It means perfect and finished. From Latin, its roots suggest something filled up and entirely fulfilled. Elsewhere, Smart writes that 'a LION roars HIMSELF complete from head to tail.' We cannot be complete unless we live our lives lightning-struck by the force of animal spirits within us and among us.

Smart tells us that his cat led to a discovery: 'For by stroking of him I have found out electricity.' This is physical and metaphysical: 'For he counteracts the powers of darkness by his electrical skin and glaring eyes.' This, says Smart, is the light of the divine: 'For the Electrical fire is the spiritual substance.' God is electric and Jove is in the lightning bolt.

Lightning features significantly in the Navajo language, which has an extraordinary feature: *animacy*. Animacy is a measure of how alive something is, expressing how sentient it is. Does the thing have a lot of sentience or aliveness, or just a little? How alive is it? Nouns are ranked by this animacy on a continuum, and the most animate is a human while the least animate is an abstraction. One thing, though, is classed, together with the adult human, as most animate. What is it? *Lightning*, by Jove, *lightning*.

In the Homeric world, a particular energy – a shining momentness – surrounds the gods: *energeia*. It is entirely vital, an intense presence of wildness incarnate. In this sense, the animals are the gods still walking – swimming, tumbling, climbing, pouncing – in the world.

A kingfisher: a bolt from the blue and a bolt of the blue. How else is summer lightning going to flash within us, except through a kingfisher? The world is charged with the vitality of animals, an electric current of life driven by such voltage that it leaps the gaps between one earthed species and another, this life force as highly charged as a volt of vultures or a leap of leopards.

The early studies of electric fish took place alongside the study of electricity, and the electricity of the fish sparked the discovery of tiny electrical currents in the muscles and nerves of all animals.[62] In an astonishing discovery, neurologists have shown that when we see animals, a specific part of the brain (the right amygdala) lights up in a flare of electrical activity.[63] Fox. Whale. Penguin. Saucepan. Mouse. Your brain lights up for them all (except the saucepan, naturally). This fact totally stops me in my tracks. We are electrified – right in the core of our brains – by animals: they, the great transformers, could transform us if we would let them. To be fully, vitally, alive, we need to be within the wild circuit of animal electricity where the jaguar with lightning in her eyes and her fur crackling with static can charge you up for your whole life for, with her, you can take the shock, let the current surge through you and vow to protect the tribe of Tiger.

~

At the heart of Chinese medicine, *qi* or *chi* energy is the vital force that circulates and flows through the body. *Prana*, from Sanskrit, is similar, the 'life force energy' or 'vital principle'. For centuries, the Western medical tradition referred to the vitalizing principle as 'animal spirits'.

Hippocrates (c.460–371 BCE) thought that three spirits (vegetative spirits, vital spirits and animal spirits) impelled the body's functioning, and of these he considered animal spirits superior and thought they came from the air and induced the development of intelligence. Aristotle (384–322 BCE) considered that the animal spirits flowed like wind through the blood and that the sensations which the body received from the outside world were transmitted by the animal spirits in the form of vibrations (ah, my treehopper friends!). The Greek physician Galen (129–c.216 CE) believed that animal spirits were the body's principal source of vitality. Specifically, he considered that food, absorbed by the liver, produced vegetative spirits which the heart transformed into vital spirits, then the brain mixed vital spirits with air in a 'marvellous net' (the *rete mirabile*, consisting of a network of blood vessels at the base of the brain). Stored there until needed, the animal spirits could move through hollow nerves to transmit muscle action or to enable those nerves to receive sense impressions.

In 1936, the term *animal spirits* was repurposed by the economist John Maynard Keynes to describe how decisions made in times of economic uncertainty are guided by animal spirits that may be pessimistic, confident or exuberant, but crucially those spirits drive impulsive, emotional and possibly irrational decision-making, in contrast with cool rationality.

When we speak of being animated, it implies activity, vigour and vitality. Animal nature is understood to be active and invigorated. In Spanish, the term *ánimo!* is used to inspire someone, to encourage, to stimulate, activate and urge by calling up, in effect, the animal spirits.

Animal spirits were explicitly linked to air: for Hippocrates, the animal spirits came from the air. For Aristotle, the animal spirits flowed like wind. The word *animal* is connected to *anima*, the spirit, the vitalizing breath, and both are related to Proto-Indo-European *an(e)*, breath or air: that which animates and gives us life. The matrix of ideas here suggests that the mind is inter-intelligent with the outer world, that the wind or air that vitalizes us all is a shared commons of spirit, in the marvellous net of the real world. There is medicine in the electric air around us.

Ánimo! Ánimo!

2

A Remedy for the Lonely

'Dogs simply can't help falling in love'
— dog behaviour specialist Clive Wynne

Lonely hurts. It just does. It hurts in particular places, on the edges of the self. All of them.

The lonely feel it at the heart's edge, a hot and searing hurt as if it has been scraped on a claw of barbed wire. The lonely feel the pain at the body's edge as it touches the void on the other half of the double bed. They feel it at the voice's edge as their words, unheard, are bruised by silence. They feel it at society's edge as they stand at the edges of rooms, and that edge is sharp as a blade, cutting them off. They feel it at the edges of the day, waking alone and falling asleep with no one in their arms. They feel it at the edges of the home, the thresholds where there is no one to greet them, no welcome at the doorway as they return to emptiness.

Loneliness can kill. Long-term loneliness increases the risk of a stroke by 56 per cent.[1] It can be more dangerous than smoking[2] and is a strong contributory factor in heart disease,[3] which is poignant as this is indeed a heartbreaking emotion. The lonely are more likely to get cancer and to suffer from serious mental health problems.[4]

I've known too much loneliness in my life, and from childhood I've felt a bereftness that I couldn't recover from — until the cats. I'm not alone in experiencing loneliness: there is an epidemic of it. In Europe, one in eight people say they are lonely most of the time.[5]

Pets offer medicine for loneliness in simple touch, which salves the loneliness at the body's edge. Psychologically, we fail to thrive at any age without touch, especially the soft, slow stroking that we mammals adore, because we need physical closeness as well as emotional intimacy.

I have never missed physical touch so much as I did in lockdown. With no partner and no kids, I was in a tiny bubble with a friend who was too vulnerable to accept or give a hug. But in those months I experienced the touch of two animals. The most unexpected was being hugged by a foal named Rocky who was only a few days old. He was lying in a sunny meadow when I walked up to him slowly. He let me sit near him and lie beside him and then, gazing at me, he lifted one leg and tucked it over my shoulder, pushing his other leg into the side of my neck. I felt flooded with bliss. The other animal was of course Otter, who was often in my lap, in my arms, rubbing my ankles and giving me nose-to-nose headbutts. Touch is primal and when I stroke Otter the feel of his fur sleeks the pelt of my first mind, for with an animal we may step into a core experience of being a cub nuzzling up in the befriending warmth of a den.

For over a decade, Otter was my light source, my shiner, my most reliable mood-lifter, but a few months ago he went completely blind. He could not see even the sun. For a while it seemed to remove all the light and lightness from him, and therefore from me, but with the sadness came one intense sweetness: the relationship of touch between us became eloquent and marvellous. Before, he was happy sleeping in the crook of my knees, but now he wants to sleep as close to me as he can, wrapped in my arms, his body pressed to mine, his cheek touching mine, his nose tip on mine, his paws each side of my neck. Then he purrs loudly enough to shake the bed. Helen Keller, blind and also deaf, would have known the astonishing communication that touch can offer, noting: 'Paradise is attained by touch.'

Last night, Otter fell asleep with his nose tucked under mine, so his whiskers lay along my top lip. It was, literally, the cat's whiskers. For a brief moment, his whiskers twitched and it felt as if the antennae of my mind widened into a different world. Sometimes he will comb my hair a little with his claws, but he will always sheath them near my skin: he knows the difference, and I trust him on this even in our sleep, much as he trusts me not to roll clumsily into a position which could break one of his legs. Falling asleep with him, and waking with him, he is a remedy for the loneliness of the day's edges.

Animals also offer remedies for the loneliness at the voice's edge through vocal communication. Cats try to 'talk' to us. Domestic cats vocalize in forms that tend to appeal to us and get a response, using sweeter, softer, higher mews and chirrups rather than the lower guttural calls of their closest wild relative, the African wildcat.[6] Animal rescue workers have long noticed that feral cats rarely mew, but after spending time with humans, they begin to do so.

Otter is a communicative cat, in body language and in vocalizations. If he wants to come in to my bedroom from outside, he climbs the cat ladder and knocks on the window in a rapid flurry of paw-strokes. He can't open the cat-cookie jar and curses the fact that evolution has not granted him an opposable digit, but he found a way round this problem. Before he went blind, he had a particular mew, a peremptory one, that he only used to fetch someone to open the jar. He's stopped making that imperative mew since he went blind (perhaps when you're totally dependent on someone, you don't chance your arm being bossy), but his blindness has provoked in him an entirely new call, loud enough for me to hear in any part of the house. He uses it only rarely, but when he does it is piteous, a huge inconsolable howl as if he's crying for all the world he's lost. It seems he wants me to hear it and come to him, because when I do he stops crying.

Otter has an antic disposition and an ability to make people laugh that he evidently enjoys. In the kitchen, above the counter, there is a shelf full of about twenty different teas. Otter (before he was blind) observed me, many times, taking a packet down for a guest. Then he started doing it too. Friends were with me, watching incredulous as he stood upright, his back legs on the counter, balancing his left front paw up on the tea shelf. He looked at us, exultant, *Watch this!* and then he walked sideways, catching the cardboard corner of a packet with the claw of his right paw and flicking down the boxes, one at a time. Liquorice? Flick. *Thuck* as it landed on the counter and he turned to us as close to giggling as a cat can. Mint? Flick. *Thuck*. Camomile? Rooibos? Flick, flick, flick, till all the packets were down. I put them all back. Otter watched our laughter with robust delight and did it all again. His communications are not random. If talking means wanting to say something, and expressing yourself in a way that will be comprehended, then this is a cat who can 'talk'.

Dogs are, of course, highly skilled communicators. Dogs understand when there is an argument going on. There is a lingua franca between us and many other animals in the emotional expression of different calls, so a growl is a warning, whoever it comes from. As Carl Safina, ecologist and utterly exquisite writer, notes: 'Whether the receiving ears belong to a human, a dog, or a horse, several short upward calls cause increased excitement, long descending calls are calming, and a single short abrupt sound can pause a misbehaving dog or a child with a hand in the cookie jar.'[7]

When looking at a human face, dogs (and humans and rhesus monkeys) automatically gaze to their left, to look at the right-hand side of the face. This is the side that most tellingly expresses emotions. Dogs don't gaze left when looking at monkey or dog faces: it's just for us, and the authors of a 2008 study suggest that they may have evolved this 'left gaze bias' in order to gauge our emotions.[8] They try to read us and our feelings. Our dogs try to communicate in ways they know we perceive, barking to us and for us, while adult wolves, by contrast, hardly ever bark, preferring to communicate through body language or scent.

The communication between Evenki hunters and their dogs is deft and precise. The Evenki (formerly called the Tungus) live in the far east of Russia, Siberia, Northern China and Mongolia, where they have traditionally herded reindeer and hunted elk, roe deer, wolverine, lynx and fox. The Evenki hunter and his dog communicate closely in a relationship that is both intricate and independent: they think separately but do so in order to coordinate their timings and actions. Evenki philosophy does not accept strict boundaries between species, and so does not expect any difficulties in people and dogs comprehending each other. Further, Evenki philosophy avoids hierarchies between species: the dog is considered equal to the man in the hunt because what is needed is not a slave but a partner who can make their own decisions. The dogs are neither trained nor punished but rather learn for themselves, sharing contexts and experiences until both hunter and dog have a deep understanding of both the environment and each other. The relationship between the Evenki and their dogs left a shaman of the neighbouring Buryat people totally flummoxed. He didn't observe the men giving any commands to the dogs, but instead noted the synchronicity and harmony between dog and man, and said he felt that an unseen thread linked them.[9]

Animals ease our loneliness in their befriending. The poet Byron had a beloved dog, Boatswain, who he called his only friend – 'I never knew but one.' Byron would have understood the feelings of elderly dog-owners living alone, of whom in one study 75 per cent of the men and 67 per cent of the women said that their dog was their only friend.[10] *Their only friend.* It is both heartbreaking and heartmending. For the poet Emily Dickinson, the relationship with her dog, a huge Newfoundland called Carlo, was a psychological consolation. He was her 'mute confederate', her companion both at home and out on long walks, and when he died she became more reclusive.

Many times as I was writing this book, people would tell me how important their childhood pets were when they were lonely. They had confided in their animals, telling them their fears and hurts, who they had fallen in love with, or who had bullied them. Children, given half a chance, will self-medicate even with a gerbil, talking to their pet, inferring their communication, finding mind-medicine for the curtains of strange sadnesses that can drift across a child's mind, often invisible to others. Children want to talk to animals, and they know the real Doctor Dolittles are often the animals themselves.

In a study of ten-year-old Scottish children, a third demonstrated that their pet was their most significant companion, someone they talked with, played with, cared for, and who understood their feelings and thoughts.[11] When a study asked eight-year-olds in the United States what their most important relationships were, the children included their dogs as often as they included their parents.[12]

Mary, the lonely child in *The Secret Garden*, is without family and unbeloved until she finds herself befriended by a robin, and this marks the start of her emotional recovery. Robins are company, the gardener's friend, a symbol of companionship in actual winter and in the winters of the soul. In the Covid pandemic, many people suffering from lockdown-loneliness found a special friendship with a nearby robin. When the epidemic of loneliness intersected with the pandemic, many people knew that an animal would be medicine and got a pet, the lockdown puppy. Sixty-nine per cent of parents said that having a pet during lockdown benefited their children,[13] although post-Covid abandonment was harsh for many dogs.

Greta Thunberg's school experience was unhappy. She was bullied, and stopped laughing, eating and talking. She cried all the time, day and night. Almost every day, her father had to take her out of school and bring her home to Moses, their golden retriever, and she would sit stroking him for hours. If she howled in emotional pain, Moses lay beside her, pressing his nose into her head, comforting her in his language.

Dawn Prince-Hughes is an anthropologist, primatologist and ethologist who, like Thunberg, has autism. Animals, she says, have 'gone to amazing lengths to find common language with our species which, to them, must seem deaf and blind to rich and healing language'.[14] Orangutans use gestures with each other and, if they are conversing with humans, will modify their signals according to how much the person understands.[15] Koko, the gorilla who was taught to use American Sign Language, communicated her thoughts to humans, including her grief at losing her mate, her own fear of death and her yearning to have a baby.[16] Such communication is unbuyable and uncommandable, an unfeigned relating as if she were in that moment — in spite of the fact that she was captive — inviting us to step across the divide.

Indigenous cultures have kept faith with an understanding that animals and birds and insects are issuing communiqués all the time, and in such a world, enriched with meaning, loneliness seems almost unthinkable. A widespread Indigenous belief maintains that long ago humans shared the language of animals.[17] Nalungiaq, an Inuit woman interviewed in the early twentieth century, said, 'In the very earliest time, when both people and animals lived on earth, all spoke the same language.' Black Elk of the Lakota people (in Dakota territory) refers to a similar time when his people could talk to the animals, and he adds tellingly, 'we all spoke the same mind.'[18]

If you own a pet, your odds of frequently feeling lonely are halved, compared to non-owners.[19] One cardiologist in Connecticut prescribes pets as he would prescribe medicine for about 15 per cent of his patients, knowing how healing they are and how necessary.[20] Several studies looking specifically at bereavement show that those who had a pet were less depressed, despairing and isolated, were in better health and needed less medication than those similarly bereaved but petless.[21]

Loneliness is a particularly common experience for people who are deaf, who may, as a result, feel isolated and disconnected. One woman who lost her hearing commented: 'Night-time was the worst: the silence of nothing. I couldn't sleep. I always felt lonely,' and getting a Hearing Dog was a lifeline.[22] The dogs are trained to respond to everyday sounds that hearing people take for granted, including the doorbell and phone. When the dog hears them, they touch their human, leading them to the source of the sound. They will also, of course, respond to danger sounds such as fire alarms, but the quotidian help these dogs can give is vital in connecting their owners to other people, lessening loneliness. One man spoke of his deafness as a 'dark and lonely world', and his isolation led to depression, insomnia and panic attacks. When he got a Hearing Dog, Clay, his world was, he said, transformed. 'I'd be like a hermit without him. My life was shattered and Clay's the one who put me back together.'[23]

It's pretty hard to feel sympathy for a psychopathic mass murderer, but I suspect Vladimir Putin must feel lonely. Puppies have a medicinal effect on him. When Putin visited Bulgaria in 2010, the prime minister there presented him with a gift, a ten-week-old Bulgarian shepherd dog called Buffy. The effect was breathtaking. Putin bowed, said that he loved the puppy and put his head on one side so his cheek was tilted to Buffy's forehead. His hands were honest; his face was open; his eyes widened and his mouth sweetened. Elsewhere, with other dogs, Putin is pictured kneeling to get down to their level, nose to nose, and in one online clip from the city Sochi in 2017, Putin is seated, ready to receive a gift from Turkmenistan's president. A puppy carrier is brought in. Putin leans forward. The puppy is brought out and swung (horribly for a puppy) by the scruff of his neck, a trophy for the cameras. Putin can't tolerate seeing a puppy held like this and swiftly, naturally, gets to his feet, taking the puppy, cradling him, stroking him, and then – quickly, shyly – he kisses him. God knows the world would be a happier place if Putin just stayed in the puppy pen, drinking their medicine.

Maybe only animals can bridge the loneliness of being a despot, emperor or queen, otherwise surrounded by posers, deposers, parasites and killers. Certainly Putin is in a long line of the super-powerful who reach for pet remedies. In second-century China, Emperor Ling invested his dogs with the rank of courtier. In seventeenth-century Japan, Tokugawa Tsunayoshi, nicknamed the 'Dog Shogun', kept some fifty thousand dogs at government expense, decreed the death penalty for anyone who harmed a dog, and declared that dogs must be spoken to with the utmost politeness. On the other side of the world, Mary, Queen of Scots, had twenty-two adored lapdogs, dressing them in little blue velvet suits. When she was taken to execution in 1587, she was denied the company of her human retinue, but her Skye terrier was huddled under her skirts, staying with her right up to the loneliest and most terrifying end.

At the other end of society's spectrum, pets were remedies for the powerless women most likely to be accused of witchcraft in the Middle Ages. Such a woman often lived on the margins of society, at the sharp edge of poverty, and was usually old, on the fringes of life. She was often without husband or children and likely sought healing for the pain of loneliness that she might assuage, perhaps, with a kitten. Sometimes, in England, this was enough to damn the woman. The iconic witch's cat is often portrayed as black, and the animal behaviourist Temple Grandin (another person with autism who is a special rapporteur for animals) says intriguingly that black cats are typically friendlier and more social than other cats,[24] a cat-characteristic perhaps especially good for the lonely. By the sixteenth century in England, simply having a pet could make a poor, elderly woman vulnerable to the accusation of witchcraft, so a black cat, often a remedy for a woman's malady of sadness, was cruelly construed as a source of toxicity.

Pet-keeping seems a human universal, although the choice of animals varies. Nemonte Nenquimo, a Waorani woman from the Ecuadorian Amazon, describes in her magnificent memoir the pets of her childhood: fireflies, tanager birds and parrots, a pet monkey, macaw, tortoise, toucan, peccary, trumpeter bird and deer.[25] In the Greco-Roman era, pets included cicadas, crickets, nightingales, parrots, partridges, dolphins, hares, pigs, goats, horses and dogs. In early medieval Ireland, the third most popular pets, after dogs and cats, were cranes, who were trained to bow for a bishop giving a benediction.[26] Traditional pets in other places around the world include fruit bats, lizards and parrots (in Fiji); pigeons and eels (in Samoa); raccoons (in Indigenous Mexico) and sloths (in Matis communities in the Amazon). The variety speaks of the profligate, gorgeous and unstoppable need to befriend animals for the psychological medicine they provide.

A pet is often treated as a member of the family, spoken to, given clothes, named at birth and mourned at death, and something profoundly intimate can happen between pets and humans. The poet Mary Oliver, as a child seeking solace, suckled milk from her family's cat as she lay with her kittens.[27] For the Barasana people of eastern Colombia where pets are part of the community, women, in particular, tame the animals into pethood, including tapirs, peccaries, ocelots, dogs and parrots, and the women may suckle puppies and masticate food for the birds.[28] For Native North Americans, traditionally, pets could include tame moose, bison calves, wolves and young bears, the latter suckled by women.[29] In Guiana, women would breastfeed young animals, including dogs, monkeys, opossum, acouri and deer, as they would their own babies.[30] The Bible tells a poignant story of a poor man who had a little ewe lamb who ate with him and drank from his cup: the lamb was 'like a daughter to him'.

I have no child of my own. I dearly wanted a child, but it wasn't to be, and the hollowing hurt lasted for years. For me, caressing and cherishing a cat remedied the pain of childlessness to the point where it dissolved. My feeling seems widespread. In ancient Greece, pet dogs could be referred to as 'foster children' (*trophimoi*). For the Indigenous people of Canada and Alaska, sledge-dogs could be treated harshly, worked hard and kept outdoors, but if a couple were childless, everything changed and they might adopt a puppy, who could be treated as lovingly as a baby.[31] For the Dyaks of Borneo, childless adults are sometimes named as the parents of a beloved pet.[32] In a study from 1998, childless women considered their cats offered them more companionship and emotional support than women who were mothers felt that their cats gave them.[33]

Animals can be substitute siblings as well as substitute children. Geoffroy Delorme, who lived with roe deer, found their company healing in the face of 'the inhuman human world', turning instead to what he calls 'my real family, the roe deer'.[34] One fawn, who he names Chevy, becomes particularly close to the man and they play together, walk together and eat blackberries together, while Chevy licks him in clear affection, tasting him, licking his eyes, ears and nose, and then, taking off the man's hat, sniffing his hair and licking his neck. Delorme learns to speak in a deer's whispers and grunts, and he sings and talks to the fawn, who is 'more than a friend, he's a brother'.

~

It is dawn and Odysseus is returning home to Ithaca after his twenty-year odyssey. Suitors are swarming over his wife, Penelope, and she is demonstrating resolute and ingenious fidelity. Athene, goddess of wisdom, has disguised Odysseus as a beggar so that he can clearly assess his situation: as no one will try to ingratiate themselves with a beggar, Odysseus will be able to see people in their true colours, though no one can see his.

At his home, Odysseus passes unrecognized, but there is one who sees him and knows him truly: his dog, Argos. When Odysseus had left Ithaca, Argos was a fine young dog, a keen hunter, but twenty years on, Odysseus sees a dog utterly changed: old, neglected, lying in cow dung and full of fleas. Odysseus, though, recognizes the dog, and Argos, in turn, recognizes the man, greeting him with the very last scrap of his energy, lowering his ears and wagging his tail. The man weeps for the love and loyalty. The dog doesn't see a beggar but his beloved Odysseus, in an intimate acknowledgement, apparent only to the two of them, of his real identity.

Pets recognize our faces, bodies and smells, information available to the exterior senses. But they offer more than just identification; they offer exactly this *acknowledgement*, a key medicine for the psyche, an essential gift that strengthens our dignity and selfhood as we are properly seen for who we truly are.

The dog meets Odysseus at the threshold of his home, at the threshold of the day. Thresholds are literal places of transition, the doorway where you cross between a public street and a private home. They are places of jeopardy and chance, sites of change, of strangers, risk and opportunity. Odysseus' return is an epic threshold moment when liminality edges everything and, with perfect mythic pitch, Homer knows there must be a dog in the scene: Argos is charged with the cargo of significance.

After the waiting and the welcome, the dog's last duty of care is done and Argos dies. As Odysseus stands at the threshold of his future life, his dog crosses over that other threshold into death, and the greeting of a lifetime transects with a heartbreaking farewell.

Pet-owners repeatedly say that the most valuable moments of interaction with their pet are the greetings at the threshold, the edge, returning home after the day's miniature odyssey. The tender – touching – greeting between Odysseus and Argos is a magnified version of what pets always do for us as they recognize us and acknowledge us at the edge-places of doorways and at the edge-moments of time.

Dogs cry tears of joy when they are reunited with their guardians and specifically for their guardian, not for another familiar human.[35] Their greeting is love-in-ecstasy, devotion gone wild, tail-wagging, ears lowered, eyes part closed, little yelps as if the delight has intoxicated them and they are hiccuping with love. Cat-love comes in soft chirrups of greeting and high-tail-in-the-air excitement as if a cat is a tram getting energy from an invisible feline power line.

Greetings. A pet's compulsion to greet us seems such a simple thing, so easy to overlook. The word *greet* is from the Old English *gretan*, and it means 'salute' (itself from the Latin *salutare*, 'to wish health to someone') and also means 'welcome', as Argos welcomed Odysseus with all his heart. Wellness and health are encoded in greetings. But there's more: *gretan* also entails a sense of 'contact' and 'touch', and it recalls how vital is our pets' tactile comfort, particularly for the lonely. When our pets greet us, they do it in Old English.

~

In the Netherlands, a project called One Against Loneliness was launched in 2013 and a key part of its work is to matchmake an elderly person with a dog as a part-time pet. While many older people say they want the company of a dog, they often cannot handle the cost and they worry about the pet outliving them. One man, a 74-year-old called Theo Nienhujis, had been lonely, saying, 'When you get to your mid-70s, you can lose your connections.' He now shares a dog: 'Bickel is the sweetest little dog and draws people in. People recognize me now and say hello.'[36]

When people feel loneliness at society's edge, the threshold between self and other can be astonishingly hard to cross, but animals, especially dogs, connect people to each other. A pet can be a common denominator between family members: families who get a pet tend to argue less and play more.[37] Dog-walkers tend to know more people in the immediate locale than those who don't walk dogs, and dogs are often the spark that lights a conversation with a passer-by.[38] A stranger with a dog is widely perceived as being more socially attractive, more trustworthy, friendlier, happier, less threatening and more approachable than someone without a dog.[39]

Writing is lonely work, and sometimes when I feel lonely in the middle of a working day, I go for a short walk in nearby woods where there are almost always dogs. I greet the dogs, and talk with their guardians, always about their dogs, and it is a sweet, precious and ordinary thing. A little dog-stroking, a little chat – I invariably feel better after this simple and congenial activity. On these walks, I have rarely felt motivated to talk to strangers who don't have a dog. Studies back up my experience: pets make a community feel healthier because they facilitate social interactions and are associated with exchanges of favours and greater civic engagement. Their presence strengthens people's belief that a neighbourhood is friendly, which can be a self-fulfilling prophecy, because if you think a neighbourhood is friendly, you're likely to be friendlier yourself.[40] Children with disabilities are noticed and talked to ten times more often when they are walking with a service dog compared to walking alone.[41] Studies in the USA demonstrate that passers-by offer substantially more frequent acknowledgements to wheelchair users, in the form of friendly glances, smiles and conversations, when a service dog is present compared to a situation without a dog.[42] The animals are bridges, enabling us to reach across to others.

Animals can comfort us – and in certain cases deliberately reach out to offer their consolation. I think most dogs have taken the Hippocratic oath. So have some chimpanzees. In the 1930s, a Russian primatologist called Nadezhda Ladygina-Kohts raised a male chimpanzee named Joni. The pair were very close, and he would offer her comfort if she was distressed. Seeing her crying, she recalls, 'he hastily runs around me, as if looking for the offender; looking at my face, he tenderly takes my chin in his palm, lightly touches my face with his finger, as though trying to understand what is happening, and turns around, clenching his toes into firm fists.'[43] To comfort her, he was preparing to fight for her. The *fort* in *comfort* is a fortification for you in adversity. This is the fierce comfort that says, 'You are not alone with this. I've got your back. I'm on your side.'

We need to be defended from emotional jeopardy as from physical threat, and animals are there for us, many demonstrating empathy.

Animal-studies scholar Mariam Motamedi-Fraser told me about her dog's sense of empathy, including one occasion at the vet's, where her dog, Monk, was usually disinclined to approach strangers. But on this particular day, a couple were talking in the waiting room and Monk began pulling at the lead to go to them. When he approached the woman, she started to cry, and he licked and nudged her in her distress. She was glad for his being there, she said, explaining that their pet had just had to be euthanized. On another occasion, Mariam and Monk were out walking, when the dog began following a woman, and would not come back when called. (It was highly unusual for him to be disobedient.) The woman – who was really pleased he was there – described her simple and devastating situation. 'My mother died this morning.'

Dogs experience empathy physiologically, so when dogs hear a human crying, the dogs' cortisol levels increase.[44] One-year-old children, dogs and cats all attempt to comfort distressed family members who seem to be crying, and they do this by, for example, putting their head in the lap of the person who is upset.[45]

A 2013 study showed how dogs empathetically reach out to help humans. In this study, an experimenter expressed to a dog that they wanted to get into a particular compartment and to do this they needed the dog to press a button. When this wish was expressed naturally, with no sense of a command, the dogs would press the button, and would do this for no reward and do it for strangers.[46] Just to be nice. Similarly, chimpanzees will spontaneously help humans, including strangers, if the person looks as if they are unable to do something that the chimp can assist with.[47]

The chimpanzee Washoe had given birth twice, but both her babies had died. In 1982, Kat Beach, one of the long-term volunteers at the institute where Washoe lived, had become pregnant and Washoe was enthralled by her belly, signing 'BABY'. But Kat miscarried and didn't appear for some days. When she returned, Washoe greeted her but then seemed to be upset that she'd been away. Kat 'spoke' with Washoe, to tell her what had happened. 'MY BABY DIED' Kat signed. Washoe first looked down at the ground and then gazed into Kat's eyes and signed

'CRY', touching her cheek. When Kat was leaving that day, Washoe clearly didn't want her to go, and signed 'PLEASE PERSON HUG'.[48] That incident was reported by Roger Fouts, Washoe's key trainer, who noted that 'she had an uncanny knack for seeking out and comforting those who were sad or hurt.'[49]

Melanie Bond, a biologist and ape-keeper, had been working closely with an orangutan in a zoo in Washington in the 1970s. When he died, she was in acute distress, crying inconsolably. A chimpanzee called Ham was watching her, and she spoke to him, saying, 'Yes, Ham, I am very sad.' The chimpanzee tenderly and slowly reached a finger through the bars of his cage, and touched a tear on her cheek. He brought his hand to his own face, smelled the tear and tasted it. 'I felt empathy,' Melanie recalled precisely: 'someone understands.'[50] Someone understood, perhaps because he'd experienced trauma too. First when he was snatched from his mother as a baby, and then, having been terrorized with electric shocks, being forced into a rocket and flung into outer space as part of the US space programme.

Koko the gorilla was once shown a picture of a cowboy on a horse with a bridle and bit. Koko signed 'POOR HORSE'. When her trainer Dr Patterson asked 'WHY POOR HORSE?' Koko gestured at the horse's head and signed 'MOUTH HURTS'.[51]

Dawn Prince-Hughes's childhood was often unhappy: human communication baffled and wounded her. In pain and lonely, she went to spend time with the gorillas at the Woodland Park Zoo in Seattle where one gorilla in particular was important to her, a silverback male called Congo. He had, she said, a kind face and liked people and would 'try to coax them close so that he could have conversations with them. He softened hard people and made sensitive people come alive.'[52]

Feeling desperately distressed at one point, and close to breaking, she turned to Congo for help:

> I looked up into his huge warm face . . . He rushed over and searched my face intently. My vision blurred, and tears spilled out of my eyes . . . Congo moved toward me, put his massive shoulder against

the window, and motioned with his hand for me to lay my head there. I let my head fall softly on the place where his shoulder had been offered and cried silently . . . It was the foundation of his inner dignity to care.[53]

Animals not only express empathy but are perceived to nurture empathy in us. Innate in most humans, its development is vital for well-being. Studies show how young children's experience of helping to care for animals deepens their ability to empathize.[54] In Croatia, a study showed that children who lived with dogs were more empathic than those who did not.[55] What researchers are demonstrating today has long been intuited by poets. When Christopher Smart considered his cat Jeoffry, he remarked: 'For he is an instrument for the children to learn benevolence upon.'

From the eighteenth century, in childhood literature, anthropomorphic and affectionate animals were seen as the ideal medium for cultivating children's compassion, with one anonymous anti-hunting story narrated by a hare. Prominent humanitarians have often been animal lovers.[56] For theologian Albert Schweitzer, humanity could not find peace until the circle of compassion was drawn to include all living beings. In the words of Mahatma Gandhi, 'The greatness of a nation and its moral progress can be judged by the way its animals are treated.' William Wilberforce, a campaigner against slavery, co-founded the RSPCA.[57] Maybe it was the animals who came first: maybe in childhood these figures learned good lessons from the animals themselves – the influential seventeenth-century philosopher John Locke believed that pets helped children develop kindness and sympathy. Animals seem to increase the ability of adults, too, to be empathic, perhaps because, not sharing words directly, we have to pay more curious and careful attention to the experience of that other creature. It is, of course, possible that people who are naturally more empathic may more readily include animals within the curtilage of their care.

When it comes to empathy, we try to sympathetically project, or we may guess at someone else's experience, but then the dolphin comes along and puts us in the shade. Dolphins get much of their information about their world through echolocation, and they can eavesdrop on each other's echolocations so, by listening to another dolphin, they can share that other dolphin's experience far more closely than a human could share another's. The eavesdropping dolphin is not only hearing but experiencing that heard-object within itself.[58] United by feeling, they are right inside each other's minds, and they can't help but be empathic. 'I hear you,' we say, or indeed, 'I feel your pain.' A dolphin might say not 'I feel you' but 'I and you are feeling the same thing at the same time. You are in my thoughts.' Literally so.

Spindle neurons, brain cells associated with empathy, were previously thought to be present only in humans and great apes. We now know that they are also found in baleen whales, including humpback and fin whales and likely others, and they are found in exactly the same place in baleen whale brains as they are in human brains.[59]

The most basic building block of empathy is emotional contagion, for example when one person yawns in response to another's yawning. Dogs and horses experience yawn contagion in response to human yawns,[60] and lions have been observed doing the same.[61] Pigs also demonstrate the arousal of emotion in one individual on beholding the same emotion (being stressed and on alert, with their ears back) in another pig.[62] So do woodlice.

Woodlice. Curled up, generally mooching around, or trotting off at a good lick if they are disturbed, woodlice had never given me pause for thought until one morning I saw one at its breakfast, nibbling a fallen leaf, and heard its soft and rhythmic bites, as if it were crunching a Weetabix. That encounter, tiny though it was, attuned me to the woodlice world, so when I read about them experiencing emotional contagion, a primal form of empathy, I was delighted. If you disturb a nest of woodlice, they disperse. But if there is a particularly calm woodlouse in the nest (I'll call him Thich Nhat Hanh: he was a Buddhist monk, so I doubt he'd mind) then all the others are influenced. Thich Nhat Hanh, calm, will move more slowly than the others, who will notice and become calm in turn, dispersing more slowly than a nest without a Thich Nhat.[63]

~

What is love? Wanting to be close to someone, physically and emotionally. Missing them if they're not there. Delighting in seeing them again. Love is an alliance of time, asking us to lay our hours in the lap of another's life. Love means wanting to defend someone, it means recognizing them, acknowledging them, choosing them and staying loyal, dwelling with them, delighting in them, intensely and ceaselessly.

If we feel lonely at the heart's edge, animals may offer their love. When a twelve-year-old Russian boy called Vadim Veligurov adopted an abandoned baby sparrow, the bird never flew away but stayed by his side, perched on his shoulder. In photos, you can see the love in the boy's gaze as he tilts his head to the bird, while the bird nuzzles and rubs the boy's face with her head. Beak to lip they kiss, and she eats from his hand.

Vicki Fishlock, an elephant researcher, describes how, after an absence of several months, she re-met a family of elephants she'd known well, including one named Enid. When she met them again, 'suddenly Enid's head *swept* up, and she gave this *huge* rumble; her ears were flapping and they all came around, close enough that I could have touched them, and the glands on all their faces were streaming with emotion,' writes Fishlock. 'I felt as though I was getting an elephant hug.'[64] I think that is love.

For conservationist Damian Aspinall, it was a gorilla. He'd raised Kwibi before releasing him into the wilds in Gabon, and hadn't seen the gorilla for five years. Other humans had been attacked by Kwibi, but when Aspinall found him, they shared food, the gorilla hugging the man tightly, gazing deeply into his eyes, in a moving piece of footage online.

The nineteenth-century French author Anatole France wrote: 'Until one has loved an animal, a part of one's soul remains unawakened.' I'd add: until one *has been loved by* an animal, a part of the soul is still dormant.

I had a cat called Tom, originally a feral cat, who loved me heart and soul for every minute of his life. He was a deep soul, capable of empathy and demonstrations of devotion. Tom never hunted in all his ten years of life, except on two occasions, and each time occurred when I had been sobbing uncontrollably. One was when another kitten had just been killed on the road. I held Tom in my lap, crying and hugging him close. He let me do that for a while, then jumped down, went outside and came back within an hour and a half with two mice and a dead bird – a huge haul for a cat who had never hunted. There was intention in this, not chance. In cat language, bringing fresh kill is a gift, and this felt as if it was offered to console me. The other time, I had been feeling low, tired and premenstrual, and had made myself even sadder, drinking red wine and watching *How Green Was My Valley*. I'd gone to bed with Tom at two in the morning, and fell asleep crying into his fur. He left, returning to my room at six o'clock with an almost – but not completely – dead rat. After that, I made myself a promise never to cry in front of him again.

He channelled his fierce love by becoming my shadow. He'd howl by the door for up to forty-five minutes if I left the house or tried to go to my study without him. My bath has a shower attachment, and if I wanted a shower, he'd get in with me, although he'd stay at the dry end. If I needed to get up in the night for a pee, he'd get up with me, sit with me and get back into bed with me. His devotion was total and only for me. His love was my refuge and it healed me, giving me the experience of unconditional love that I had not known.

Love is medicine. Love is the opposite of loneliness, that silent killer. Love touches the heart's core. It heals and makes us whole and gathers us into the wholeness of things. And because I have known the love of Tom, I realize I can never be unbeloved.

3

Untangling the Psyche

'There's no psychiatrist in the world like a puppy licking your face' – philosopher Bernard Williams

I love horses, but it was a donkey who stole my heart. Leo, chocolate-brown with a nose of cream, gazed at me as if all the tenderness of the world lay in his eyes. He came to me the moment I entered the field he was in. He snuggled, rubbed and leaned into me, and if he could have hugged me he would. In fact, most of the donkeys came to sniff me and nuzzle up. The staff at the sanctuary said they were amazed at how many of the donkeys were drawn to me – 'They seem to really love you!'

'Ummm,' I said, 'actually I think it's because of my jumper.'

When I was dressing that morning, knowing I was going to meet donkeys, I had chosen to wear a jumper I thought they might like. It was old and woolly with bobbly bits that they could nibble with their sensitive, curious lips. It undoubtedly smelled of a horse-friend of mine, Herbie, and likely also of the foal Rocky, certainly of a cat or two, and it probably also smelled of my god-dog Fflos and perhaps a few puppies, compost, leaves and general gardening. I don't know when I last washed it. It just isn't a jumper that has ever asked to be washed. And I doubt I'll ever wash it now, as it seems to be just too enticing for animals. It was absolute catnip for the donkeys at the Donkey Sanctuary in Sidmouth, Devon.

This chapter looks at animal-assisted therapy, how different creatures from donkeys to doves, and skunks to parakeets, have been seen to have healing effects, something that Indigenous cultures have long known. The chapter explores how animals can help people to speak, and how service dogs can save the psyche and the life.

So, Leo. When he snuffled me, nose to nose, I felt euphoric. Rinsed with bliss. I was as giddy as an eight-year-old when I stroked him and rubbed him. A donkey is the perfect height for a shortish woman or a child to hug, while a donkey's neck and head are exquisitely tailored for a person's arms to wrap around. I held him and nuzzled him, put my nose to his fur and smelled him.

With your cheek against a donkey's neck, you feel as if you could befriend the world. Happiness spilled out across my face with ripples of smiles in rings of bright water. The donkeys filled my eyes and my arms and my heart brimful. The fullness of their eyes, deep, dark wells of pure kindness, ten thousand fathoms deep, seemed to gaze ever beyond, seeing further than petty human concerns.

Donkeys are the archetype of gentleness, the holy animal of the Christ story twice over, once at the beginning and once at the end, and they seem to meditate by default as they are animals of endurance, patience and tranquillity.

'Be More Donkey' is a line I hear a lot at the sanctuary. I spoke to a district nurse recently whose experience of the pandemic had left her suffering from devastating anxiety and depression, extreme exhaustion and chronic stress. She told me how donkeys were medicine for her because they modelled a healthier way to be, breathing a sweet and serene peace, their presence 'so simple and straightforward and honest'.

Staff and visitors tell me how calming it is to be by donkeys and how, once someone feels calm, other changes can take place. Kids who are excluded from school and shun other interventions may be referred to these donkeys by their teachers, and the time they spend with the donkeys gives them huge gains in life skills such as the ability to manage emotions, along with greater self-awareness, self-belief and confidence. The sanctuary offers their service free to anyone who needs it.

Donkeys are sensitive. Equines, who are both herd animals and prey animals, need to be reactive as quicksilver to a flicker of fear in the herd, or to aggression in the body language of a potential predator. Their survival depends on it,[1] and that sensitivity can be put to therapeutic use.

At Green Chimneys, a farm in New York State that cares for troubled kids, one therapist was working with a thirteen-year-old boy who had anger issues and difficulty making friends. She placed him with donkeys so that he could clearly see how his body language was having a negative effect. At first, his movements were quick and jerky, and the donkeys first stared then moved away from him. He, though, wanted to stroke them, so he shoved out his arms, chasing them. They fled. The therapist asked the boy if the donkeys liked him being with them. No, he said, ruefully, they looked as if they were unhappy and frightened. Over time, he learned to move more slowly, gently and smoothly – and never to chase them. He altered his behaviour for the donkeys and from this experience he learned to adjust his body language for other humans.[2]

Horses read our body language and do so even when we don't think we are speaking it. 'Clever Hans' was a horse famous in Berlin in the early twentieth century. When he was given sums, he would tap his front hoof the correct number of times for the answer, and people thought he could do maths. But if the questioner didn't know the answer, Hans could not respond correctly. No one saw what the horse saw, which was the almost imperceptible and entirely unconscious body language from the questioner as Hans approached the right number of taps, cueing the horse to stop. Hans could read humans better than they could read themselves.

Equine therapists say that if a person's body language is not consonant with their emotional state, a horse is jangled by the disparity and finds it inauthentic. American horse-trainer Ginger Gaffney says bluntly that horses need honesty from us. 'If you are truly honest about how you feel, your body will show it. The horses know the difference,' and your body language 'tells them whether you are trustworthy or a fake. Believe me when I tell you, they know the difference.'[3]

There is something going on here, in the between. Between Leo and me. Between donkey and exhausted nurse. Between the donkeys and the troubled teenager. Further inside, though, too: between psyche and body, because some of the healing happens at the impossibly delicate interface between body and mind. Equines, exquisitely sensitive to a range of emotions in others including fear, anxiety, anger and sadness, ineluctably resonate with others on a direct, physiological level. Equine therapist Louise Reynolds, working on Dartmoor, explains that horses, donkeys and alpacas can regulate each other's heartbeats and calm each other at quite a distance. Horses can sense ours and calm us too. 'Literally standing by a horse,' she tells me, 'healing happens.'

Horses can sense the heart rate and stress level of a human rider, and the horse's own heart rate and stress levels alter in sync with the human.[4] This is crucial. Horses and donkeys clearly dislike feeling stressed, and when people speak of equines disliking inauthenticity it is perhaps because masking one's feelings is stressful for the human and therefore, by emotional contagion, stressful for a horse in close proximity. Stress feels bad, and horses would want the pain to stop in themselves and in the source.

Dr Hannah Burgon runs Sirona Therapeutic Horsemanship in Devon and also researches how horses are psychologically healing. One of her studies shows how horses can affect young people, improving their resilience and positivity. After therapy with horses, they said that they felt calm, happy, relaxed and, poignantly, loved.[5] Another of her studies shows that therapy with horses builds self-esteem, improves mental health and encourages positive behavioural change.[6] Therapists note that for someone on the autistic spectrum, intimacy may be easier with a horse than with a human.[7]

The human mind seems to have surmised a healing ability in horses. In ancient Greek myth, the centaur (half horse, half man) Chiron learned medicine and herbs from his foster-father, Apollo, the god of healing. Chiron discovered the science of pharmacy and tutored Asclepius, the god of medicine. Chiron, who was an immortal, was accidentally wounded by a poisoned arrow and it caused him terrible pain which, despite his medical skill, he couldn't heal. As he was immortal, nor could he die. Chiron was a wounded healer.

~

Dr Ange Condoret, a French veterinarian, worked in a children's nursery during the 1970s, introducing animals to preschoolers with psychological issues. One of the girls in his care, Bethsabee, had had a cruel start in life. At birth, she lost her mother and was sent to a foster home. There, she was locked into a room and usually tied to a bed. Then she was drugged. The severe effects of this abuse, coupled with having autism, resulted in her being locked in to herself. She refused all contact from humans and if someone forced touch on her, her body stiffened in rigid protest.

Bethsabee arrived at the nursery aged six. She would not meet anyone's gaze. No one had ever seen her smile. If she played, she chose hard things like boxes and blocks, manipulating them with stiff, outstretched arms. As a result of her incarceration, she could not bear to be left in a room with a closed door. She never spoke, although she would hiss at people and make clicking noises. She ignored the animals – a dog, cat and other small animals – that Dr Condoret introduced to her. Nothing could break down the prison door. Nothing could free her spirit.

Until the dove.

Condoret was filming the children's interactions with various creatures when he caught the moment a dove perched in front of Bethsabee.[8]

Suddenly, right there and then, it opens its wings. Bethsabee looks directly at the bird and it takes flight – an ordinary miracle. To the child, it has the impact of an angel. Bethsabee's body loses its rigidity and her expression softens into the first smile of her life. She is radiant. Her arms flutter up, as if her mind is finding its wings. When the bird perches again, she stops smiling. It takes wing once more and a smile flits again like a rainbow across the girl's face.

Humans had harmed her so badly, and it is a dove, that quintessentially harmless creature, who brings healing on its wings. She reaches out to it, touches it, strokes it and then, with her silenced lips, she kisses it. At this point, I see Picasso's *Child with a Dove*, the little girl alive in the bird, and the bird in her. Maybe it could only have been a dove, who wouldn't force touch on her, and couldn't abuse her, that could have worked that therapeutic miracle.

After the dove, everything changed. She began to allow people to touch her. She held the teacher's hand. She started to imitate speech, to join in with the games of the other children, and finally, she began to speak.

It is almost always humans who make humans feel distressed and traumatized. It is often animals who remedy the pain. The psyche can hurt in countless ways: you might be vacant with blunt misery, wracked by bad memories, contorted by humiliation or knotted with anguish, anxiety shrilling along your nerves. Sometimes, if you're asked what hurts, you can only say, *Everything*.

I've been moved to tears by people's experiences of animals helping them. As well as these testaments, though, formal research and studies are golden and necessary, offering solid evidence of the vital role that animals can play in psychological health. Forgive the blizzard of note numbers in the next two paragraphs: I think it matters to show how animals can offer remedies for very specific psychological ills.

Animals as therapy can lessen depression and anxiety,[9] aggression,[10] bullying,[11] trauma symptoms,[12] anger,[13] social withdrawal, feelings of helplessness,[14] and the perception of pain.[15] They can reduce violence and suicide attempts, together with lowering the need for tranquillizers.[16] They aid in what has been called 'emotional dysfunction',[17] and help with alienation,[18] the distress linked to neurodiversity,[19] isolation,[20] crime[21] and agitated behaviour.[22]

Therapy animals also improve the following: self-control and autonomy,[23] honesty,[24] concentration, motivation and calmness,[25] the ability to make friends,[26] responsibility and loving caregiving,[27] cooperation and negotiation,[28] rapport, communication and benign behaviour,[29] learning skills,[30] social skills,[31] self-regulation,[32] self-respect,[33] independence and self-confidence,[34] emotional bonding,[35] attachment,[36] morale,[37] well-being,[38] trust,[39] mental functioning,[40] empathy[41] and even the ability to ask for help.[42]

~

In the 1990s, Dr William Thomas wrote a unique prescription. He had taken up the position as head of the Chase Memorial Nursing Home in New Berlin, New York, and on his arrival he saw a lifeless, joyless place suffering from what he called the plagues of loneliness, helplessness and boredom. So he prescribed two dogs, four cats, several hens and rabbits, a hundred parakeets and a bunch of children. The presence of so many animals broke state law at the time but worked as pure medicine for what ailed the residents. Morale, happiness and independence all shot up and many of the residents began dressing themselves, eating again and taking an interest in life, leaving their rooms and interacting with others. The animals deinstitutionalized the place. Drug costs were cut in half, saving $75,000 a year. The infection rate at Chase was 50 per cent less than that of a similar nursing home, and the death rate was 15 per cent less than this home in the first year and 25 per cent less in the second year.

It could be a bird who heals. Dr Thomas believed that a parakeet at the nursing home saved a woman's life, after she had suffered a stroke and was unable to speak. Her relationship with this bird gave her 'a reason to fight through a terrible illness and come back and recover and be stronger than she ever was: I could never have given her a drug that would have caused that reaction.'

It could be three kittens. In the 1970s, also in the United States, a frail and elderly man in a residential centre was refusing to eat. One day, an aide discovered that the centre's kittens were curled up in bed with him. If staff took the kittens away, he got distressed, so they cut a deal with him: he could have the kittens if he ate. It worked and the man survived, even thrived, gaining forty pounds in weight and beginning to interact with other residents. The director of nursing said she believed that without the kittens, he would have died.[43]

It could be a dog. In Caulfield Hospital in Melbourne, Australia, a dog called Honey (a former guide dog) was introduced as an unofficial therapist and resident mascot in 1981.[44] The staff watched the Honey effect and noted that within six months the residents were happier, smiling and laughing more, and were more alert, more relaxed and demonstrated a greater will to live.

It could be an owl. Jan Parker, a systemic family psychotherapist, told me of a fourteen-year-old client, Grace, who attends farm-based alternative education and spends time with the owls on-site, finding solace there. When she is with them, she feels they 'know everything, all the shit that's happened in my life, but it's calm, and it's just me and them and we're happy. It's like a comfort, like a connection. Everyone says when I'm at the farm I'm like a different person. Or maybe it's that the birds can see me in a way that most people don't.'

It could be a skunk. Dale Preece-Kelly is an animal-assisted therapy practitioner. He often works with rescue animals, many of whom have disabilities – something that, he says, helps the patients as they may more readily identify with the animals and bond with them. He has a therapy skunk and believes that a skunk is better than a cat as a therapy animal because cats often refuse to approach a stranger, which can have a detrimental effect on a client's self-esteem, making them feel rejected.

Despite their bad reputation, skunks are sweet and affectionate. They may get results. Preece-Kelly reports how one client, diagnosed with paranoid schizophrenia, would spend a session with the skunk, and for that hour and a short time afterwards, the voices in his head would stop. Without the cacophony, he could talk to people, including his psychologist, with calmness and clarity.[45] Preece-Kelly notes that skunks may be highly effective for people with mental health issues because both mental illness and skunks carry a certain stigma and both are at the mercy of people's judgement.

From childhood, many of us suffer from the feeling of being judged – by the unsatisfiable parent or the critical teacher. Exposure to social media leaves people exposed to the malicious judgements of others. People frequently say that in their experience of animal-assisted therapy, they are helped because they don't feel judged by animals. One child who had been badly bullied and had sought help from horses at the Fortune Centre of Riding Therapy in Christchurch, UK, picked this quality as a reason for their effectiveness, saying the horses 'made me so confident . . . no one's going to judge me cos the horses don't judge me.'[46]

The clinical psychologist Dr Boris Levinson, the father of animal-assisted therapy, wrote, 'When a child craves a close, cuddly, affectionate, nonjudgmental relationship, the dog can provide it.' He could see that dogs show an unconditional positive regard for others, the gold standard of therapeutic practice. His words are furry with understanding, warm as a puppy den.

In his influential 1961 article 'The Dog as a "Co-Therapist"', Levinson describes the accidental way he had stumbled on the importance of pets in therapy some eight years previously. A boy had become so withdrawn that hospitalization had been recommended, and Levinson had agreed to see the family urgently. They arrived an hour early for the appointment, and Levinson was in his study with his dog, Jingles. When the family entered the study, the dog ran up to the child to lick him and the child cuddled up with the dog. It was the presence of Jingles that opened the child up to Levinson, 'as some of the affection elicited by the dog spilled over onto me'. He alerted the listening world to the importance of animals in therapy, particularly for children, noting: 'In many ways, the relationship between man and dog, especially between child and dog, can be more salutary than one between two human beings.'

Levinson concluded his article with a telling thought: 'Maybe some day,' he wrote, 'we shall be able to prescribe pets of a certain kind for different emotional disorders.'

Ah, dear Levinson, some have been doing so for aeons. Indigenous cultures have long been considering the medicine brought to us by different animals. The lore of the Haida people of the Pacific Northwest coast, for one, includes the healing gifts of the animals. When the Rediscovery International Foundation takes young people to wilderness camps for therapy, the programme introduces them to the native traditions of that land. The first camp was in British Columbia, where the organizers based the therapeutic work on Haida culture.

The kids were set an exercise. First they were sent to find fourteen small pebbles, and asked to paint each stone to represent a different animal. Then, as the camp progressed, each day, the kids would pick one of these pebbles and try to take the psychological remedy offered by that particular animal on the pebble. The wolf's medicine is self-esteem. The raven's healing gift is curiosity. The salmon teaches generosity, the spider patience and the bear inner strength. The healing guidance of the hummingbird is joyfulness, of the squirrel assertiveness, of the deer peacefulness, while the frog offers self-expression, the goose cooperation, and the mosquito tolerance. The beaver teaches self-control, the eagle teaches long vision and the loon guides people towards spirituality. The children move through all the pebbles over two weeks, practising those different qualities each day, and when they get to the end they begin again.[47] I love this idea so much: I'm going out now to get pebbles.

Influenced by Indigenous therapeutic wisdom, psychologist Dr Darline Hunter and Professor of Counselling Cheryl Sawyer, based in Texas, blend Native American spirituality with academic child psychology to facilitate counselling. They show how children may be invited to consider animal abilities and then to map those strengths on to themselves as a tonic for self-esteem. The children make a mask of their chosen animal and write a poem or essay about its qualities, then wear the mask and share the words.[48] I instantly think of every child I have known (including myself) and how this would have been rich and powerful mind-medicine.

~

Dozer and Lupe, two black Labradors, are members of the Special Victims K9 Unit, in San Bernardino County, California, and their job is to comfort children who have been witnesses to, or victims of, crime. Being in a courtroom can be terrifying for children, and the content of the cases may be fearful, embarrassing and traumatic. The dogs are 'courthouse facility dogs', taking the stand alongside children, particularly those who are giving testimony of physical and sexual abuse. In one case, a boy had been raped from when he was four until he was ten and had been unable to speak of it. In court he was very nervous and stressed, finding it too hard to give evidence, until Lupe, with a serious gaze, nudged the boy's leg and the boy began rubbing the dog's ears and became able to speak.[49] The support provided by the dog was more effective than anything else for the boy, and it reminds me of one remarkable study of work with children who had been sexually abused which showed that children rated their pets as more supportive than people.[50]

Animals such as Lupe can make humans feel safe enough to speak.

What is it with words? They can cure, soothe and delight. They can also hurt, harm and humiliate. For some, after the wounds of words, falling silent is a defence, sometimes the only fortress for the injured psyche. Silence, of course, is the response of many animals when they fear being made prey. When frogs don't croak and small birds seal up their song, it is often because there are predators about. Humans, feeling themselves to be prey, often do the same.

Therapy with horses improves clients' relationships with their therapist,[51] and the presence of animals makes psychotherapy progress faster[52] as the animals encourage spoken language between humans. In one instance of animal therapy in an old people's home, an elderly man spoke a coherent sentence for the first time in twenty-six years, reported by psychiatrists at Ohio State University in 1980.[53]

'Mr Koehler, he chewed my socks. What should I do?' This was the first time Joey, an eleven-year-old boy with autism, had ever spoken to a human in his whole life. Not one word. His therapist had arranged for Joey to have a dog, and the boy was taking the dog to training classes, led by Dick Koehler. In the third week, the boy spoke for the first time in his life, saying to the dog, 'Jason, heel! Jason, sit. Good dog!' About halfway through the thirteen-week course, he spoke to Koehler.[54]

A study of children with autism who were given therapy llamas suggests that the presence of the animals encouraged greater use of language and social interaction compared to standard occupational therapy.[55] Michael Morpurgo, the children's author, runs a charity called Farms for City Children, and reports how a boy called Billy, who could barely speak because of a terrible stammer, was found one day talking and talking and talking – to a horse. Billy needed to speak and the horse gave him the gentle audience he needed, the gift of listening.

The same thing was noted in the Bethlem psychiatric hospital in

London when, in 1860, the *Illustrated London News* described the men's ward where some patients would 'pace the long gallery incessantly, pouring out their woes to those who will listen to them, or, if there be none to listen, to the dogs and cats'.[56]

The therapeutic use of animals has long been intuited, often by poets. James Hadfield, a poet inmate in Bethlem Hospital from 1800 until his death in 1841, kept two dogs, three cats, birds and a squirrel, writing verse epitaphs for them when they died. The poet Christopher Smart was an inmate in mental asylums from 1757 to 1763, from where he wrote his praise-poem to creation, *Jubilate Agno*, which included the ode to his cat Jeoffry, who accompanied and attended him in hospital. Various psychiatric institutions in history also understood that animals could help treat the mentally unwell: seagulls, hawks, rabbits and poultry were a key part of the treatment at the York Retreat in England from the 1790s.[57]

In the 1770s, the poet William Cowper suffered from devastating depressions and surrounded himself with a menagerie of animals including rabbits, guinea pigs, goldfinches, canaries and dogs. He prescribed hares for himself, because they were amiable and affectionate and took great enjoyment in life (something much needed by depressives). Beguiled by the hare's fur, quivering nose, and ears soft as sage leaves, he found that the hares would 'engage my attention without fatiguing it', an attentive definition of the lightly focused state of mind now called 'soft fascination'. He had three hares, named Puss, Bess and Tiney, all males. They encouraged him outdoors insistently. One hare, Puss, 'would invite me to the garden by drumming upon my knee, and by a look of such expression, as it was not possible to misinterpret. If this rhetoric did not immediately succeed, he would take the skirt of my coat between his teeth, and pull it with all his force.'[58]

Hare medicine may help someone out of the grave of depression. Donkey medicine is excellent when you need tranquillity, and horse medicine may spur someone into authenticity. Kitten medicine is indisputably good for instant distraction and humour. Bird medicine harmonizes the psyche and may be a tonic for someone who needs to know freedom. Dog medicine reliably offers devotion and total acceptance. And dogs, of course, are the animals most commonly chosen as therapy animals and service animals.

~

Service dogs can stitch a life and a mind back together, offering the handiwork of daily care, fetching, telling, finding, reminding, and mending one need after another.

In Uganda, the Lord's Resistance Army has been operating since the late 1980s and has abducted tens of thousands of children in one of the most gruesome wars of recent times. The effects of war have left no one unhurt, but for some, dogs became rescuers. One child, Francis, was blinded by a bomb-blast and although he continued attending his boarding school in northern Uganda, he faced numerous difficulties. If he needed the bathroom in the night, it was hard for him to find the toilets, which were some distance from the dormitories, so he would stumble, get a bit lost and bump into things with no one to help him. Or so he thought. Actually, two dogs living next door to the school began to notice the child's difficulty and made a habit of watching out for him. Whenever he left the dormitory, the dogs would run over to him, letting him know they were alongside him, and would guide him to the toilets. It happened every night for years, and as a result, Francis said, he felt he could navigate the world.

Francis's story was the inspiration for the Comfort Dog Project,[59] a programme set up in northern Uganda using dogs to help the victims of the war. Each person is paired with a dog, and takes a vow to be the guardian to that dog for life, to give them healthy food, shelter and companionship. The key to the programme's success is that what the traumatized humans give to the dogs they also get back, as the dogs offer them companionship and emotional shelter and act as a guardian for the spirit. One man's wife and two children had been killed in front of him during the war. It left him with devastating depression and flashbacks. He began drinking heavily. When he was paired with a dog from the Comfort Dog Project, they became very close, but one day the man fell seriously ill, unable to leave his house or raise the alarm. The dog went and got help for him and the man eventually recovered, believing that the dog saved his life twice over because the dog hated the smell of alcohol so much the man had to quit drinking.

One US army veteran, who had done eight years of active service by the time he was twenty-five, was left traumatized and sleepless, with a seriously irregular heart rate, bad headaches and suicidal thoughts. (In the USA, more war veterans of Vietnam have died by suicide than were killed in the war.) Then he got a service dog, Birdie, and when she was with him his heart rate shifted into the healthy zone for the first time since he'd joined the army. More than that, he could finally — with Birdie at his side — sleep.[60]

A service dog can pull a wheelchair, find lost things, put laundry in a machine and take it out when the wash is done.[61] A dog can help their human to get up from the floor, or walk upstairs, bracing on command to steady them.

One of the most famous service dogs was Endal, a golden Labrador, who worked with Allen Parton. Parton had served in the British Royal Navy in the Gulf War in the 1990s, where he was horrifically injured. He lost the use of both legs, leaving him in a wheelchair. He also sustained devastating head injuries, involving severe memory loss. He couldn't talk, read or write, and suffered serious depression. Endal's interventions, initiative and intelligence were magnificent.

In 2001, Parton and Endal were invited to take part in Crufts dog show, in Birmingham. They were outside a hotel when a speeding car hit Parton, knocking him out of his wheelchair and leaving him unconscious. Endal pulled Parton into the recovery position, retrieved his mobile phone and pushed it under Allen's head. He got a blanket from the overturned wheelchair to cover him, and then alert-barked at the nearby hotel. When no one responded, he ran to the hotel to get help.

Endal could follow over a hundred instructions, including retrieving certain items from supermarket shelves, and if Parton became unconscious in the bath, Endal would pull the plug out and then go to fetch help. He could use the emergency button on a phone to summon help, and he learned to use an ATM, inserting the card and retrieving the card, the money and the receipt, and returning the card to the wallet.[62]

Endal is not alone: service dogs can do far more than offer their company and love. Service dogs can retrieve a medical bag and drag-deliver it to their human, fetching a drink to help their human swallow medication: if the cupboard or fridge has a strap the dog can pull, then the dog can be trained to pick up the drink before the door swings shut. If medication leaves someone unresponsive to a caller, a service dog can be trained to jump on their bed and lick their face until they wake, then the dog can turn on bedroom lights with a floor pedal and escort their human to the caller.

They can fetch an emergency phone, answer a doorbell, open the front door and escort emergency personnel to their human. They can carry a note to another person on command, or bark to summon help in a prearranged way.

Guide dogs for those who are blind are trained to obey a command to help their handler navigate the world by walking centrally along pavements, avoiding obstacles, stopping at kerbs and steps. They must also be on the lookout for something amiss, for potential harm to their human, and must make some decisions on their own: if, for example, the handler indicates that they want to cross a road, the dog must decide if it is safe to do so and, if it is not safe, disobey the command. Obedience matters, but this – intelligent disobedience – is more important. Like the dogs of the Evenki hunters, service dogs must be able to think for themselves.

A psychiatric service dog can notice the difference between healthy sleep and a dizzy faint and, in the latter, fetch medication. The dog can note mood swings and alert their human early, by staring, nudging or barking and refusing to stop until their human has taken note. A dog can also drop a big hint, bringing medication to a person on the edge. This ability is a godsend, according to Dr Mark Smith, a psychopharmacologist specializing in mood disorder, because those with bipolar disorder may often lack insight when they are moving into manic mode. As he says tellingly: 'Mates are never believed. Doctors are often doubted. Whereas the messages of the pet are taken as bedrock truth.'[63]

As a guard dog at the threshold of home keeps you safe from danger outside, so psychiatric service dogs at the threshold of the psyche guard you from demons within. The unwell mind can be a hideously complicated knot, a cat's cradle tripwire multiplied by tangled string theory, intricate in sickening complexity. The dogs gently tease out the knots, unravel the complexities and untangle the psyche, as various specialists including Joan Froling reveal.

In high anxiety, a dog may offer deep pressure with their paws, calming their human. If someone has nightmares, night terrors or unshakeable horrifying memories, the dog can start a game of tug-with-toy, or turn on bedroom lights or bring the television remote so that the sudden effect of a game with light and sound can disrupt the toxic trance.

If someone suffers from hallucinations of a potential intruder, their dog can be trained to establish what is real. On an instruction such as 'Go and say hello', a dog will check out whether there is actually someone there. If so, the dog will greet them, but if there is no one there the dog will return to their human, which lets the person know it was a hallucination.[64]

If their human is becoming withdrawn, a psychiatric service dog can initiate interactions. If someone is self-harming, the dog can deliberately interrupt. If someone has a dissociative episode or panic attack, the dog senses it and nuzzles, nudges or licks them to reorient them to reality. If someone is disoriented by a dissociative episode, the dog can guide them back to the place where the dissociation began.[65] The dog may always guide their human home and, once there, a dog can be trained to tug their human's socks off, gently, and without biting their human's foot.

In August 2015, Maria Colon was asleep in her home in Holmesburg, Philadelphia. She had been blind since 1992, and had a service dog, a golden Labrador called Yolanda. On that August night, Maria was woken by the smell of smoke. She shouted 'danger' to her dog, who immediately went to the specially adapted phone and dialled 911. 'I hear the phone – *tke, tke, tke*. And she's growling. And I said, *Oh my lord, she called the police*.' Both were treated for smoke inhalation and recovered.[66]

Sometimes a person in psychiatric crisis may need help but be unable to summon it, perhaps because of a tranquillizer overdose, or perhaps because they are in a state of PTSD-terror. In such a case, the dog may be given hand signals to bring a speakerphone and, if their human cannot speak, the dog will bark for them, alerting the person on the end of the line. If there is a psychiatric crisis, a service dog in the USA can call 911. Some dogs may instinctively sense a crisis while others may be trained to recognize one and to touch a screen, placed at dog height, which shows three separate large circles, with a *9*, then *1* and another *1*. If the dog presses these with their nose, in the right order, a message is automatically sent to the emergency services. (They may also use a specially adapted K9 rescue phone, pushing a large white button with their paw.) 911 computers can be programmed to tell the operator that if there is no human voice, they need to assume that a service dog is placing the call as an emergency.

For some people with psychiatric conditions including PTSD, gatherings of any kind may feel stressful, and they may become distressed or panicky and want to leave, but they may not want to explain why they need to. A dog can provide a perfect exit strategy. First, the dog is taught a surreptitious hand signal (a tiny movement of one particular finger, perhaps) and then the dog is taught to respond by performing attention-seeking behaviour, disrupting the situation, whining, vocalizing as if they urgently need the toilet, jumping up and pretending to hassle their human, thus providing them with an urgent and plausible excuse to leave the situation.[67] They are acting.

If you are at an ATM in a wheelchair, you'd need eyes in the back of your head to protect yourself if you're vulnerable to robbery, so service dogs can be trained to follow the command 'watch my back'. But service dogs must have a friendly nature and are trained not to attack. What if there is someone menacing near that ATM user? There's a conundrum.

The answer? The dog is trained to *pretend* to be aggressive, trained to act the role well enough to see off a potential attacker. I salute the dogs who've done drama classes and majored in improvisation.

It is as if the dog provides a prosthetic mind, a healthy psyche that can take over when the human mind is out of action. The dog is the epitome of clear thinking and wellness, orienting the person in place and time (be here and now); finding, balancing, focusing, grounding, calling for help if necessary and clarifying the reality of a situation. The dog is the guide, the doctor, the helper and the friend.

Donkeys, horses, doves, kittens, parakeets, hares, skunks, llamas and owls all play their parts in healing the human mind, but dogs seem to be the ones we lean on most readily. We humans have been living alongside them for some thirty-two thousand years and they give us a deep sense of safety as they can smell and hear far further out into the world than we can, so in the ancient memory of our atavistic genes, we know that they are offering us rings of protection wider than we can provide for ourselves. When a dog is there, calm, happy, maybe snoozing, an ancient part of the psyche knows 'the camp is safe.'[68]

Safety spreads in wider rings around our campfire selves. A physical safety – *no danger about* – yields to an intellectual safety – *don't worry about a thing* – yields to emotional and psychological safety – *everything's going to be okay*. And this safety carries further, wider than us and the campfire, out into the sleeping birds and waking mice, out into that fundamental bond of all that is co-living, life safe in the arms of life.

4

Oh God, Get That Young Woman a Dog

'I think he is The Friend who never gives up on me'
– Arwa Omareen

Picture it. 15 June 2021. A melting-hot day. The sun is nearly at the top of its game, streaming towards the summer solstice, pouring gold across the gorgeous western counties of England.

This is the kind of day that mocks the sad. Depressed people may loathe the difference between the outer sunny weather and their inner grey misery because the contrast increases the disconnection: all the world seems happy while you alone are not.

A young woman, Sally (not her real name), was caught by more than depression that day: she had become suicidal.

I don't know – can't know – her exact reasons for being in this situation, but the pandemic had been raging for more than a year and many people's mental health was in tatters. Loneliness and depression were rife. People's relationships with their family, friends and partners were under strain. For many, too, the work environment had become difficult with job losses, job alterations and, for some, the loneliness of working from home. Many of us suffered. Some of those who suffered stepped towards the abyss.

Sally went alone to a bridge over a main road, outside Exeter in Devon. And she stopped there.

In depression, we can feel an unbridgeable isolation. Nothing and no one can reach us. Depression is not only about sadness but also about feeling beyond communication, unable to bridge the gap between one's own psyche and another's.

Bridges connect. They are intended for crossing over, for walking across. To go to a bridge and stand still is different. The span of a bridge is designed to be crossed completely, as the span of the human life is to be lived out fully. Stopping in the middle of a bridge is like ceasing in the middle of a life. There is something about bridges for the suicidal psyche because for a person in suicide's grip, a bridge is no longer a link, nor a way, nor a route, nor a path. It is not a place of connection, as you walk or cycle across, but a point of cessation. There, in a dangerous psychological place, the bridge can morph into a cliff to jump from. Not the sweet ordinariness of the horizontal passage, but the vertical scream. The suicide's bridge is between worlds. Neither still in the land of life nor yet in the country of death.

I know.

I've been to The Bridge. Many of us have. And we can come back.

One time, in an agony of pain, I ran without knowing where I was going, trying to flee my mind through my body's flight. I stopped on a bridge over a river, my elbows on the stone parapet, my hands cradling my head. Going to that place felt like a compulsion to find the most accurate symbol of how I felt.

The Golden Gate Bridge in California draws people who are suicidal and *The Bridge* is the name of a documentary film that discusses this, recording some of the hundreds – perhaps now even thousands – of lives ended there, lives that did not have to finish like that. One of the rare people to have survived a suicide attempt at the Golden Gate Bridge says of the moment in mid-air, 'I instantly realized that everything in my life that I'd thought was unfixable was totally fixable – except for having just jumped.'[1] Suicide, says a friend of mine who has also known The Bridge, is a long-term response to a short-term problem.

People patrol the Golden Gate Bridge to prevent suicides, and police, volunteers and bridge workers try to talk people down, hoping to reach them in their devastations, doing so with some success but not enough. Huge efforts have been made to put up suicide barriers, to

Oh God, Get That Young Woman a Dog

make hotline numbers readily available and to try to put other people on the alert for warning signs. Saving lives is hard and sometimes it is not people who do it.

On 25 September 2000, nineteen-year-old Kevin Hines jumped from the Golden Gate Bridge, suffering from bipolar disorder and serious psychosis. He survived, later recalling how as he leaped, 'my first thought was that I had made a terrible mistake.' Although he lived, he was severely injured, and on resurfacing in the cold waters, he felt something brushing his legs. 'I feared it was a shark come to devour me whole. I tried to punch it, thinking it might bite me. However, this marine animal just circled beneath me, bumping me up.'

It was a sea lion.

Someone saw what was happening, realized that the sea lion was ensuring that Kevin's head was kept above water, and called for help. Kevin was pulled from the water, alive.

Back on the bridge outside Exeter, someone noticed Sally's intense and hovering stillness and felt it presaged badly. Worried for her welfare, they reported it and emergency services were called to the scene just before 11 a.m.[2] The response was rapid. The road was closed, an ambulance was on hand and the Devon and Somerset Fire and Rescue Service were at the incident as part of this multi-agency response. Police negotiators began trying to talk her down.

All the right people were there, doing all the right things, trying to communicate with Sally, hoping to establish some rapport to build a bridge, no matter how tenuous, across that gulf between them. But she couldn't respond. On the wrong side of the safety barriers, she was looking over the edge, in both senses. She was also unable to make eye contact, that other bridge between mind and mind.

The day was getting seriously hot as the emotional temperature was rising. It is hard to talk someone down when you have no thread, no link, and the police negotiators spoke into Sally's far darkness without a response. Hours passed like molten lead. Noon came and went. One o'clock and then two o'clock passed. The tension and worry were increasing.

Eventually, Sally managed to say one thing – she told the police that her family's dog had died. It was the only piece of information that the negotiators had to go on, and it turned out it was the only bit they really needed.

The death of a pet. Most people just don't understand. 'You can get another dog,' people will say brightly or, worse, you can hear them think: 'It's only a cat.'

But this animal may have been your best friend, your tell-first and witness to your childhood. They may have soaked up your tears, a tender, living lachrymatory, gazed into your eyes in unflinching adoration and indeed already have saved your psyche from collapse. The loss of a pet has resulted in suicides,[3] severe psychotic depression, intense sadness and that slow, heartbroken and fatal illness called Just Giving Up.

The police negotiators now knew about the death of Sally's dog, but what could they do with that information?

~

Arwa Omareen has shining eyes. They shine with love and intelligence and they shine with tears, as she has lived through more sadness than anyone should have known. Emotions stream through her in rivers. 'I'm thirty-six, and the last time I was happy was when I was twenty-four, when I graduated, when I had family and friends,' she tells me in an interview.

She is Palestinian, but her grandparents had to leave Palestine in 1948 for Syria, where her parents were born and where Arwa in turn was born: three generations of refugees from their homeland. 'I was born with this curse.' A year after losing her father, her brother died, and then her beloved grandmother. 'I have suffered loss,' she says with precision and dignity.

As a young child, she was close to animals and had a special relationship with a neighbour's dog who was her friend and who she trusted absolutely. 'I had secrets I couldn't tell anyone except him. This cute thing, he can't tell anyone but he can understand.' (She had been speaking to me in the past tense but slips into the present tense as the little dog of her childhood seems conjured into life again in her mind.) In Syria she first studied law and then drama, and as a student she was very close to a friend's dog, Jacko, a husky. Arwa graduated in 2011 and was building her life when suddenly the war came and tore up everything she knew and everything she was. When the war started, Jacko's owner couldn't look after him and he was put in a shelter. One night shortly after, Arwa dreamed that Jacko had come to her and hugged her. Afterwards, she was told that on the night of her dream, Jacko's shelter had been bombed and Jacko was dead. She weeps and weeps as she talks to me, speaking of her love for Jacko and his for her: 'He could understand my feelings and he came to my dream to say goodbye.'

The war left her deeply depressed, alone and psychologically vulnerable. She decided to get a golden retriever puppy. 'I believe in destiny, and when I saw him, I knew he was The One.' The puppy transformed her. 'Mentally I became super happy. I felt there was something that I could live for.' In honour of the husky she had previously loved, she called her new puppy Jacko.

But Syria was becoming too dangerous. Because of the war, she says, 'I lost my friends, my future, I lost everything.' She fled Syria, forced to leave Jacko behind with her family, a decision that broke her heart. She knew he would suffer and that, unlike humans, he wouldn't even know where to flee.

She headed for the UK, a journey that began by crossing the mountains from Damascus into Turkey with a group of fellow refugees, walking for nine hours without water, in forty-degree heat, so difficult that she felt she could not breathe. On the way, already exhausted and frightened, she was threatened with rape. She cries talking about it.

At one point, they had to cross a river, and one of the men in the group had an iron leg and was terrified of doing so because the leg would weigh him down, and he couldn't swim. So Arwa carried him across the river.

Arwa arrived in the UK in October 2018 and claimed asylum. 'I came here mentally and physically done in,' she says, but she tried hard to survive. The Home Office sent her to Rotherham, where she volunteered with the Red Cross, opened a drama class and took an interpreting course to help refugees. She volunteered with a dentist, and worked as an actor on a BBC documentary. 'It had its ups and downs but I did my best. Most refugees want to prove ourselves to the country that welcomed us, so we want to build and to help and to be part of it.' In 2019 she was given the right to stay for five years and permission to work. She moved to London, found a home and in 2020 got a waitressing job.

When her formal papers arrived, she saw that she was officially registered as stateless because the UK does not recognize Palestine in its ID system. The passport code that the Home Office gives to a refugee is XXB, and she repeats that 'XXB' like the bitterest axiom of despair. 'In the UK I am stateless, and this traumatized me more. To be unknown as a human is hard.'

Although she held herself together, had a home and a job and was trying to cope, she was swimming against the tide and losing strength. She became reclusive and deeply depressed, isolated from all those she had loved, both human and animal. 'For a long time, I kept myself alone in my room. I didn't have family and friends and I was going down deep and dark.'

In her despair, she made a decision which she felt her life depended on: to rescue her dog, Jacko. But how do you rescue a dog from a war zone? And even if she did, could Jacko rescue her in turn?

~

Sally's family dog may have similarly consoled her; a dog by whom she felt understood and loved. Perhaps if Sally's dog had not died, she would not have been on that bridge outside Exeter on that hot June day.

There, the police negotiators were at their wits' end. The ambulance team could only feel tension and worry. Despite all the humans at the scene, despite their care, training and skill, the situation was getting more concerning and anxiety was rising.

Then a member of the fire crew said the magic words: *I think we should call for Digby.*

Digby, a Labradoodle born in 2018, is the Devon and Somerset Fire and Rescue Service 'defuser', whose work usually involves helping crews who have been in traumatic situations. Asking for Digby was a stroke of genius. Digby's handler, Matt Goodman, took the call. Yes, he felt, Digby just might be the answer.

Digby is the first UK-based therapy dog in the fire and rescue service to be used specifically for psychological well-being among emergency personnel who have attended a traumatic incident. 'Digby just naturally defuses situations. I didn't teach him,' says Goodman. In the defusing process, as members of the crew articulate their own experiences, they may find it hard to continue speaking, and may call Digby over, breaking the tension. Goodman notes how the positive interaction with Digby means that people feel more fully present in the moment, and their heart rate and blood pressure are lowered. After the dog's intervention, the more formal aspect of the process can begin. 'Digby is a bridge between the incident and the process of defusing.' A bridge again. This is the site dogs can occupy, bridging the gap between past and present, bridging psyches.

When Digby arrived at that critical incident on the bridge, what would Sally have seen?

I've met Digby, and I can take a guess. Digby is a living, scruffy teddy bear. Clear eyes. Straight gaze. Uncomplicated heart. His expression is kind, concerned and implacably patient. Being with him is like stepping back into the simplest and happiest moments of childhood.

When Digby arrived, the Devon and Somerset Fire and Rescue Service said, 'The woman immediately swung her head round to look.' She had been looking towards the abyss, but Digby turned her attention back towards life and the living. She smiled, that involuntary smile that a dog can elicit, and that must have looked like a miracle to the observers. Although she had previously been unable to make eye contact with humans, she now locked eyes with the dog and was saved by the look in his eyes. When even the love of friends and family may fail to reach a psyche in anguish, an animal may be a living bridge, able to draw humans – even those on the brink of forever – right back into the heart of now.

Sensitive to the thinnest filament of communication with Sally, the negotiators chose not to speak to her about her own situation, as physically dangerous as it was psychologically terrifying. Instead, they began to tell her about Digby and his role at the fire and rescue service. The sudden freshness of that conversation for Sally must have been totally unexpected. It would have rewritten the script that her psyche had been writing.

The negotiators asked Sally if she would like to come and meet Digby.

She said yes.

Only, said the police, if she came back over to the safe side of the railings.

She said yes.

She climbed back over the barrier.

Sally patted Digby, stroked him and talked to him. The relief among the rescuers was palpable and their pride in Digby was immense, this first responder for the psyche. Sally had a few minutes of Digby-time, and then was taken into the care of mental health professionals.

Time is on a terrible pause during a critical incident like this, with the wait, the tension, and the awful changelessness of a person hopeless in their pain. But all the responders commented on how time changed when Digby arrived. Sally 'immediately' swung her head to look at him. The emergency had lasted about four hours and Digby sorted it out in five minutes. They work quickly, these animals.

~

Crisis dogs have been used in the USA in emergencies and trauma situations. Twenty teams of dogs went to help after the Oklahoma City bombings in 1995. Dogs worked with survivors at Columbine High School in 1999 and Ground Zero after the 9/11 attack. Dogs were sent in to help console people after the deadly massacre at a gay nightclub in Orlando, Florida, in 2016.

Therapy works only if and when trust is established between client and therapist but developing such trust may take a long while. In the most urgent of crises, rapport has to be established almost in an instant. That's where the dogs come in,[4] working at the speed of instinct, seeming to have an inborn sensitivity to seek out the people who need the most support in an emergency.[5]

One of the dogs attending the survivors of the Thurston High School shooting in Oregon in 1998 was an intuitive, kind-hearted dog called Bear. On the scene, one girl was in such shock that she was frozen into a paralysis. It was dangerous to stay like that and Bear's therapist-handler needed to establish communication fast. The dog approached the girl, making a soft sympathetic little noise. It caught the girl's attention and broke the awful spell. Grabbing Bear, the girl pulled the dog on to her lap where she hugged her and burst into tears. After tears, words. The therapist commented: 'Bear was like emotional search and rescue. Go in and bring the emotions out.' Then Bear could hand over to humans for slower healing work.[6]

Dogs can work so fast that a new term has been coined for it: *rapid rapport*.[7] Digby was a quick antidote to anguish partly because animals live in the moment and draw us there. 'Live vastly in the present,' says poet Gary Snyder. Although some animals can remember the past and anticipate the future, they are remarkably good at living both vastly and intensely in the present and they influence us to do the same.

A fascinating study examined the role of pet dogs in the casual conversations of older people (aged sixty-five to seventy-eight, some of whom were dog-owners and some not) while out walking. Without a dog, people's conversations focused on past events, whereas conversations in the company of a dog concentrated on current things happening in present time. *This* stick, *this* tree, *this* rain *now*! As the study authors say: 'when speaking to dogs or to people, owners generally avoided the past tense, whether or not their dogs were present.' The dogs, they note, 'played a role in capturing attention on the here and now'.[8]

~

Digby is not alone in preventing suicide.

Maddalena Bearzi, who studies the ecology of marine mammals, recounts a dolphin rescue in her 2012 book, *Dolphin Confidential*. Bearzi had been out on a boat near the Malibu Pier, Los Angeles, taking notes on a familiar pod of nine coastal bottlenose dolphins happily feeding on a school of sardines. All was normal. Until it wasn't.

One of the dolphins suddenly switched its behaviour, changing direction sharply and heading out to deep water. A minute later, the rest turned and followed. These coastal dolphins don't normally abandon a meal and re-route for the deeps, so Bearzi and the other researchers, surprised by this abrupt decision, followed the dolphins. The dolphins sped up. So did the boat. Then, nearly three miles offshore, the dolphins stopped and formed a circle in the water. At the centre of this ring of bright dolphins was a dark shape.

'Someone's in the water,' yelled one of the researchers. They saw a young woman, apparently dead. Bearzi slowly took the boat closer. The girl was pale, blonde and fully clothed and had a sealed plastic bag tied around her neck. But she was not dead. She turned her head to the boat, weakly raising her hand. The team pulled her on board where one of the researchers, a trained lifeguard, saw she had severe hypothermia. They took off her wet clothes and wrapped her in a blanket, huddling with her in turns, as they steered the boat to Marina del Rey, where there was a hospital.

Once back on land, the girl was given emergency medical care and one of the doctors told Bearzi that she was a German girl, on holiday in Los Angeles. The plastic bag contained her passport and a folded, handwritten note that explained she was trying to commit suicide. As Bearzi says: 'If the dolphins hadn't led us offshore when they did, to that specific place, she would have died.'[9]

A huge number of people I happened to talk to while I was writing this book, both friends and strangers, wanted me to know how animals had saved them when they felt suicidal. The psychological medicine of animals was of such enormous and life-saving power that they felt everyone should be aware of it.

A friend of mine, an Italian vet, Nicoletta, told me of feeling dangerously depressed in her early twenties and thinking she wanted to end her life. Her dog, her 'funny, intelligent, beloved dog Flip', came up to her and did something that he had never done before, putting his face on her knees and staying there. She felt overcome by this intervention from a 'furry angel'. In gratitude and amazement, she whispered to him: 'You can feel what I am feeling,' and the sense of being understood and loved saved her life. I think of the painting *Fidelity* by nineteenth-century artist Briton Rivière, with a dog whose eyes are streaming concern, compassion and love.

Mary, now in her fifties, had reached a crisis in her life when she had become unable to work and was going through a divorce. Then came the most savage blow. Her mother cut Mary out of her will to favour her other children. Such an act, often intended to express that the child is of no worth to their parents, has driven people to suicide.

'Everything came crashing down. My heart hurt so much: to the point where I was googling *heart attacks in women* but it wasn't that. It was heartbreak.' Mary went into a spiral of depression, and one midwinter day she went to bed. She describes it simply but profoundly as 'That day when I lay down.' She did not want to live. 'I thought I would just lie here and never get up again.'

Her cat Cleo, though, seemed to sense something. Cleo leaped up on the bed, then began jumping on Mary's chest. 'That made me sit up again,' she says. The realization that if she died, Cleo would die too, brought her round. 'She cared so much about me. She absolutely was my saviour.'

In August 2015, a young man called Byron Taylor from Slimbridge in Gloucestershire was in a dark place. He was working as a dispatcher for the ambulance service, but his partner had left him, he couldn't afford the rent and he was falling into a serious depression. One day, when he'd been drinking heavily, he became suicidal. He got a rope and made a noose but his dog, a six-year-old bull mastiff called Geo, took it in his mouth and when Taylor tried to get it back, Geo started growling at him. Byron was shocked. Then Geo tore the noose to bits, shredding it. 'He never growls, but each time I tried to take it off him, he would snarl. In a way, I think Geo knew what I was going to do. They have a sixth sense about this kind of thing. He knew something was up.'

One study with adult pet-owners who had become suicidal identified three things about having a pet that protected them from actually committing suicide. One was the comfort and emotional support that the pet gave them. A second was the way that a pet may demand attention and distract them from suicidal thoughts. A third was that the owners felt obliged to care for the pet; the animal gave them quite literally a reason to live.[10]

Almost 80 per cent of people on the autism spectrum suffer from a diagnosable mental health problem, compared to 25 per cent of the general population, while suicide is a leading cause of premature death in those with autism. In a study of adults with autism, an incredible 16.7 per cent said that their dog prevented them from taking their own lives, mainly due to the dog's affection for them and their need to care for the animal. Cuddling, stroking, walking the dog and simply having their dog near them lifted people's mood. One person in the study described how a dog is a protective factor: 'I have attempted suicide before, and he has helped it stop happening again. I feel that I'm a burden to my family but I don't feel the same about him because I think that I meet his needs pretty well. That gives me confidence, and keeps me going in a way that my family don't.'

The study authors give a quick scale-up from their data:

> If we assume 1% of the 52 million adults in the UK have autism and that dog ownership among this population is as popular as other adults at 26%, then dog ownership would be responsible for preventing around 22,000 suicides among 135,000 autistic adults in the UK alone. We do not claim this is the actual figure, but do believe this rough exercise highlights the importance of this.[11]

~

I heard about Digby on the radio as I was in my kitchen cooking supper. My eyes filled with tears and a huge smile lifted like sunrise across my face. I went to my phone, googled Digby and felt a wave of empathy for the young woman on the bridge and a rush of gratitude for all Digbys.

I was not alone in my passionate reaction. Devon and Somerset Fire and Rescue had put the word out to show the benefits of animals in supporting mental well-being. The story swept through the media, first in Britain then out to India and the USA. It was a sensation. And then the responses flooded in, many underlining the message that animals can save the psyche in crisis.

One person on social media posted a picture of a dog, writing: 'This is Lucky my toy poodle, he has stopped me from taking my life on a number of occasions.' Another wrote: 'Digby rocks. There's something about a dog that can pierce the greatest fog of despair.' A third: 'Oh god, get that young woman a dog.'

I wish that there were teams of Digbys on paw patrol, kind, furry paramedics at the parapets of sites such as bridges that broadcast that terrible siren call. When the suicidal mind wants to finish its life sentence by reaching a full stop, the animals can step in, suggesting a comma.

~

Meanwhile, what of Arwa, searching for her dog, Jacko?

Arwa was told about a charity called War Paws, which reunites people with their animals, bringing the two together so they can save each other. She spoke to War Paws about her situation as a refugee and about Jacko's in a war zone. In Syria, dead bodies were piling up in the streets, unburied, and the starving dogs were eating the bodies, so the government started poisoning whole areas to kill the street dogs, making it too dangerous for Arwa's family to take Jacko out for regular exercise. They managed, though, to get Jacko out of Syria, to a charity in Lebanon, while War Paws prepared to bring him to the UK.

On 13 June 2021 (two days before Sally's anguish on the bridge), Arwa had Jacko in her arms. The recognition, the tears, the immeasurable rapture were caught on film and posted online. War Paws had rescued the dog, and the dog could now rescue the woman. With

Jacko, Arwa felt she had something to live for: she cared for him as he cared for her. Her happiness, though, did not last, for reasons way beyond Arwa.

A new blow struck her. As for so many people, housing problems can devastate a life. Arwa's landlord sold the flat she was in, and due to the stress of imminent homelessness, Arwa lost her waitressing work. Stateless, jobless, homeless, the one thing she had left in her life was Jacko.

She tried to reach out for help but the local council gave her two choices. Option one: take Jacko to a dog shelter and then the council would put her up in a hotel. Or option two: keep the dog and sleep on the streets. They wouldn't – or couldn't – find a solution for her to be housed with Jacko. The choice was punitive, the impact terrible. 'I wanted to end my life when I was told I couldn't take him. This life isn't worth it.'

Arwa and Jacko became rough sleepers. She chose staying with Jacko on the streets over staying in a hotel without him, because, she says, 'I had already lost everything else, literally everything. I had nothing left to lose, only him. Without him I'm a stateless person, a homeless, jobless number in the world. With him, I have a reason to live. He's more than a home, more than a country, he is the world to me.'

Many homeless people are forced to make that heartbreaking choice between accommodation and their pet. Large numbers of people choose the streets rather than betray someone who may have been their only friend, knowing that their pet is more important for their well-being than anything else, including shelter.

For some, they are more important than life itself. John Chadwick moved into a rented place in London in 2007, and a dear friend of his, Dee Bonett, gave him a kitten. Then another friend gave him a Jack Russell puppy, and a year later he adopted a second Jack Russell. But at the end of 2016, Chadwick's landlord decided to sell, and Chadwick was evicted. He was temporarily sent to a bed and breakfast where his pets were barred, and then he was told he would be moved to a high-rise flat with a no-pet policy. Ten days after that he killed himself. In her grief and anger, Dee Bonett set up a campaign to allow people to be housed with their pets, calling it the John Chadwick Pet Policy.

Perhaps unsurprisingly, up to 25 per cent of the UK's 300,000 homeless people have a pet. When you are on the streets and society has told you that you don't matter, *Bollocks* says the dog. *You are everything to me. Everything.* And signs it with a lick. A dog can transform a doorstep into a hearth. A dog can provide a home because the dog *itself* can be a home, giving emotional comfort, stability and shelter. With a dog, you have a protector, an ally and a comrade. You have someone for whom you are precious and beloved.

One woman (interviewed by the Simon Community Scotland and the Dogs Trust, which support homeless people with their pets) had experienced the devastation of losing her baby to cot death and had spiralled down, splitting up from her partner, turning to drugs and suffering from mental ill health. Her family gave her zero support. Within a year of her child's death, she and her dog, a white Staffie, were alone and sleeping on the streets. The Staffie saved her.

> I honestly don't think I would be here today without her. She is the only family I have. Aren't family meant to be there for you? Well, mine weren't, but she's always there for me, no matter what. It means everything to me to know that there is still someone who loves me and I know she'll never leave me. She makes me feel like life is worth it all.[12]

Aaron, who has been homeless in Edinburgh, spoke to me about his two-year-old dog, a collie crossed with a black Labrador. He called her Sky 'because she's black like the night sky' and he credits her with saving his life. He was, he says, living like a recluse, isolated and lonely. He is guarded in his phrasing, but it is suicide he is talking about. 'Put it this way, I wasn't going to get any better. I was in a bad place in my life. I had nothing to live for.' Sky gave him that reason to be alive. 'From when I got her there was no more loneliness,' he says. 'I don't feel I had a lot of love in my life. When I realized she actually loved me, it was overwhelming. It was a few weeks after I got her. I was sitting on the couch and she sat facing me. And I felt it.' I can hear his tears over the phone, as if love is a miracle and Sky his salvation. Exactly as it is. Exactly as she is.

He notes that in Edinburgh there is only one hostel – the Hub in the Haymarket, run by the Bethany Trust – that lets people bring dogs with them, and only one medical surgery for homeless people, where the writer and GP Dr Gavin Francis has worked, where dogs are welcomed. For homeless people, owning a pet is powerful medicine, reducing depression and substance abuse, loneliness, isolation and suicidal thoughts.[13] Dr Emma Williamson, Principal Clinical Psychologist at the Maudsley, who works with homeless people, notes: 'Many of my clients have confided that without their dog they may have committed suicide already. Anything that places people at risk of losing their dog – such as being separated in order to access housing – could increase the likelihood of suicide and self-harm.'[14]

Street sleeping ravages a person's health, physically, mentally, socially and emotionally. The psyche is exposed to all the ill winds that can knife you on the cold night streets. People on the streets have to live their lives in public, sleeping, eating, talking in a piece of raw, ineluctable theatre where they are exposed to the cruelty of strangers and the judgement of anyone.

Even with Jacko, Arwa was vulnerable in the aggravated jeopardy of the streets. One night she woke up with a man trying to touch her up. Jacko leaped to defend her. On the streets, Arwa reached the lowest point of her life and became suicidal. Someone, concerned for her safety, called the police. When they came, they prevented her from killing herself, with a quick and profound reading of the situation. 'The police came and said I should live for him, for the dog. Then they said he was my therapy dog, and I had to keep him. I didn't know you could have that, but he is, he's helping me to overcome all the issues I have mentally and physically.'

Jacko is also a bridge in time, from her past self forward. The dog, so alive to the moment, brings her to the present and indeed the future. 'He is part of my past when I was happy. He's part of nice memories.

He's my present now.' When we first spoke, Arwa and Jacko were being looked after together by the homeless charity St Mungo's. 'I kept him and he kept me. I think he is the hope I had that I can fight to the end because of him and for him. I think he is The Friend who never gives up on me.'

As I was finishing this book, I got back in touch with Arwa and her story has a very sweet ending. After we'd spoken, she had fallen in love with a good, kind man called Jonathan. They had married, found work, made a home together and had a baby. They had met in the garden of St Mungo's, where Arwa had been sitting with Jacko when Jonathan had come out for a cigarette. Jacko padded over to Jonathan and started playing with him. The dog's actions had been an icebreaker, facilitating the communication of strangers and metaphorically bridging the gap between them. Arwa picked herself up, walked across that bridge and stepped into a new life.

PART TWO

How Animals Heal the Individual Body

This section looks at how animals have saved lives physically; how dogs can raise the alarm in certain medical emergencies, alerting their owners to an incipient seizure or diabetic low; and how dogs can be trained to detect the presence of particular diseases, including Covid and some cancers. It explores some of the history of animals in healing, and looks at their beneficial physiological effects on us, lowering blood pressure, heart rate and stress hormones. It then considers how animals provide a hospice for the heart, accompanying the dying and sometimes being able to give medics advance warning of a death.

5
Emergency Services

*'To know even one life has breathed easier because you have lived.
This is to have succeeded'* – Ralph Waldo Emerson

On 9 June 2005, a twelve-year-old girl was walking back from school, that utterly ordinary event in the everyday life of a child. The dusty afternoon sun fell across a landscape of flat scrubland on the outskirts of a small town in south-west Ethiopia. Even though the town, Bita Genet, is a provincial capital, it is set in vast rural environs, remote from any cities, and consists of just a few streets and a few hundred buildings, with occasional dirt roads and patches of forest.

On her way home, the girl was pounced on by seven men. The gang kidnapped her, wanting to sell her into a forced marriage. They attacked her, trying to beat her into submission, and kept her captive in the forests. Her terror and vulnerability must have felt almost unbearable: a minute would have felt like a day, and a day like a lifetime. Her family, meanwhile, raised the alarm and, together with the police, had gone out to find her. In spite of their desperate search, they couldn't locate her and days passed. The seven captors held her for a week, then tried to move her to another site. The traumatized girl must have been praying to be saved.

She was rescued – not by her family or the police but by three lions. When the lions arrived at the scene, they instantly drove the men away but they didn't touch the girl. They were ferocious, but never towards her, instead staying beside her and keeping her safe.

Ethiopian lions have large black manes haloing their heads and, like all lions, greet each other by rubbing their heads together with their tails looped in the air. These three lions would have been pride-mates, most likely females, who cross-suckle their cubs, one female letting another lioness's cubs feed from her. Stuart Williams, a wildlife expert with Ethiopia's rural development ministry, said that it was likely that the young girl was saved because she was crying. 'A young girl whimpering could be mistaken for the mewing sound from a lion cub, which in turn could explain why they didn't eat her. Otherwise they probably would have done so.' This only goes so far as an explanation, though, as no lion would actually have mistaken a child for a lion cub.

The lions protected her for half a day, until police and relatives tracked her down, and when they did, there were no kidnappers in sight, just the girl and her three lion guardians. One of those who arrived was Police Sergeant Wondimu Wedajo, who described what he saw. 'They stood guard until we found her and then they just left her like a gift and went back into the forest.' It is as if the lions were fully aware of her anguish and fear, and could not only tell the difference between her response to the kidnappers and her response to the police, but crucially could take an active role in protecting her from the kidnappers before happily relinquishing her safely to the police and slipping back into the forest.

She was left needing medical attention as a result of the beatings but, as Wondimu Wedajo says: 'If the lions had not come to her rescue then it could have been much worse. Everyone thinks this is some kind of miracle because normally the lions would attack people.'

Angels with black haloes.

~

This action was outside the lions' normal behaviour, and beyond humans' usual experience of these animals. Did the lions feel a sense of pity, perhaps? Did they feel a sense of wrong when they saw seven men terrorizing a child? Did they dislike the aggression and feel that they would show the men who was really in charge, in lion territory?

In emergencies, animals may step forward with a spontaneity and a willingness to help which is very touching. They have saved lives, like an extra emergency service. This chapter explores real-life examples of this and then looks at the myths that are the shadow-truths of the literal rescues.

~

Operator: Emergency Services. Which service do you need?
Woof!
Police?
Fire?
Ambulance?
Lion?
Pot-bellied pig?

On 4 August 1998, Jo Ann Altsman from Pennsylvania was on holiday with her husband, staying in a vacation trailer near Lake Erie. While her husband had gone fishing for the day Jo Ann was in the trailer with their pet, Lulu, a Vietnamese pot-bellied pig who she doted on, giving the pig attention, food and treats including sweet ice in the summer and jelly doughnuts in the winter.[1]

Pigs can be clever creatures with individual personalities, and they are able to solve challenging problems. Highly emotional, they can pick up on the emotions of others.[2] They can recognize their own names, use tools, learn tricks, make friends with other pigs and form close bonds with humans. They have good memories, love snuggling and play-wrestling, and are good at finding their way home.[3] Their effervescent playfulness is contagious.

Quite suddenly, on that day, Jo Ann began feeling acute pain in her chest and her left arm went numb. She shouted out, but no one heard her and she was terrified, unable to go for help, in increasing pain and fearing she would die. Lulu, though, became her first responder, noticing the situation and working out what to do. She forced herself out through the dog flap, designed for a 50-pound dog not a 150-pound pig, which scraped her sides so badly she was bleeding. Then she charged out of the trailer-yard, through a dog gate, battering at it until she could get out on to the public road.

Jo Ann could hear the pig crying and then she heard those cries getting fainter, but she couldn't work out why. What happened, it transpired, was this: Lulu went to the crossroads of the campsite, which was the place likely to have the highest volume of traffic. When the first car came along, Lulu walked out in front of it and lay down in the road. The driver did see her but, frightened of an unfamiliar creature, swerved and drove on. Lulu got to her feet, went back to check on Jo Ann, saw she was still needed and returned to the crossroads to wait. No cars.

A second time she went back to Jo Ann, saw help was still required and once more returned to the crossroads to wait for a car. When one came, she walked right in front to block it, and this time it worked. The car stopped and a young man got out, bemused. Seeing the cuts on her body, he became worried for the animal. Lulu scrambled up and began to move off, checking the man was following. She led him directly to Jo Ann's trailer, where the man knocked and shouted, 'Lady, your pig's in distress!' Jo Ann, inside, feebly called back: 'I'm in distress too.'

The man called 911 and when an ambulance came for Jo Ann, Lulu tried to get in the ambulance with her. The woman was hospitalized and given open-heart surgery. It had taken Lulu forty-five minutes to bring help and it was only just in time. The medics said that if Jo Ann had been left without help for only another fifteen minutes, she would have died.

There's empathy going on here, perceiving that help was needed, and intelligence too, in knowing how to get that help. Behind them both was the willingness that loyalty and love provoke. What I find so moving about this is not only the devotion that prompted the pig to help, and the intelligence of her plan, but the perseverance. Even though her first attempts failed, she kept trying, and this persistence underlines how her aid was deliberate. This was not chance: she chose to come to the rescue and chose to do so repeatedly.

~

Emergency Services. Which service do you need?
Woof!
Police?

Emergency Services

Fire?

Parrot?

Parrot?

Parrot.

Putting you through now.

In Denver, Colorado, Megan Howard owned a pet Quaker parrot called Willie. Megan worked as a babysitter, caring for children in her own home, where in 2009 she was looking after a two-year-old called Hannah. She'd given the toddler some breakfast, but then needed the bathroom, so she left Hannah for a moment. The baby began to choke. Megan, in the bathroom, could not hear the child.

So the parrot raised the alarm. 'Willie started screaming like I'd never heard him scream before,' Megan said later. He flapped his wings, frantically and noisily, and screeched 'Mama! Baby! Mama! Baby!' over and over again until Megan heard, came out of the bathroom, took one look at Hannah, saw she was turning blue and performed the Heimlich manoeuvre.[4]

The parrot understood the urgency and knew the human words he needed to use. It makes me wonder: surely animals wish we understood their talents and indeed their motives more: they try so hard to communicate, learning our languages and gestures. I'm also struck by how badly the parrot wanted to help: he became frenzied, physically and vocally, desperate to do what he could to rescue the child.

~

Emergency Services. Which service do you need?

Bodyguard.

On 16 August 1996, a three-year-old boy climbed the wall of the gorilla enclosure at a zoo in Brookfield, Illinois, and fell twenty feet on to the concrete floor. The fall left him unconscious. Binti Jua, an eight-year-old female gorilla, immediately approached him, which made the other visitors scream, thinking she might harm him, but her intention was the reverse. She lifted him and cradled him in her arms, growling at any other gorillas who came close. Then she took the boy to an access gate and gently handed him over to the staff. She was a nursing mother herself, and was demonstrating what primate researchers identified as good gorilla parenting.[5]

Like the pig and the parrot previously, the gorilla answered the emergency call and also knew what to do. She actively wanted to help, and her wish to help was so strong that it overcame the fact that she was unwillingly imprisoned: she could have taken revenge on this tiny segment of humanity accidentally appearing in her enclosure. She didn't. The desire to protect was stronger.

Elephants have been known to guard humans. In Kenya, an elderly and half-blind Turkana woman, tiring towards the end of the day, had lost her way and, as night fell, settled herself under a tree and slept. In the middle of the night, she was woken by an elephant sniffing her all over with her trunk. Other elephants gathered around, and the woman felt terrified and vulnerable, with her strengthless legs, tissue-paper skin and almost sightless eyes. But the elephants were looking out for her. They broke branches, brought them to where she lay and covered her, possibly trying to make a shield to protect her from hyenas and leopards. In the morning, her faint calls for help were heard by a passing herder who found her. Carl Safina, who reports this story, comments, 'if compassion is a desire to act toward easing another's suffering, an elephant who protects a lost old woman feels – and wields – the full range from empathy to sympathy to compassion in action.'[6]

Also in Kenya, a herder was involved in an accidental confrontation with a matriarch elephant, and the man's leg was broken. He was in pain and unable to walk, but the elephant chose to take care of him, gently moving him with her trunk and front feet, shifting him to a tree that he could lean against and be shaded by. To the heft and the tenderness, she added patience, staying with him even though her family walked away, leaving her alone. She stood guard over him, occasionally touching him softly with her trunk, this elephant guardian spreading a protecting veil over him, all through the night.[7]

The elephant distinguished between accidental confrontation and deliberate hostility, and wanted to help, a wish made more evident by the kindness of her approach. All of us know that feeling when, bodily injured, someone offers us emotional tenderness alongside physical care, and we feel the healing of this remedial gentleness.

~

Emergency Services. Which service do you need?
Coastguard.

Nan Hauser has terrific presence, ocean-swum, sea-salted, with that sky-and-sand, blue-and-blonde thing going on. She is a marine biologist and has spent decades protecting whales, little knowing that she would herself be saved by one.

On 14 September 2017, she was swimming in the waters off Rarotonga, an island in the Pacific where humpbacks frequently visit. Out in the water, one whale began charging towards her. She tried to get away, but he was far too fast and strong. The whale tried to tuck her under his fin and then at one point he lifted her right out of the water, holding her on his long head, which is very strange whale behaviour. 'He was trying to tell me something and had an eye that was so wide it was like he had just seen a ghost, so I knew something was up.' Suddenly he turned and in a brief moment she could see past his head, to another whale who was tail-slapping the water. Nan was in shock from having been tossed around by the whale for ten minutes, and it took her a moment to realize that there was a third huge creature in the water with her. 'It was the largest tiger shark I've ever seen in my entire life and it was coming right for me.' A tiger shark is perhaps fifteen feet in length. And they are killers. Nan panicked, but the whale was determined. He came up behind her and, as she says, 'put me on his head and just pushed me as fast as he could to the back of the boat'.

Once she was safe, and as the shock receded, she was overcome by gratitude and love. 'I love you and thank you,' she kept saying to the whale.[8] Humpback whales are known to be altruistic across species as they often save seals from orcas,⁹ but it is a rare and precious thing for a human to experience. Altruism, as Nan points out, 'is a true act of kindness when you protect someone without asking or expecting anything in return'.

He could have ignored the situation completely and swum away, but he didn't. The humpback wanted to help so much that he moved out of his normal behaviour, holding her on his head. There's more. Nan never expected to see the whale again as, in her twenty years of research in that exact spot, only two whales had ever returned. But one year and fifteen days later, she was out in the same area doing research and the whale did return – she recognized him by the notches in his tail fluke. 'The next thing I knew, the whale came up next to the side of the boat, ignored everyone else and stared directly at me.' She slipped on her wetsuit and slid into the water, swimming down next to him. 'He opened his eyes and he just looked at me and kept nudging me and nudging me and nudging me with his head and he was just nuzzling and moving his head in my belly.' It was quite clear he recognized her too and felt a bond with her.

She wanted to hug him but didn't know how. He did. He put his pectoral fin right under her (the fin's length is about four times her height) and he held his fin to the surface of the water so she could breathe. 'I laid on it and I hugged it and I lay there forever and I just lay there,' she says, the repeated phrases conjuring an eternity of bliss. The impression it made on her was profound: 'I was blown away. I felt love, I felt happiness. I was speechless for the longest time. I couldn't even really call people and tell them, it was too *sacred*. I can say that he will always be a part of me.'

~

Emergency Services. Which service do you need?
Lifeguard.

On 30 October 2004, a lifeguard called Rob Howes was swimming near Whangarei, New Zealand, with his daughter Niccy and two of her friends. Seven dolphins appeared and began behaving strangely.

They herded the swimmers, pushing all four together by turning in tight circles around them. At one point, Howes and one of the girls drifted away from the other two and immediately two of the bigger dolphins drove them back, first swimming straight at them, and then diving down right in front of them. As they did so, Howes spotted a ten-foot great white shark heading towards him.

'I just recoiled. It was only about two metres away from me, the water was crystal clear. They had corralled us up to protect us.' The scene was witnessed by another lifeguard, Matt Fleet, who was on patrol in a lifeboat and saw the dolphins circling the swimmers and slapping their tails on the water to keep them in place. He too had a clear sighting of the great white shark which glided around Howes and then headed for two of the girls.[10] 'My heart went into my mouth because one of them was my daughter,' Howes noted. 'The dolphins were going ballistic.' For about forty minutes, the dolphins swum on guard, protecting them until the shark gave up and the group could swim the 100 yards back to the shore. The dolphins were the lifeguard's lifeguard.

Like the lions, the pig, the parrot, gorilla, elephants and whale, the dolphins recognized an emergency and knew how to help. The dolphins here were so eager to help that they kept up the emergency procedure for an hour or so in total. They acted beyond their normal behaviour, offering to save humans in a situation that is not without stress for the dolphins: great white sharks can and do kill individual dolphins – this was a tough shift.

~

Emergency Services. Which service do you need?
Ocean guide.

The whale researcher Ken Balcomb found himself out at sea off Washington State when a thick fog enveloped his boat. He and his companions had a rough compass bearing but it was a tricky stretch of water. Then a pod of orcas arrived, setting themselves just ahead of the boat's prow, and Balcomb took the decision to follow their lead, doing so for two hours as the whales swam slowly, inches from the boat so the crew didn't lose sight of their protectors. And so they went for fifteen miles. At that point, the fog lifted and Balcomb could see the island where he was living. Home. It piques my curiosity: did they know where Ken lived? Why else pick that particular island? In this rescue, it is clear that the whales not only knew their way, but crucially seemed to know that in those conditions we humans won't know ours. As Balcomb says: 'They knew absolutely that we had zero visibility.'

There is more. Ken Balcomb's experience happened only a year after whale-captures had ended in that area. Orcas were chased and brutalized to take them to aquariums where one, Lolita, was imprisoned for over half a century, crying out all her life for the family she had known, with calls only her family used. Ken and his crew had never been part of it and the whales had noticed, often coming to his boat and staying close. It implied, said Ken, that the whales had 'a consciousness of what's going on'.[11] Was it only his boat they would have helped? Or perhaps it was only a good whale-noticer who would have attended their communication and trusted their guidance? Have whales perhaps offered other fog-bound boats help but found their offers unnoticed and unaccepted?

It makes me wonder if the animals are offering us their help far more than we know. Maybe they come laden with gifts of care and we, for the most part, reject them.

When orcas saw Alexandra Morton in trouble, they were certain that she would understand that they were offering to help: they knew her. Morton, also a whale researcher, was out one day in an inflatable boat in Queen Charlotte Strait in Canada, tracking and following orcas who had been swimming west towards open ocean when a thick fog descended. It was, she said, like being 'in a glass of milk', and they were right out at sea. This was bad enough, as she and her assistant had nothing to take directions from, nothing was visible. There were no waves either, just flat water and white air. It got worse. A huge cruise ship was coming towards them. She couldn't see it but she could hear it, although in that kind of fog even the sense of hearing is confused, as sound bounces, seeming to come from everywhere and anywhere. The cruise ship couldn't see them either and the two vessels could have been on a collision course. They needed something like a miracle.

And they got one.

Some of the orcas that she knew personally came to her boat, gathering around it and setting a course for her to follow. 'I never worried. I trusted them with our lives.' The whales took them south and twenty minutes later the fog lifted as they neared land, and it was not just any land but her home. They had guided her precisely to where she needed to be and they had clearly gone out of their way to do it. They had been heading west but had turned to the south to take her home. Leaving her, they started back out again, returning to their earlier plan.[12]

It was, once more, a deliberate act to save someone. Messaging takes two: one to send a message and one to receive. The whales knew Morton, knew she'd receive the message they were transmitting. *We want to help you. Over. Follow us. Over.* I wish we humans could have our mind-radios more often set to 'receive' and a little less often set to 'transmit' so we might perhaps hear the myriad messages from the animal world saying, *We're here for you. Over.* Perhaps these messages are being sent – over and over – but we are routinely not reading them; are we ignoring the messages, to our own cost? I wonder whether our inability to pick up on messages from the animals is linked to the fact that we are so flooded by messages from other humans that we have insufficient bandwidth to receive messages from all the others, the animals.

~

Emergency Services. Which service do you need?
Fire? *Woof!*
Ambulance? *Woof!*
Lifeguard? *Woof!*
Police? *Woof!*
All the above? *Woof! Woof! Woof!*

They are there, the dogs, waiting patiently all through this chapter. *Dolphins? We'd do that if we could swim like them. Lions? We do that all the time.* The dogs have a point.

Dogs' caretaking behaviour doesn't surprise us so much because we share our lives with them, recognizing their communication more often than other animals'. Even so, their willingness to rescue, even to the point of self-sacrifice, is profoundly moving.

Search and rescue? *Woof!*

In the First World War, the Red Cross used dogs to find wounded soldiers. The dogs would be equipped with saddlebags stuffed with first-aid supplies which they would leave with the injured, and they were trained to take something from the soldier back with them to the Red Cross field hospital, to alert staff.[13]

We humans have a history of getting lost in snow in high mountain passes and we are more or less helplessly hapless with our unfurry bodies, without the hooves of goats or wings of condors. We can lose our direction in an instant in a blizzard. One bar left in your body-charge and your core temperature plummeting.

Over a thousand years ago, St Bernard de Menthon established a hospice and a monastery to look after travellers as they crossed the Alps at the St Bernard Pass, once the main route from Switzerland into Italy. From the late seventeenth century, the monks began to breed the massive, intelligent and loyal mastiffs known as St Bernards. Their heyday was around 1750, and the last rescue they helped with was in 1975. During this time, they found and rescued about two thousand people. They were renowned for sensing impending avalanches. Their wide chests acted like snowploughs, easing the way for any human companions. They had a near-infallible sense of direction, a resistance to cold, and an extraordinary sense of smell, enabling them to track people even buried deep in snow. The dogs worked in teams of three and when they found a lost person, two dogs would lay beside them to keep them warm, while the third dog would return to the hospice, alert the monks and bring help. Intriguingly, the task was considered too complex for humans to teach, so the dogs trained each other, with a young dog running with older dogs out in the mountains, seeing what the experienced dogs did, and copying their behaviour. Each dog would in time decide for themselves whether their role would be to stay with the lost person or to leave and get help.[14] St Bernards have now been replaced by helicopters, but these dogs are still the icon of search and rescue.

Emergency carer? *Woof!*

A friend of mine was living in Sydney, Australia, about twenty-five years ago, and recalls an old man who lived alone and who had fallen one day. He had hurt himself, possibly with a hip injury. No one knew about the accident. He couldn't move and it was the middle of an Australian summer when the risk of dehydration is serious. But he had a pet collie dog and within a few hours of the accident, the dog had worked out what to do. He went and got a towel from the bathroom, pushed it into the toilet to soak up water and took it to the man, so he could drink, saving his life.

That is a dog who can show initiative, as well as a huge willingness to help and save. Sometimes a dog's intelligence comes from senses beyond ours.

Emergency paramedic? *Woof!*

Duke was a rescue dog living with the Brousseau family in Portland, Oregon. In the middle of one night in October 2012, he seemed to sense something was wrong with the family's nine-week-old daughter, Harper. Although Duke was not sleeping near the baby, he was clearly aware of danger and went to the parents' bed, jumping up and down, shaking uncontrollably. Duke was normally 'insanely obedient', according to the parents, and he had never acted like this before, so they responded instantly, going to check on their daughter. She was not breathing. They called an ambulance and the baby was revived by paramedics. If the dog had not been so scared and raised the alarm, the parents would have slept through the night and Harper would have slept forever.[15]

Coastguard? *Woof!*

Dogs don't only save 'their' pack-humans. They may also take extraordinary measures to save strangers. One, a Rottweiler called Orion, became a kind of canine lifeboat when torrential rains in Vargas, Venezuela, in December 1999, caused flash floods and mudslides. Tens of thousands of people, perhaps 10 per cent of the population of the state, were killed – entire towns were swept into the ocean. Orion began saving lives. He repeatedly swam out to people in the sea and dragged them in, one a little girl trapped by swirling water, and he also helped children climb to higher, safer levels of dry land. In total, he rescued thirty-seven people in twenty-four hours, a Guinness World Record for a dog,[16] and became known as 'El Perro Valiente', the valiant dog.

Some dogs, such as Orion, are honoured, but I wonder whether we are unappreciative of the fact that animals help and save so widely? Do we think they are simply guided by instinct and a modicum of training? Do we take for granted the fact that dogs surround us with a rescue service, saving us even at terrible risk to themselves?

~

Sometimes the devotion that a dog may feel for their human may be so great that they do put their own lives in jeopardy. In May 2012, CBS News Boston reported on a woman, Christine Spain, and her dog, Lilly, a pit bull therapy dog who had helped Christine in combating chronic depression and alcoholism. On 3 May, Christine was walking back from a friend's house with the dog and their route took them over a railway line. When they were crossing, Christine collapsed, just as a train was coming down the tracks. The train engineer saw Lilly going into saving mode and trying to pull Christine off the tracks, but the dog was not able to get the woman completely clear. The train crew tried desperately to stop the train, but they couldn't. The dog then came around between the train and Christine, 'and took the hit of the train', said the engineer. Christine's son, a Boston police officer, said, 'She saved my mom's life. But Lilly, she didn't fare as well.' She had a broken pelvis and her right front leg was so severely injured it had to be amputated.

The primate researcher Roger Fouts tells a devastating story from his childhood, when his family had a dog called Brownie. The family had been out for the day and were returning home in their truck, down a dirt road. Roger's brother Ed, nine years old, was cycling ahead of the truck, with the dog. Brownie began barking more and more intensely, snapping at the wheels of the vehicle. The track was so dusty that the driver couldn't see what was ahead. Quite suddenly, Brownie dived in front of the truck tyres, and shrieked as they drove over her body. The driver slammed on the brakes, and they got out to find Brownie dead, and Ed stuck in a deep tyre rut, unable to get out of the way in time. Brownie had seen that in another two seconds the truck would have run him down. 'No one doubted for a second that Brownie had sacrificed her own life to save my brother's.'[17]

~

Legends speak of dogs who give their lives guarding their charges. The tragic ones relate that dogs are sometimes wrongly accused of killing those they were in fact protecting.

There is a legend from Lyons, in France, where a medieval knight went out hunting for a day, leaving his greyhound, Guinefort, to look after his baby. The father returned to find the greyhound drenched in blood beside the child's empty, overturned cradle. The man, traumatized and raging, assumed Guinefort had attacked the child and he killed the dog. Only then did the father find his child, alive, sleeping under the upturned cradle, where, close by, the real culprit lay dead: a huge snake torn to pieces by the faithful dog. In a state of agony and guilt, the knight buried the dog and planted a grove of trees around the grave, to honour the greyhound and commemorate the dog's actions while wanting, if he ever could, to atone for his own.

In the thirteenth century, Guinefort's grove became the centre of a healing tradition, and people would bring their sick children to the grave as to the shrine of a martyred saint. The Church, though, was furious that a dog was receiving this level of veneration, and a Dominican friar, Stephen of Bourbon, had the dead dog disinterred, and the sacred grove cut down and burned, along with the remains of St Guinefort. An edict was also passed making it a crime for anyone to visit the place in future. (There is a certain irony in the fact that it was a Dominican friar who was so enraged by the greyhound: the name of their order in Latin, *Dominicanus*, named after its founder, St Dominic, has been playfully rendered *Domini canis*, meaning 'Dog of the Lord' – it was said that St Dominic's mother dreamed that a dog leaped from her womb just before she became pregnant with the saint.) Until the 1970s, St Guinefort was honoured in the living memory of the local elders, who remembered people going to the shrine before the Second World War to seek the dog's healing for their sick children. Images, ancient and modern, show Guinefort with a halo.

The Welsh legend of a dog called Gelert is similar to Guinefort's. The story tells how Llywelyn the Great returned home from hunting one day to find his baby missing, and the cradle overturned, while his dog, Gelert, had blood all over its mouth. Llywelyn assumed that the dog had attacked the child and, in grief and fury, killed the dog. But as the dog lay dying, Llywelyn heard the baby's cry from under the upturned cradle. He went to the child and found there a dead wolf. The dog had protected the child and killed the wolf in doing so. Llywelyn felt the anguish of utter remorse and buried Gelert with ceremony, raising a cairn of stones to mark the grave, while the town was named Beddgelert, the 'grave of Gelert'. Llywelyn could always hear the dog's dying yelp, and for this, Llywelyn never smiled again.

It isn't exactly true. David Pritchard, who came to Beddgelert in 1793 and became landlord of the Goat Hotel, wanted more customers. So in an imaginative solution, he began telling tales, apparently inventing the name Gelert and much of the story.

What matters, though, is not the factual truth of the story but what it reveals. It tells us, as so many myths do, how important the animals are to us, and how we will grieve for them if we do not appreciate and look after them in turn. It also cautions us to pick up messages properly, and warns that sometimes we don't even understand the language of dogs, the animals we know the best.

Myths and legends do not tell literal truths but augmented truths; they do not jar with what is known but amplify it. Myth has its own subtle, metaphysical validity and its wisdom is not arbitrary. It advises and reminds us of things we must not forget. Contemporary society can be sceptical of the importance of myth, as if it fails the critical threshold of literal credibility. This may be a terrible mistake: myths often tell how the animals are on our side and stress that we need to acknowledge their care, healing and saving because if we don't, we will be the sadder – and the iller – for it.

Arion was an ancient Greek singer and lyre player whose voice was honey and whose songs were lanterns of the soul. They say that he played his lyre to the dolphins of the Mediterranean, who would come when he played, delighting in his music. Arion left his home in Corinth and set sail for Italy and Sicily, where his music was prized and won him wealth and renown, but after some time he wanted to go home, and hired a ship and crew to take him back.

At sea, though, his story darkens. The sailors knew of his fame and learned of his treasure. They were gold-thirsty. They plotted to throw him overboard, steal his wealth and then, concocting a shared backstory, planned to claim that his death had been a tragic accident. Arion caught wind of their strategem and begged them not to kill him, offering them all his wealth if they would grant him life. They refused. If he had to die, he then pleaded, could he have a dying wish? All he asked was to be allowed to put on his full singer's attire and play his lyre before he jumped to his death.

The sailors agreed. So he dressed, robed for the performance of his life, took his lyre, stood on deck and sang his heart out to the sea.

The dolphins heard him and, magnetized by the beauty of his song, swam to him, gathering around the ship. When Arion jumped, one of the dolphins carried him safely to the shore.

What is treasure? the story asks. For Arion, both music and wealth. For the sailors, money, money, money. For the dolphins, song and the pleasure of rescuing those in peril.

Stories of animal guardians are widespread in the traditional spiritual lore of different cultures. According to Old Testament belief, Elijah was saved from starvation in the wilderness by ravens who fed him. St Cuthbert, each dusk, would wade into the sea at Lindisfarne, to pray all night long, his voice a sea-chant until dawn, when he would walk out of the ocean back to the shore, drenched and frozen; two otters would then approach him, warming his feet with their bodies and trying to dry them with their fur.[18] There was a traditional belief in Aceh, on the Indonesian island of Sumatra, that guardian tigers known as 'follow tigers'[19] would accompany people in the forests, to save them from harm.

Among the Eveny people in Siberia, most people had a 'guardian reindeer', reports anthropologist Piers Vitebsky. This reindeer was specially consecrated to protect their owner. If a person was at risk of serious harm, the reindeer would place themselves in front of the person, dying in their stead, and only a reindeer could make this intentional sacrifice. Afterwards, another reindeer had to be consecrated to maintain protection, 'like renewing an insurance policy', Vitebsky is told.[20]

A similar belief is found among a linguistically related group, the Evenki, who consider that a young child is vulnerable as they have an 'open' body, and need to be guarded because they may be attacked by malevolent spirits. If this happens, the child's *khavek*, or 'double soul', steps forward, and this is a reindeer, who will disguise themself as the child and stand in their place, taking the wounds and prepared to sacrifice themself for the child.[21] Two other animals, a dog or a horse with a strong 'spirit charge', may sacrifice themselves to save humans.

These beliefs tell us how the world could be a healthier, kinder, sweeter and happier place if we recognized and acknowledged the enormous circle of healing surrounding us, if we accepted the more-than-human circle of tenderness that may wish us well. Mythic imagination, ancient wish or modern whisper may concur that the border between humans and the world is porous and protected, and certainly our lives feel warmer and safer when we open ourselves to the possibility that animals can be our guardians.

Many stories tell of neglected and rejected children, and how animals save them. These stories tell us that, thankfully, we are not condemned to the care of our parents. There are glimpses throughout the world of an age-old fear that a child may not be cared for by their own parents, and there is an age-old consolation: the animals may step forward.

'Bears take better care of their offspring than do some parents.'[22] This is the moral of a traditional story, in the Great Lakes area, according to an Ojibwe commentator. In the story, the parents are unkind to a child, so the child runs away, gets lost and is taken care of by a bear, suckling, eating and sleeping in the den. It is reported by Professor Michael Pomedli, of the University of Saskatchewan, who explores the profound healing power that the Ojibwe have attributed to animals. In another Ojibwe story, a male owl comes across a young person shivering (physical cold symbolizing emotional cold) and the bird is warm to him, calling him 'grandson', wrapping his wings around the boy and sheltering him all night in his thick down-feather warmth.[23]

In the Celtic legend of King Cormac, a baby is suckled by a wolf who guards the child as if, we are told, he were the eye in his head.[24] Medieval folk tales tell of 'swan-children' and children suckled by a hind, a goat, a lioness, a wolf, a raven or a rat.[25] When Chronos threatened to kill his infant son, Zeus, his mother, Rhea, hid their baby in a cave on Crete where the bee-guardians cared for him, feeding him honey. In Shakespeare's *The Winter's Tale*, the crazed king orders that his baby daughter, Perdita, be taken away and abandoned in the forest. Antigonus, charged with this horrible act, beseeches the animals for help, asking for kites and ravens to come to her aid.

> Wolves and bears, they say,
> Casting their savageness aside, have done
> Like offices of pity.

In ancient Greek myth, Paris, as an infant, was left exposed on the slopes of Mount Ida and was suckled by a bear. In *The Jungle Book*,

Mowgli, lost in the forest, is adopted by the Wolf Mother and Father Wolf; Kipling's fiction is based on stories of abandoned children raised by wolves.

Do these stories have real-life counterparts? Often the so-called true stories don't stand up to scrutiny, but some of them do, revealing a depth of care surrounding children, like the lions stepping in as guardians for the little girl in Ethiopia.

When I was young, I dreamed of Atticus Finch being my dad. That's idealism. Children need a parent who is a watchful and judicious social guardian, and without such a figure, a child is at risk, likely to be prey for others. In one instance, a dog, Laddie, was able to safeguard his human child, Gina Griffith.

Griffith grew up in West Virginia in the 1960s. She was not abandoned, but she was a fatherless child. The family dog, a border collie called Laddie, read the emotional situation and adopted her, stepping into the role of her absent father. As a child, people would ask if Laddie were her dog and she always felt the correct response would be to say: 'I'm his child.' Richard Louv in *Our Wild Calling* reports a particularly telling incident when Gina had been invited by other kids to go with them to smoke cigarettes and, she recounts, Laddie did not approve and stood in her way, his head low, giving her a long stare. When that didn't work, the dog picked up her hand in his mouth, pushing his teeth to the initial pressure point but without breaking her skin, and still giving her that stare. She turned back with the dog and headed for home. Once back, Laddie went to find Gina's mother and did something he would never normally do: he jumped up on to a coffee table so the mother and dog-father were at eye level and he stared into her eyes. 'Mom let him outside, turned to me, folded her arms, and said, *Laddie tells me that you need to tell me what you were getting into.*' It was true, she felt, to say she was a border collie's child. 'And he raised me right.'[26]

Sometimes animals guard us from our own kin. Family brutality has thrown children into the arms of animals who can be kinder than humankind in protecting the very young, as if demonstrating the truth of the legends.

Emergency Services

In the Siberian region of Altai, Andrei Tolstyk was three months old when his mother walked out, leaving him with his alcoholic father. Sometime later, his father left as well, and the baby was entirely abandoned. Except he wasn't. The family's guard dog cared for him and the tiny child survived, taking on the dog's habits, walking on all fours, sniffing his food carefully and (with justification) being afraid of humans.[27] He was found by social workers when he was seven and taken to an orphanage where he would at first bite and attack humans, but gradually learned sign language and elements of human behaviour.[28]

In Chile, in 1996, a five-year-old boy called Axel Rivas was thrown out by his abusive parents and ended up in a children's home. He hated it and, when he was eight, he ran away and lived with dogs in a cave, on the outskirts of Talcahuano, scavenging for food with a pack of about fifteen dogs and suckling on a nursing bitch for some of his sustenance. He was recaptured and escaped again a couple of years later, after begging to be allowed to return to his dogs because, he said, they were his family.[29]

In Moscow, in 1996, a four-year-old boy called Ivan Mishukov left home and lived on the streets. His mother had not looked after him and alcohol was wreaking its havoc in the home. For Ivan, the streets looked a kinder option. He begged for food and shared what he had with one particular pack of street dogs. The dogs, who he named Jesse, Goga, Masha and Seva, trusted him and befriended him and returned the favour so when the animals scavenged food, they shared it with Ivan. He slept with them during the long winter nights and their heat kept him warm and alive. If anyone tried to steal from Ivan or threatened him, the dogs would immediately attack, and when the police tried to take the child off the streets, the dogs would defend him fiercely.

He lived with the pack for two years. During that time, the dogs were his 'only family'. Ivan later told social workers: 'I understand that if it wasn't for those dogs I wouldn't have survived on the street. I loved the dogs and they loved me.' They kept him physically and emotionally warm as he cuddled up with them. 'They gave me a lick on the face – that's how dogs give kisses,' he explained. The police did eventually capture him, and social workers put the child in a grim orphanage near Moscow. Incredibly, his beloved dogs sensed his location and waited in vain for him at the institution's gate. Officials ordered that the dogs be killed.[30]

The true stories are, in their way, as consoling as the myths. We yearn to know that if as infants we are abandoned in a forest, or given parents who desert us, we may be taken care of by animal guardians casting a blanket of soft protection around us. If our parents throw us to the wolves, the wolves may well take a dim view of our parents. Wolves of mercy. Dogs of pity. The animals who answer the call to care, to protect and rescue, right up to the ultimate heroism if necessary, are angel paramedics, animals with scruffy haloes.

6

Dog Doctors

'The dog's nose is the only thing on the planet that knows what cancer smells like'
— Dr Claire Guest, Medical Detection Dogs

This nose was born for sniffing. It's off the leash, smelling everything it can with delighted dedication. It twitches, half crazy with illuminated enthusiasm. Actually, 'twitch' doesn't begin to cover it. This nose wobbles, it trembles, it bounces, it quivers, it cavorts with curiosity till it seems like it will spin right off its face. It is the picture of ecstasy, as tiny as it is bright, in this exorbitant world of smells. I would be that dog's nose if I could. Luminous-verging-on-psychedelic smells make his brain ripple and tingle, while engagement and total attention hold his body still.

The nose belongs to Asher, a working cocker spaniel, and Asher belongs to Dr Claire Guest, dog-listener. In 2008, Guest co-founded the charity Medical Detection Dogs (MDD), of which she is Chief Scientific Officer and CEO. All the work of MDD comes down to the dog's nose. Dogs have around twenty-five to forty times more smell-receptors than humans and their sense of smell may be ten thousand times more accurate than ours.[1]

Guest has made it her life's work to bring the skills of the dog's nose to the public, showing how they can detect disease and be trained to tell us. For this, she has been given an OBE, and her work demonstrates enormous intellectual courage, following the trail of a scent that has led to extraordinary results. Her own life was saved by a dog's sense of smell.

I visited the MDD centre, near Milton Keynes, eager to know more. Comprising a series of low white buildings set around three sides of a square, the centre is the size of a large primary school, and indeed this is a school, training the canine elite. Most of the staff foster dogs or socialize them, and as there is a no-kennel policy there are dogs everywhere, young dogs, retired dogs, dogs of many breeds, colours, shapes and sizes, in the grounds, in the corridors and in the offices. Some of the dogs are sleeping, some playing. I'm told the dogs listen to classical music, mostly Classic FM, and seem to like it. (Studies show that dogs like reggae, too.)[2]

I went to MDD during the pandemic, so I'd offered to do a Covid test before I arrived, but a smiling email came back. *Don't worry, one of the dogs will check you out.* Instead of the gagging experience of having a swab poked down your throat and up your nose, I had the fastest, sweetest screening ever. 'Please step forward,' said the doctor's assistant. The screening doctor approached, wearing a special harness. He walked towards me then speedily trotted around me, quickly sniffing me at about knee-height, probably catching scents of cats and honey in my bag and then, with a flick of his tail, Storm, a Labrador/golden retriever cross, tossed his head and rejoined his assistant. 'That's it, you're clear.'

The Covid dogs passively screen, meaning that the dog makes minimal contact with people, rather like a search dog sniffing for drugs at an airport. Their best-performing dogs can detect Covid with a sensitivity of up to 94 per cent and specificity of up to 92 per cent. (High sensitivity means fewer false negatives, i.e. when the test says you don't have it but you actually do. High specificity means fewer false positives, i.e. when the test says you have it but you actually don't.) Dogs trained to detect diseases are known as bio-detection dogs. As well as Covid, they can sniff and give a 'Tell' for other diseases including certain cancers, E. coli and more.

Illness is a funny thing. It can be lurking inside your body unbeknownst. It doesn't always show its face. Your eyes may be just as bright and your tail just as bushy and yet a virus or disease could have crept stealthily across your borders and be breaking into your system, burgling your wellness.

Storm has been in training for eighteen months. For this work, says Storm's handler, the charity chooses dogs who have natural drive, good use of their noses and are naturally inquisitive. Storm has an excellent reputation, correctly identifying people with the virus, whether or not they are experiencing symptoms. Dr Guest's partner had come to the centre with others during the pandemic feeling entirely well, but Storm picked him out from the rest, detecting Covid. Dr Guest's partner took a conventional PCR test which confirmed the diagnosis of asymptomatic Covid.

Outside, some dogs are being taken for a walk or led over to the training area. They look like they are on a mission, each one alert, utterly and manifestly aware: the very atmosphere seems bright, as if you can smell intelligence in the air. Storm is being led to a nearby field. His head is held high and he looks elastic with health. There is something else about him and the other dogs pictured on the MDD website – they look proud, proud of themselves, proud of what they do and proud perhaps that they have convinced these humans to listen to them.

Inside the centre, the walls are filled with life-size photos of dogs on hospital visits, and there is a sculpture of Daisy in the central reception area, and postcards with her portrait. She is the dog who saved the life of her owner, Dr Guest.

Some years ago, while working with Hearing Dogs for Deaf People, Dr Guest met Gill Lacey, their placement counsellor. When Gill was in her late teens, she had been very close to her family's pet dog, a Dalmatian called Trudie. Gill had had a tiny mole on her leg, and Trudie began licking it, repeatedly, obsessively, irritatingly. Gill went to see a GP, who told her there was nothing wrong, but the dog's behaviour made Gill seek a second opinion. The mole was removed, and lab tests showed it had been a malignant melanoma that would have invaded her body had it not been for Trudie.

The minuscule mole was not sending out any alarm signals; its message was coded surreptitiously and a dog was needed to decode it and send an alert. But this was only the first part of the undertaking. What was also necessary was that someone paid attention to the dog's message, and Gill did.

Her story had a huge effect on Dr Guest, already an innate dog-listener, and her life changed course as she devoted herself to attending to what dogs might smell, detect and tell. Dr Guest had a dog, Dill, who was an early detector, but only unofficially so, in her kitchen. 'I soon had him sniffing out Earl Grey teabags when I hid them around the room, ignoring the PG Tips teabags, in order to get him used to the idea of being alert to something different within a set of similar samples.' Another dog of hers, a spaniel called Tangle, was superb at detecting: trained to sniff for bladder cancer among healthy control samples, he would alert her by lying down at the one that contained a positive sample. 'Time after time after time he got it right.'

In 2004, the *Lancet* medical journal published a lengthy letter from a surgeon, Dr John Church, reporting some thirty anecdotes of dogs detecting different cancers and alerting their owners. Dr Church made an appeal on BBC Radio Four for anyone who could work with dogs on cancer detection, because all the stories at that point were anecdotal and involved dogs with close relationships to the individuals concerned. He was keen to know if it was something dogs could be trained to do, in order to help a wide variety of people, and he knew it needed to be done under rigorous scientific conditions.

Dr Guest teamed up with Dr John Church. Tangle was trained to detect bladder cancer and this work resulted in the world's first study of canine detection of bladder cancer, published in the *British Medical Journal* in September 2004.

The training involved Tangle smelling all the samples he was offered and when he found the cancer scent he had to drop to the ground. At the trial, there was a line of seven stainless-steel dishes at intervals on the floor. 'All I knew,' said Guest, 'was that there was one sample from a patient with cancer among the seven, and the other six – the control samples – had been donated by healthy volunteers.' Tangle kept finding the right sample, the cancerous one. But then something odd happened. He was *also* stopping at one of the control samples, refusing to pass by a sample from a patient who had been cleared of possible bladder cancer. Tangle kept going back to it. He was, well, *dogged* about it.

The consultant urologist took note. The patient had been cleared but because of Tangle's behaviour the urologist called the patient back in for further testing. An ultrasound scan showed he had a tumour on one of his kidneys. Luckily it was at an early stage, and his kidney was successfully removed. 'Incredibly, Tangle had been telling us the right thing all along: there were cancer cells in the urine, although not from bladder cancer. A few weeks later, a letter arrived, addressed to Tangle. *Dear Tangle, thank you for saving my life . . .*'[3] It was from the patient.

These are the good-news stories, but for Dr Guest they have a very personal shadow. She had a colleague, Lydia, who had died of breast cancer at the age of thirty-eight only a short while before I interviewed Dr Guest. Lydia had been working for the charity but off-site and not alongside the dogs. Medics had said her symptoms were nothing to worry about, but, says Dr Guest, 'One day she came on-site, and one of our dogs kept sniffing at her, and I said she should see my doctor. It was cancer. But it was then too late.'

Too Late. That phrase dwells with its anguished cousin *If Only*. How many diagnoses happen too late? If only we'd known. If only we'd had it checked earlier. If only it had been detected – like looking through your fingers at glimpses of another future. If only. Too late.

Dr Guest makes it clear that this is not a criticism of the doctors concerned with Lydia's case. 'We're not in any way trying to say they missed that. We know how complex disease-diagnosis is. We've never been critical of conventional diagnosis.' Then she leaves a pause, into which I read a plea to anyone listening to heed the dog-doctors, to help this charity scale up its training and research, to let the dogs perform their healing roles.

We go to the training area where the dogs learn which scent they are being asked to detect. Almost always, with very few exceptions, each dog is trained to detect one single thing: Covid, breast cancer, E. coli or UTI infections. Each dog, like a trained medic, then keeps to their speciality.

A black Labrador called Viking is being trained to detect E. coli ('which is very smellable and dogs love smelling it', says Guest). There are various pots in stands set by a wall, each of which contains different scents. The dog is asked to approach the stands, sniff each one in turn and give a positive indication when he reaches the E. coli sample. (The experiments are being run as a double-blind.)

To see this is to watch with the eyes of the body first and then with the eyes of the mind. The dog approaches so efficiently and confidently, and indicates so surely. A couple of times, once the dog gets to the target, he seems to forego visiting the others, as if to say, *I've found it! It's this one!* but the trainers insist that the dog tests all the stands because, in real-life situations there may be more than one of the target scents. Tangle's life-saving refusal to stop at one target, when he knew he was smelling two, stays with me.

With the eyes of the mind, I see each pot as a stand-in for a person, and one of them has a life foreclosed, though they don't know it. You can imagine a mute, desperate plea to the dog: 'Find it, please, find the Thing that will otherwise kill me.'

Different diseases create different odours. To pick up those odours, what is needed is the best kind of bio-sensor, highly tuned, sophisticated, and calibrated to a tee. The dog's nose. Specially trained dogs can sniff out a 'signature' of volatile organic compounds (VOCs) associated with disease growth. 'The dog's nose is the only thing on the planet that knows what cancer smells like,' says Dr Guest.

They can smell the signature odour of bladder, prostate and kidney cancers as well as breast cancer. Similar successes with dogs are being found across the world. In Italy, when German shepherd dogs were trained to detect chemicals linked to prostate cancer in urine samples, the dogs were correct in 90 per cent of cases, whereas the standard blood test is not considered reliable enough for screening.[4]

German shepherd dogs at the In Situ Foundation in California are trained to detect the smell of various types of cancer in the very early stages or in recurrence. A schnauzer called George has been trained to find melanomas undetectable by a hand-held microscope.[5] A study has shown trained beagles correctly identifying lung cancer samples 96.7 per cent of the time, and correctly identifying normal samples 97.5 per cent of the time.[6]

In Florida, a company called BioScentDX is trialling dogs to detect breast cancer from smelling a woman's breath. Guest comments, 'In the UK, more than 50,000 people a year are diagnosed with breast cancer, and 12,000 of them die. Women over fifty are screened with mammograms, but they cannot routinely have these more frequently than every three years because of the radiation dangers, so a simple non-invasive breath test would be a major breakthrough.'[7]

Medical Detection Dogs, in collaboration with Manchester University and Edinburgh University, has been working on a groundbreaking study showing that dogs can detect Parkinson's disease, possibly years before symptoms begin. Currently, Parkinson's is often diagnosed too late for treatment to be effective. Dogs can also detect (by smelling socks) whether people are carrying malaria parasites.[8]

~

When I visited the centre, a photograph caught my eye. A woman lies in a hospital bed with her dog by her side. The woman, Claire Pesterfield, a paediatric diabetes nurse, is herself diabetic and she had just been hospitalized after a serious hypoglycaemic incident (when the body's glucose levels crash). Her dog, Magic, is a male golden Labrador, with his forepaws up on the bed, as if they are holding hands and he is giving her all the love and kindness in the world.

Magic has an extraordinary skill: he knows before Pesterfield does that her glucose levels are going awry. Trained to alert her to the situation, he can give her as much as forty minutes' warning, and does this by thrusting her diabetes kit at her.

'Imagine life with an incurable disease that impacts every minute of every day of your life,' says Pesterfield. 'Imagine the exhaustion of waking every hour, night after night, in the hope that you will prevent the episode that may otherwise kill you . . . Now imagine a four-legged friend jumping on your bed at 3 a.m., warning you to take action now, before it is too late. Imagine a dog saving your life, day after day, night after night.'9

This is the second aspect of the work carried out at MDD. The centre trains and certifies Medical Alert Assistance Dogs, who can give warnings of an impending medical crisis. The centre then matches up the dogs with a human who has complex health conditions with crisis episodes that can be life-threatening. These include severe allergic reactions as well as Addison's disease, where sudden drops in cortisol may lead to fainting and hospitalization: a dog can detect changes in cortisol levels more quickly and efficiently than any test yet devised. They can give warnings of seizures and postural tachycardia syndrome, or PoTS, a condition where your heart rate shoots up as your blood pressure plummets, often leading to physical collapse.

As Magic does for Claire Pesterfield, dogs may alert for diabetes when blood-sugar levels move too high or too low. Giving their early warnings, the dogs can help people avoid some of the effects of diabetes, including blindness, cardiovascular disease and kidney failure.

Diabetes in childhood takes a heavy toll not just on the sufferer but on their parents, as they have to wake every hour or two to monitor their child's blood and can spend hours in hospital with their child after a collapse, dwelling in that exhausted groggy fog of the underslept.

Cerys is a diabetic child. Her parents, Debbie and Hywel, were doing everything they could, but the condition needs relentless vigilance and they were suffering. Then, when Cerys was almost five, MDD paired her with Wendy, a black Labrador trained to scent a diabetic event. The dog sleeps next to the girl's bed, and if her levels are moving away from the norm, she wakes Debbie or Hywel. The dog's senses are finer and faster than a glucose monitor, and the dog alerts them two or three times a week.

Dogs sift the air for signs, the telling emergency signal in the breath of the child, and will then alert their owners for diabetic events in different ways according to their training, so one may pick up a blood-testing kit, and another may have a toy bone that they take to the parent. If the parent doesn't wake, the dog will jump on the bed, or lick their hand or nudge them until they respond. The dog unfurls a parachute of silken safety over the lives of a whole family.

Cerys can now do things she couldn't safely do before, including going to football training, where her father coaches the team. From the touchline, the dog has alerted her father to Cerys's blood sugar moving out of safe levels; while at home the dog, even from downstairs, can give an alert if Cerys, playing upstairs, is under threat. As Debbie comments: 'Wendy is Cerys's guardian angel.'[10]

By the end of 2015, MDD had seventy trained and certified dogs working in the community, with five more in training and forty puppies. Everything depends on funding, as it costs about £12,000 to train an alert dog, but considering the amount that each dog saves the NHS it's cheap at the price.

~

Some people – and Elizabeth is one – can warm a room with their personality alone, even over the phone. Her spirit, soft as alpaca, spills with love. I have to remind myself we've never met in person, so strong is her presence even months later. She's someone who stops for injured birds, looks after puppies in distress and once took a dog and a horse together to church on the Feast of St Francis of Assisi.

Her Catholic faith and her love of animals are braided together in a golden strand through her life, and she's needed both. 'When I'm talking about animals, especially Lucy, I feel different inside, I feel as though I'm in heaven. I tear up.' Lucy, a golden Labrador, is a Medical Alert Assistance Dog, able to perceive a seizure in advance and give Elizabeth a warning.

Twenty years ago, Elizabeth began having these seizures and sought help. Medics described them as 'epileptiform' episodes (like epilepsy but not quite the same). Then Elizabeth was told the words no one wants to hear: 'There was nothing they could do for me.'

The seizures could spring on her anywhere and at any time, such as crossing a busy road or when alone by a hot stove. It is, she says, 'as though the brain's gone to sleep but I'm awake', and she can't speak or walk, or get up if she is sitting or lying down. A condition like this flings booby traps in your path, making every inch of life dangerous. It also appals the life slowly, silting up independence and congealing confidence. Many people are frightened to go out alone and become increasingly housebound.

After the seizures began and before she had Lucy in her life, Elizabeth had become unable to go anywhere without a human companion, most often her mother (who is also on our video call). Elizabeth alludes to the social isolation of those years, as the blackouts came like bad Jokers. The emotional effects were terrible.

'Oh heck. How would I describe it?' She has tears in her eyes, thinking of that time. 'You just don't know what would have happened. I'm not saying I would have killed myself but I think I would have gone downhill. If it hadn't been for Lucy, I wouldn't have been the same person, would I, Mum?'

About ten years after her seizures began, she got married briefly and unhappily. Her husband decided to get a puppy from a puppy farm, a decision which Elizabeth would not have supported had she known. (Puppy farms are notorious for forcing the females into repeated pregnancies without recovery time and removing the puppies from their mothers far too early.) At the farm, the owners picked up a puppy and shoved it into Elizabeth's arms. The puppy, Lucy, smelled terrible and was cold and filthy but Elizabeth brought her home, bathed her, warmed her and mothered her. Elizabeth shows me a little white teddy bear. The toy bear is small but the puppy had been even smaller and would curl up between the bear's paws as if looking for her mother's fur.

If Elizabeth saved Lucy from squalor and motherlessness, Lucy, even when very young, saved her, co-miraculant. 'Lucy is like an angel dog,' says Elizabeth. Without any training, Lucy began noticing the patterns of the seizures quite intuitively and started alerting Elizabeth to them. She would come to Elizabeth about fifteen minutes before one struck and 'she would give me a *look* that was not *just* a look, but a *worried* look, and that was when she was only young.' If Elizabeth didn't take any notice, Lucy would bark at her, telling her to sit, and when she did, Lucy would stop barking and sit with her. The puppy did this for a while before Elizabeth saw what she was doing. Lucy was alerting her when no one else, not Elizabeth, nor her mother, not the doctors nor indeed any medical equipment, would be able to tell that a seizure was imminent.

Before a seizure, there is some abnormal activity in the brain which can result in sweating or another kind of secretion which a dog may smell,[11] and Lucy is on a sniffing brief. 'She is always following me, always protecting me,' says Elizabeth, gratitude and astonishment ringing through her at this daily domestic miracle, as if she had found Our Lady of Lourdes doing the washing-up in the kitchen.

'When the medical people can't do any more, then the animals take over,' Elizabeth says.

It reminds me instantly of a line I know well.

'The humans have tried everything. Now it's up to us dogs and the twilight bark,' says the Great Dane on Hampstead Heath in the film *101 Dalmatians*. He has just heard the message barked by the Dalmatian father. 'It's Pongo. Regent's Park,' the Great Dane says. 'It's an All Dog Alert. Fifteen Dalmatian puppies stolen.' He booms out the message and it is relayed dog to dog, across all the dogs of London: the dogs sound the alarm. It's just one scene in just one story, and yet it has roared through the imagination of so many childhoods, wonderstruck and leaving us longing for there to be truth in it. And there is.

One day, as Elizabeth was taking Lucy for a walk in a large park, the dog gave the warning that a seizure was coming, so Elizabeth had time to sit down, leaning against a tree, but it was a particularly bad one and she was, she said, 'poorly'. Lucy needed to send out an alert, not an All Dog Alert but one specifically to another dog, Brandy, who belonged to friends of Elizabeth. Though they were too far away to see each other, Lucy knew by scent and sound that Brandy was also in the park that day. And she knew she needed back-up.

So she barked to Brandy, and Brandy recognized Lucy's bark and responded. Elizabeth's friends said later that Brandy's bark was different from normal, and that was what alerted them to something being wrong. Knowing their dog well, they could see that she wanted them to follow, so they did, and Brandy went straight to Lucy. Brandy's owners were then able to give Elizabeth the help she needed.

'There's more to animals than people know,' Elizabeth comments. 'In fact, I think Lucy knows more than I know she knows.'

Elizabeth contacted Medical Detection Dogs with the information on how Lucy was correctly alerting her and, after their tests, Lucy qualified as a certified Assistance Dog.

~

A dog can restore a sense of freedom, so someone can take the stage in the theatre of their own life. In the States, Mike Lingenfelter knows this well. He has severe coronary heart disease and frequent attacks and his golden retriever, Dakota, alerts him when one is imminent, warning him so he can take medication swiftly. The dog has saved the man's life countless times. Mike's cardiologist thinks that Dakota smells an incipient heart attack because when the heart muscle is damaged, enzymes start to build up in the blood, and this is what Dakota is smelling.[12]

To emphasize how important it is to pay attention to the dog, Mike tells this story against himself. One day, Mike was giving a talk about Dakota and the steadfast obedience of service dogs with Dakota obediently sitting at his feet. Until he wasn't. He stood up, laid his head in Mike's lap and gave him The Stare. Mike gave him the 'sit and stay' command, embarrassed, as he said later, that Dakota was undermining his talk. Dakota wouldn't sit and stay. He started poking Mike with his nose till Mike had to stop and leave the stage. Within moments he was felled by an almighty heart attack.

~

Through MDD, I also met Jess, with a background in geology and geophysics, two debilitating medical conditions and a dog called Dougie. Jess, a horse-rider and a long-distance runner, lives life in italics with a glorious *don't-fence-me-in* energy. She has postural tachycardia syndrome, PoTS, where a crisis leaves her with an adrenaline-fuelled feeling that can sometimes cause her to faint.

PoTS affects approximately 0.2 per cent of the population, about one in every five hundred people. It's sudden and it fells you. Side effects range from headaches, breathlessness and heat intolerance to fainting and collapse. The condition frequently leaves a patient anxious and afraid, not knowing when the next strike will come, and sometimes housebound by it, or even wheelchair-bound. Medical Alert Assistance Dogs are currently the only way PoTS patients can receive a warning, and the dogs can give them up to five minutes' grace before an impending crisis.[13]

PoTS is bad enough but Jess also has mast cell activation syndrome (MCAS), which means the cell walls that hold histamine are too readily activated and can burst, flooding the body with histamine like a severe allergic reaction. There can be many triggers, including acute emotional stress, a sudden change of temperature and certain foods or medications, but sometimes it's hard to tell why or when it will happen. Jess has flare periods when she can have hundreds of incidents in a month, then periods that are far easier.

At worst, she would go into full anaphylaxis, her airwaves would close, her face would get swollen and she could have gastro-intestinal disturbance, and the condition has landed her in hospital many times. She suffered with extreme insomnia because she could have these reactions in her sleep. 'My worst nightmare is what happens if I don't wake up.'

It meant a circumscribed daylight life of anxiety for Jess and her family, while insomnia took her to that netherworld of night ghouls many of us know.

Enter Dougie.

On New Year's Day 2020, Jess and her fiancé brought a puppy home. With no training, on that very first day, aged only eight or nine weeks, Dougie stepped up to the plate. He had been playing with his dog toys but, says Jess, he suddenly 'broke off and came and plonked himself right on my lap and sat and looked at me, and then I fainted, because of PoTS'.

So it began. When a PoTS episode is imminent, before Jess's heart rate spikes, Dougie alerts her. 'He presses his head on me, and if I'm standing he'll paw my leg and press on to me, on to my thighs, and if I don't pay attention he'll escalate by becoming quite vocal and jumping up.' She then has a minute or so, a short time but long enough to get herself into a position sitting or lying down, so that when it strikes she won't injure herself falling. 'Once I'm sitting, he presses his head on me, like he's telling me not to get up until he sees it's safe.'

When Dougie was six months old they approached Medical Detection Dogs, and he was certified as a Medical Alert Assistance Dog. He could alert her to an imminent PoTS episode, but could he also do it for mast cell activation?

It turns out he could. The difficulty was that at first Jess couldn't get the message. 'You just wish they could talk. Looking at him, *he* wishes he could talk, like *why aren't you listening to me?*' The main problem was timing. For PoTS, Dougie would alert her about a minute before the attack, making the connection between his behaviour and the cause for concern very clear, but with MCAS, Dougie would alert her up to forty minutes in advance and the gap of time meant that it was initially hard for Jess to see the pattern. Also, his alerting behaviour was very different for the two conditions. With PoTS he'd come close, while with MCAS, says Jess, 'he'd move away from me and *stare*. One time, I was in my study and he was in the doorway incessantly staring at me, then tapping his feet to make me look at him, and I thought he was in a mood and I didn't understand what he was trying to tell me. That was the worst allergic reaction in my life and I ended up in intensive care for a week.'

She talked it over with Gail, a gifted dog-trainer from MDD, who asked the crucial question.

'Is Dougie ever disobedient?'

This matters immensely. A well-trained and normally obedient dog who suddenly disobeys is trying to give you a 'Tell', a specific message of alarm.

'Yes,' Jess said. 'He stands off and stares, and if I give him a command, he won't do it.'

'That's it,' said Gail. 'That's his Tell for mast cell.'

Bingo.

They were away.

Now they both do the things they love. On walks, Dougie is 'a tornado of energy. He's high on life. If I blow-dry my hair he has to come and be blow-dried too as if he's saying: *Now me, now meee.*' Jess can safely go long-distance running, her fiancé bringing Dougie to check her over and see if she's ready for the next stage. She can go horse-riding too, with Dougie sitting on the mounting block and watching her, as he can sense an impending PoTS or MCAS incident at a distance of thirty yards.

She can sleep well, knowing that even if both she and Dougie are asleep, he will wake and come and alert her if necessary. Her mum is happier too. 'Now that I've got Doug, my mum is not exactly at peace – because she will always worry – but she can finally take a breath because it's not all on her.' When Dougie gives a Tell, she can take medication which works much better with the extra time that she gets after his alerts, so much so that Jess's consultant has made the dog part of her treatment plan.

From their research, the team at Medical Detection Dogs comment that PoTS is the condition that their dogs seem to detect most intuitively and with extremely high levels of sensitivity. Data from a survey of their clients showed that their dogs had a 96.7 per cent sensitivity before a collapse. (Sensitivity in this instance means the accuracy of the dogs' ability to predict an episode is about to happen.) PoTS clients averaged twenty-four injuries a month before having their Medical Alert Assistance Dogs and afterwards the average number of injuries was just three – a reduction of almost 90 per cent. There are remarkable financial advantages for the NHS. The costs associated with assessing and treating injuries for each PoTS client without a trained dog averaged £26,288 each year, but with a Medical Alert Assistance Dog that amount dropped to £3,392 – a reduction of 87 per cent.[14]

~

That dogs give alerts is well documented.

How they do it is pretty much knowable. (Smell mainly, perhaps temperature, maybe other senses.)

But why they do it is an open question.

Why does anyone, puppy or eighteen-year-old medical student, want to become a doctor? Maybe to heal others and to gain respect? Likely a dog wants a role beyond subjugated pet, that undignified position. Possibly they want a sense of purpose. Maybe they want to matter to the pack, and want acknowledgement for their intelligence. Most pet dogs are bored, their gifts wasted, and perhaps they want to be more than just a dog-bowl belly.

I asked Dr Guest about the possible motives of dog doctors. Dogs are pack hunters, she points out, and it could be that dogs smell to check whether the other members of the pack are strong enough and well enough to go out hunting, or if they are carrying a disease or are suffering a medical incident that might weaken them. 'The domestic dog is a protector, and they want to protect their humans: they quite clearly take us into their family. We have clearly selected for guarding and caring, and therefore part of their wanting to keep us safe is transferred into giving warnings when we are ill.'[15]

Dogs want to be part of the pack by warding off danger, even when the enemy is within, insinuated in the cells and circuits, blood and brain, of a pack member. They are also excellent messengers, twilight-barking, pee-sniffing, clue-collecting with the delight of the clever kid in the classroom, crying out, *I know! Me! I know!* The dogs seem to really like the role, says the centre's receptionist, adding, 'They get completely serious and seem to take on full responsibility, giving their client a sense of total assurance, as if the dog is saying firmly, *I've got this. I'll handle this.*'

Around the time that Dr Guest set up MDD, her dog Daisy, a fox-red Labrador, totally changed towards her. 'She started to behave strangely around me, to be wary of me,' Guest tells me.

One day, taking the dogs for a walk, Daisy, an otherwise scrupulously obedient dog, refused to get out of the car. 'She stood there in the boot, nudging my chest with her nose and staring up into my face intently with her big brown eyes, forcing me to pay attention to her. That evening I noticed that my chest was sore. I thought she had bruised it with her persistent nudging. But when I rubbed it I detected a small lump in one of my breasts.' She was not too worried, she says, as it was tiny, but Daisy had made her take it seriously, so she got herself tested and the lump turned out to be a benign cyst.

That, though, was not what had troubled the dog. Something else showed up on the mammogram, much deeper than the little cyst. That Something Else was cancerous, and was surgically removed. But it had been so deep within her breast that, she was told, by the time she had been able to feel it, it would almost certainly have been too late. 'If you hadn't come in for a check-up . . .' the consultant had said gravely. Dr Guest continues: 'As the consultant said the words, I remembered Daisy nudging me, I could see the pleading look in her eyes, and I knew that, without her, I was unlikely to have ever noticed the small benign lump that led to the much deeper cancer being caught. She had saved my life.'[16]

In the USA, Dr Marty Becker, author and a professor of veterinary medicine, reports a similar situation where a woman's dog began repeatedly sniffing at her right breast, licking at it and not leaving it alone. When the woman, Nancy Best, touched the area, she felt a lump and sought medical advice. It was a Type 2 oestrogen-positive invasive ductal carcinoma, an extremely fast-growing cancer that, undetected, can kill in six months.[17] She listened to her dog.

The scientific rigour of MDD's trials and the data produced has overwhelmingly persuaded people of the dogs' abilities, including Dr Alan Makepeace, a consultant oncologist specializing solely in the treatment of breast cancer, who began from a position of scepticism and is now a highly supportive trustee of the charity. But in the early years, Guest tells me, the very idea that dogs could have this level of perception was mocked. 'Why would you believe what a *dog* says?' one person asked her. 'It's foolish to listen to dogs,' said another. 'The dogs are telling us something incredibly important,' was Dr Guest's response. 'We are fools if we *don't* listen. And I'm still alive to tell the tale.'

She was listening. As Gill Lacey was listening. As Nancy Best was listening.

It's as if, comments Dr Guest, the dogs are saying, *We've been sitting here for ages knowing this and when are humans going to get it?* She mentions untrained dogs (like Elizabeth's dog, Lucy, and Jess's dog, Dougie) who alert their owners to a medical crisis, and comments that the dogs were confident enough to tell their owners. That's the first half of the process. The second half is humans being willing to listen.

I'm struck that all the people I hear or read about who noticed their untrained dogs trying to give a Tell were women. I was told that when Dr John Church's *Lancet* letter listed people who had experienced their own dog, untrained, detecting their cancer, all bar one were women. 'We think what happened was women noticed that the dogs were trying to communicate,' says Dr Guest. This makes me pause.

Women, it seems, may be more ready to listen to what animals are saying.

I'm not saying men don't listen to the natural world. They do, and I honour them: Bernie Krause (we'll meet him later) listening to the plays of sound across landscapes; David Rothenberg jamming with anyone, human or animal, who'll play with him; musician Paul Winter's lifetime of natural inspiration, Roger Payne so powerfully listening to the whales, and Chris Watson, musician and sound recordist to the natural world. Yet many of those who pioneered studies on the communication of animals, particularly primates, lions and elephants, were women, including Jane Goodall, Dian Fossey, Biruté Galdikas, Joy Adamson, Temple Grandin, Sue Savage-Rumbaugh and Dawn Prince-Hughes.

Perhaps it's scale: do men listen large while women listen small? Irene Pepperberg listened for a lifetime to her African grey parrot Alex (who we'll also meet later on) and gave the human world a new understanding of their communication. Safe to say no film-maker has listened to a single cow as astutely as Andrea Arnold did. I've long seen that my cats have always communicated more when they know they are being listened to, when a human attends to them as a creature capable of communicating. Men visiting my house have too often brushed off the cats' communications as some basic demand for food, whereas women visiting tend to listen for a 'conversation' and, when they do, the cats indeed communicate, in play, in gesture or in chirrups.

If women pay more attention to the possibility of animals communicating, women may be more likely to notice when they communicate life-saving diagnoses and detection.

As I leave the centre, I notice a photograph on the wall of the late Queen Elizabeth II with Dr Guest and Queen Camilla (the current patron of the charity). There is a dog (Florin) just out of shot and all their gazes are directed towards Florin. Dr Guest comments of the late queen, 'She was very invested in this work, and very interested. She wasn't in the least bit surprised at the dogs' ability to do this work. She knew their potential.' In no other photograph have I ever seen the queen's face like this. She looks unmasked, undefended, and there is nothing aloof or stiff in her expression. Her face is lit up, entirely captivated, careless of the camera, smiling down as she only has eyes for the dog. A cat may look at a king, but a queen may listen to a dog.

7

The Animal Apothecaries

The root of the word doctor *is* docere*, 'to guide', 'to teach',
and 'to show the way'.*

If I had to choose one place where the landscape itself feels like medicine, it would be Epidaurus on the north-eastern Peloponnese, in Greece. Swept with sunshine and sea breezes, wooded peninsulas touch the shores of the Aegean and the air is full of the scent of pine, lemon and orange trees.

The elements ring out their healing, from the scented air full of bees, to the salt sea waters and the earthy woodlands. The ancient Greeks understood that harmony between the physical body and the natural environment was a crucial aspect of health, and for them Epidaurus was a perfect site for what was known in Latin as *vis medicatrix naturae*, the 'healing power of nature', a key part of Hippocratic medicine.

A healing temple was founded here, dating from the fourth century BCE. It was dedicated to Asclepius, the Greek god of medicine, who, according to legend, was abandoned as an infant and protected by a dog. He was a wounded healer who had known anguish and had consequently dedicated himself to its remission through medicine. While Asclepius was the god of medicine, his father, Apollo, was the god of healing and associated with animals including the crow of cleverness and the dolphin. Asclepius' healing ability also included creatures at a time when medicine was an art of the gods and a gift of the animals. In one statue, Asclepius looks strong, healthy, kind and profoundly confident, sure of his cures, the sort of doctor who would make you feel better the moment you entered his clinic. He holds a stout staff with, proudly curled around it, a snake.

Patients in need of healing would come by ship, donkey or on foot to this sanctuary. Priest-medics would attend them but much of the power to heal, people said, came from sacred dogs and snakes. Dogs were said to cure people by licking them, and stone tablets were inscribed to evidence the effectiveness of their medicine. 'Thuson of Hermione, a blind boy, had his eyes licked in the daytime by one of the dogs about the temple, and departed cured,' said one.[1] Another temple story was of a man whose foot was badly injured after an attack by a wild animal and, after the wound was licked by a sacred snake, tame and non-venomous, the man was healed.

Barefoot by twilight, the sick would approach a dormitory area where they would sleep on a couch and wait for a dream that would guide them towards healing. The dream couch that they slept on, often covered in animal hides and fur, was called a *klinē*, which gives us the English word *clinic*, the 'doctors' surgery', and here the clinicians were animals.

During the night, priests would softly tiptoe among the sleepers with sacred snakes and, under the guidance of the priests, the snakes would gently slide across a patient's slumbering body and were said to whisper the correct remedy into their ear. In sleep, the psyche may be highly receptive, and patients at the temple would likely be in an even greater state of sensitivity, at a sacred site and in a dedicated time when they were committed to getting well. Added to this, they would experience the delicate and unusual feeling of being kissed by iridescent and sensual snakes. Perhaps this extraordinary combination of feelings in their sacred sleep activated a deep inner knowledge within the patient of what they must do to get well.

Women unable to conceive would visit the temple and were said to be impregnated by a sacred snake. The Freudian interpretation is obvious, and the possibility of a priest impersonating (as it were) a serpent does of course spring to mind, but there is a serious possibility of the power of belief, the placebo effect, and of the psychological benefit of arriving at a place new to the woman and set aside as holy. Belief would have intensified the natural remedy of the location. The body is never separate from the mind, and perhaps a woman's subtle, sensitive mind-body would be influenced by the fresh experience, the lush and verdant fertility of the setting and the shimmering presence of the snake such that she became ready to conceive the next time she made love.

~

When I was very ill, once, my doctor told me the etymology of *doctor*, which I had not known. It is from the Latin *docere*, meaning 'to guide', 'to teach' and 'to show the way', an etymology which offers insight into healing not only in the form of treatment but also through guidance, teaching and cautioning. I found it very moving, as that doctor had been a guide to me, through months of serious, frightening sickness. This chapter considers how animals may be our doctors, how they can heal the individual body physiologically, how they work like doctors to cure us, and reveal remedies to us. Like good doctors, they guide us by their influence and they also sometimes literally guide us to safety, like wise doctors alerting us to public health crises.

The idea that animals are doctors – of divine power – is rooted in antiquity. The Asclepian temple speaks of it. So does ancient Egyptian symbolism, where the invention of medical science was ascribed to the god Thoth, who was usually drawn with the head of an ibis, a bird with a long, curved beak, symbolic of probing thoughts, examining things deeply, exactly the attitude of mind needed for medical curiosity, precision and exploration. Contemporary scientific studies also show how animals heal our bodies. (We'll be coming to that later.)

There are many different ways of knowing. Sources of wisdom include myth, literature, ancient healing practices, direct observation and scientific research, and they all have their strengths. When it comes to animals' ability to heal, these wisdoms often seem to agree. Taken together, they create a sensibility that tells us that we humans have believed for aeons, sometimes with exact demonstrable evidence, and sometimes with intuition, that they are our apothecaries. Of course, different ways of knowing express themselves differently. Scientific studies offer evidence in the language of cold fact. Direct experience speaks in warm tones that the heart hears. Religious lore offers its evidence in another dialect. Myths speak metaphorically. Historical practices use another register. But they all matter. Listening to them all, I hear the same things being said, albeit in such varied voices. It is easier for modernity to trust most the empirical status of science, but there are good reasons to attend to other ways of thinking as well, because the beliefs that surround one's view of animals affect one's sensitivity to their actions which, in turn, may save one's life. Those who listened to the animals as guides before the Boxing Day tsunami in 2004 were the ones who lived.

The snake, crucial doctor at the temple of Asclepius, has long been associated with medicine across the world. In Ojibwe tradition, all remedies that come from the earth – roots and plants – are said to have been given to the snake, who, as their keeper, must be addressed by medicine men and women wanting to use these to make remedies.[2] The Amazon forest is a huge green temple of healing and here, too, shamans and ayahuasqueros associate snakes with curing.

The way that snakes shed their skin and live on gives rise to an almost universal association of snakes with medicinal power, one so strong they can defeat death, not by denying it but by penetrating it, sloughing off one skin to reveal another, dying to one life only to live to another. A sense of the divine surrounds their life-affirming power. Snakes are divine in many cultures: for Dravidians, a serpent god is carried in a sacred procession by a celibate priestess each year, while the 'King of the serpents', Nagaraja, was worshipped in northern India and there is a temple of pythons in Ouidah, Benin, where a python procession was said to drive out evil.

Remnants of this ancient lore are everywhere, astonishingly persistent. In fact, you may have a snake in your handbag, purse or wallet right now. Or in a drawer, or on the sideboard, or in the paper-pile in the kitchen by the kettle. Or you may have a snake in a fruitless fruit bowl, together with old batteries and a key for an unknown door, a wine cork and a pen lid, or in a scary stack, inches deep, of unsorted adminny bits teetering on the stairs (yes, my friend, you know who you are). Wherever you keep a medical prescription, in fact, you may find a snake. For millions of prescriptions are given out globally by medics who have trained in rigorously trialled medical systems and those prescriptions are printed with a snake-prayer, the predominant symbol of medicine and health care around the world.

The snake is on the flag of the World Health Organization and is the logo of the British Medical Association. The All India Institute of Medical Sciences has it and so does the Australian Medical Association. The snake is everywhere, from the American Academy of Family Physicians to the University of Copenhagen Faculty of Health and Medical Sciences; from the Royal Canadian Medical Service to the Nigerian Medical Association; from the South African Military Health Service to the worldwide symbol for emergency medical services, the Star of Life, among dozens of others.

In contemporary culture, snakes are considered to be healing by those who use them to deliver therapeutic massage from New York to Cairo and the UK. People report that after being treated by snakes, they feel both calmer and more focused: it is thought that the touch of a snake against our skin stimulates dopamine.[3] A crucial moment is when the snake is coiled at the back of the neck, applying gentle pressure, which stimulates the vagus nerve. *Vagus* is Latin for 'wandering' and this nerve is well named: it meanders around the body, reaching down from the brain to the heart, lungs, liver, gut and colon. The vagus nerve, like an intelligent snake within us, has been called the polymath of the parasympathetic nervous system.[4] It is one of the most important of the twelve crucial nerve networks connecting the brain to other organs and is involved in much of what keeps us alive and healthy, including breathing, heart rate, digestion, appetite, immune response and orgasm. It's important, too, for relaxing the body after stress. Experiments stimulating the vagus nerve suggest it can help with epilepsy, diabetes, depression, PTSD, inflammatory autoimmune conditions such as Crohn's and rheumatoid arthritis, and even possibly with long Covid symptoms.[5]

~

Historical accounts tell us how people perceived animals, from snakes and dogs to foxes and bears, to have a healing effect. Women in Elizabethan England were advised to get a 'Spaniel Gentle or Comforter' as medicine: 'It is thought of some that it is verie wholesome for a weake stomach to beare such a dog in the bosome, as it is for him that hath the palsie to feele the dailie smell and savour of a fox,' wrote English clergyman William Harrison, in his 1577 *Description of England*.[6]

Harrison's comment makes me wonder if the human mind-body does find the smells of certain animals healing. In the smallest possible study, using only my own nose and my own responses, I'd say yes. When I press my nose into the neck of a horse, or smell my cat, my nose deep in his fur, or get a hit of pure dog pelt from my god-dog Fflos, I feel a spurt of good clean joy. I have never sniffed a fox but I wouldn't rule out that Harrison was on to something. It's long known that smells can make us feel good. The temple at Epidaurus would have been steeped in the smells of flowers and petrichor, that good smell of rain-drenched earth carrying the scent of mushroom and wet leaves that is known to raise serotonin levels and be good for the health. Patients at Asclepius' clinic would have smelled the hides and fur they slept on, and also the dogs and snakes that were understood to be healing them. Could it be that smelling animals is as demonstrably healing as smelling petrichor?

The Asclepian tradition of using dogs as doctors is not the only one. St Roch, patron saint of dogs, and a saint invoked for healing, lived in fourteenth-century France. According to legend, he caught the plague and went to a forest to die but was there befriended by a dog who licked his plague sores and brought him food so he recovered. An ancient French proverb says, *Langue de chien, sert de medicine*, 'The dog's tongue serves as medicine',[7] but it's worth bearing in mind that a dog's saliva on a human wound can in fact cause sepsis.

Dogs abound in the mythology of healing. A dog was the emblem of Marduk of Babylonia and Ninisina and Gula of ancient Mesopotamia, goddesses of healing. In ancient Egypt, Anubis (doctor and apothecary to the gods) was pictured with the head of a dog. It is as if, from ancient times, people have perceived the healing of animals and encoded the belief in myth.

Letting animals be our health instructors would ameliorate some of the diseases that our caged minds inflict on our animal bodies. Bad posture, for example, often caused by desk-work, can lead to back and neck conditions, poor balance, headaches, breathing difficulties, stress incontinence, constipation, heartburn and slowed digestion. Take lessons from how your cat stretches after a cat-nap.

Animals are good yoga instructors, and many yoga poses are named for particular animals who instinctively assume certain postures: dogs, on standing up, often do the 'downward-facing dog' stretch. The cat, cow, cobra, butterfly, pigeon, camel, swan, fish, eagle, tortoise, crow, crane, peacock, scorpion, frog, lion, monkey, locust, horse, rabbit, firefly and crocodile all have their signature poses in yoga. There is a bee pose too, in which you cover your eyes with your fingers, lean forward and hum like a bee. This stimulates the brain, a yoga teacher tells me, which, we'll see later, is exactly what happens in the brain when we hear bees. Perhaps early yoga practitioners, living more closely alongside animals, watched and learned from them how the body could stretch towards health.

~

Animals, natural physicians, heal the individual in all sorts of direct, physiological ways as the medicine of their company suffuses us right into the mind-body.

Endorphins are the body's natural pain relief, and aid healing for many issues including back pain, migraines, ulcers and heart attacks. Petting a dog can raise our levels of endorphins.[8] Cortisol, the 'stress hormone', is necessary to the body's metabolism, but it needs to be well regulated not just because when it is out of whack it feels horrible, but because dysregulated cortisol levels impact brain functioning and are a risk factor in dementia and Alzheimer's disease.[9] In the presence of a dog, cortisol levels in humans decrease and stroking is also good for the dog for the same reason – lowering the dog's cortisol level.[10]

Oxytocin, the 'cuddle hormone', calms us and makes us feel happy and more trusting while also inhibiting the stress response and it is likely to help wounds heal and to promote the growth of new cells.[11] This lovely hormone can nearly double in both humans and dogs when they interact,[12] sweeping through them when they gaze into each other's eyes.

The neurotransmitter dopamine gives us feelings of pleasure and delight and though we may get a dopamine hit by buying stuff, the company of dogs gives it to us freely: dopamine is increased in humans when we are with dogs.[13] They calm us. In a study on women, the presence of a dog was shown to moderate stress responses more than the presence of a supportive friend.[14] In another experiment, patients at the University of California Medical Center in Los Angeles who had been hospitalized for heart failure, and were highly anxious, were given a dog to pet. Their anxiety levels dropped by an average of 24 per cent.[15] Stroking an animal can lower heart rate and blood pressure.[16]

It isn't just dogs. When we pet our cats, too, oxytocin is released in us.[17] When pets and other animals make us laugh, this laughter both decreases stress and improves immune functioning.[18] Watching fish in an aquarium can reduce stress and aid relaxation to such an extent that it can be as effective as hypnosis in reducing the anxiety and discomfort of patients undergoing dental surgery.[19]

Studies show that pet-owners are more likely to survive a year after being discharged from a coronary care unit than people who don't own a pet, and that this is independent of the severity of their disease and independent of other sources of social support. Risk factors for coronary heart disease (high blood pressure and cholesterol) were significantly greater among those who didn't own a pet than among pet-owners.[20]

~

What do doctors do? They attend the patient; they are physically present. Asclepian temple healing involved animal medics in close proximity to patients' bodies, in licking distance. Dog-owners say their dogs respond to their migraines or headaches, sometimes licking the side of their owner's head where the migraine is worse.

When I had Covid, I had a terrible headache that lasted for days. Nothing shifted it: no amount of pain relief worked. Otter came to me in bed and got on to the pillow, where for the most part I was sleeping on my side, my right cheek down on the pillow. Repeatedly he came and slept actually on my head, at the place of the pain, which he had never done before and has never done since. It didn't cure my headache but it made me feel better in the specific sense that I felt the awful pain was being physically attended to. I mentioned it to a friend, who said her mother had had exactly the same experience with her cat when she had Covid. Like Otter, her cat had never done it before and never since.

Animals can provide physical healing for us. Children who experience different conditions including cerebral palsy, muscle disorders and learning difficulties are physically helped by the act of horse-riding, which requires a person to continually find and refind their balance, stimulating learning receptors in the brain,[21] improving postural control and weight bearing.[22]

Animals are also healing for us in that we need to be needed: caring for others is physically healthy. If people cease to care for others, they become vulnerable to illnesses, accidents and depression as the feeling of giving up on life can result in subtle changes that disorganize the body chemistry, reducing resistance to infectious diseases and speeding up the progress of degenerative diseases including cancer and coronary-artery disease.[23] Pets require us to care for them, and this is not just a duty and a pleasure but also a medicine.

People with pets make fewer visits to a doctor than people without.[24] In a study that monitored people for ten months after they adopted pets, the results showed that they experienced significant decreases in minor health problems as soon as just one month after adopting the pet, and dog-owners maintained the decrease although cat-owners did not, which the authors say could well be because of the extra exercise that dog-owners take, compared to cat-owners. (Like good doctors, dogs promote healthy exercise.) The minor ailments included the kinds of things that are not in themselves serious but somehow make you feel your body's developed a bit of a grudge against you: difficulty sleeping, constipation, eye or ear trouble, a bad back, colds and flu, general tiredness, difficulty concentrating, sinus problems, indigestion and other stomach issues.[25]

The Asclepian healing temple put sleep right at the heart of the healing practice. We know how vital it is. We also know the most important way to ensure good sleep is to go to bed at the same time and get up at the same time: regularity is key to sleep health.

Sleeping when it's night and waking for the light is healthy for us humans and other animals of the day. These natural rhythms affect us physically and emotionally and are linked to the body's internal systems of temperature, blood pressure, heart rate, respiration, urine flow, and hormonal and enzyme levels. A disruption to those rhythms can make us irritable and low or physically ill. Animals, who naturally dwell in circadian rhythms, are healthy role models, influencing us to adhere to those rhythms. Otter is a good sleep doctor. Being a cat, he delights in the dawn and dusk hours and, in part influenced by him, I wake early. I like the regularity and shared rhythm: the sun wakes the birds, who wake the blind cat, who wakes me. Being in tune with the day feels good. Dog-owners speak of the requirement to get up early to take the dog out in the morning light and they know the positive health consequences of that regular exercise.

Some animals, including cats, also adopt seasonal rhythms. Otter turns from summer-cat to winter-cat, with more fur, more sleep, more food, more warmth, guiding me to do something similar, seeking more denning up, more sleep and more food.

Regulation is a key concept in health, from the regularity of exercise and sleep to a well-regulated diet. In traditional lore, animals have been seen to promote good habits: in Ojibwe tradition, the owl is a healer of sickness because it demands a regular, healthy regimen in life.[26] Ancient concepts of medicine understood how important for human health were the deep beats of the living world, a rhythm running beneath everything, every plant and animal. Taoism teaches that good health in all its forms, physical, emotional and spiritual, comes from being in balance and in harmony with the rhythms of nature. The Tao, the primal principle of the universe, guides all the cycles of nature, day to night, summer to winter, and aligning oneself to the Tao is profoundly medicinal. In Ayurvedic medicine, health is understood in terms of Svastha: our inner nature living in harmony with nature outside us, the plants and the animals.

~

At the Asclepian healing temple, the snakes were said to whisper remedies into a patient's ear as they slept. A good doctor tells us what medication to take, suggesting and guiding us to the right remedies. Some animals do this too. Herbalists teach us which plants may be medicinal for which specific illnesses and, just so, animals too can guide us to medications that heal certain conditions. Some animals self-medicate and many cultures believe that humans learned pharmacy from the animals. Given that animals have been around long before us, and given that some self-medicate, they may well have been our first apothecaries.

In parts of western North America there is a plant called *Ligusticum porteri*, which is a topical anaesthetic and has antibacterial properties. Navajo tradition says that the use of that plant was taught to them by the bear: they refer to it as 'bear medicine'.[27] In Ojibwe culture, the bear is a keen herbalist, rooting for medicinal plants[28] and is said to teach people their use in healing. John Fire Lame Deer, medicine man of the Lakota (Sioux), noted: 'The bear is the only animal that one can see in a dream acting like a medicine man, giving herbs to people. It digs up certain healing roots with its claws. Often it will show a man in a vision which medicines to use.'[29]

When chimpanzees and other primates have stomach pain, diarrhoea, worms, bacterial infections or suffer weight loss, they have been known to relieve the symptoms by chewing *Vernonia amygdalina*, often called 'bitter leaf', a member of the daisy family that grows in tropical Africa. People living in chimpanzee territory also use the bitter leaf to treat themselves.[30] Michael Huffman, as professor at the Primate Research Institute at Kyoto University, studied self-medication in animals. He spent time in Western Tanzania in the late 1980s and noted a sick female chimpanzee peeling the bark of a shoot of *Vernonia amygdalina*, then chewing the pith and swallowing the juice. Huffman's local collaborator, Mohammed Kalunde, was himself a herbalist, and said the plant had medicinal qualities and that his people, the WaTongwe, used it to treat stomach disorders, malaria and parasites. The day after the sick chimpanzee had self-medicated, she was seen again, no longer ill, happily eating ginger and figs.[31]

Chimpanzees can tell the difference between two hundred forest plants, are aware of their growth in which seasons, remember exactly where they can find the plants, and know what their uses are.[32] Chimpanzees sometimes combine botanical and geological ingredients to create more potent treatments. In the Kibale National Park in Uganda, they have been seen eating specific soil shortly before or after eating certain plants. A local healer noted that the soil used by chimpanzees was high in kaolinite, which local people were also using to treat diarrhoea.[33]

Plutarch knew. In *On the Cleverness of Animals*, the ancient Greek philosopher notes:

> After devouring a serpent, tortoises take a dessert of marjoram, and weasels of rue. Dogs purge themselves when bilious by a certain kind of grass. The snake sharpens and restores its fading sight with fennel. When the she-bear comes forth from her lair, the first thing she eats is wild arum; for its acridity opens her gut which has become constricted. At other times, when she suffers from nausea, she resorts to anthills and sits, holding out her tongue all running and juicy with sweet liquor until it is covered with ants; these she swallows and is alleviated.

Jaguars are known to eat leaves of the *yagé* vine (*Banisteriopsis caapi*), the primary ingredient of ayahuasca, the most powerful and profound medicine of the Amazon. In a clip from a BBC documentary, a jaguar in the Peruvian rainforest, having eaten the leaves, turns kittenish and playful, then she looks entranced as if she were dreaming her own quintessence, the vital spirit at the heart of the animating Amazon.[34] Since the jaguar evolved before we did, maybe she taught us that there was mind-medicine in the forest and showed us how to find it.

~

As we saw, the etymology of doctoring is teaching and guiding. If animals may, like doctors, teach us a healthy regimen and perhaps healing herbs, they may also be guides, quite literally so, leading us to safety and warning us of physical danger.

As *National Geographic* reports, the devastating Boxing Day tsunami of 2004 (striking Indonesia, Sri Lanka, India, Bangladesh and Thailand, among others) seems to have been anticipated by both wild and domestic animals. Elephants screamed and ran for higher ground. Dogs refused to go outdoors. Flamingos abandoned low-lying areas. Survivors reported seeing animals, including cows, goats, cats and birds, moving inland just after the undersea quake and just before the tsunami. Human early-warning systems failed to raise a clear alert. At least 225,000 people died across a dozen countries, but comparatively few animals. Many of the humans who did survive had run along with the animals – they had been guided by them.

As a dog can connect a person with hearing loss to the communication systems of doorbells, phones and alarms, just so the animals are patching us through to the communication of the Earth's systems. The Max Planck Institute of Animal Behavior in Germany studied the movement patterns of cows, sheep and dogs in an earthquake-prone region of central Italy and noted that the animals altered their behaviour up to twenty hours before an earthquake, moving more, and acting frisky and nervy. When the animals were, collectively, 50 per cent more active, for more than forty-five minutes at a stretch, a strong earthquake could correctly be predicted seven out of eight times.[35]

Diodorus knew. The ancient Greek historian reported that rats, dogs, snakes and weasels fled the city of Helike in the days leading up to a catastrophic earthquake in 373 BCE.[36]

In China, snakes are considered to be perhaps the most sensitive creatures on Earth to imminent quakes, in another iteration of their power to save us. Authorities evacuated Haicheng in 1975, just before a major earthquake. They did so having noticed the sudden changes in the behaviour of snakes, who will move out of their nests, even in the cold of winter, when an earthquake is about to occur.

Dogs may deliberately intend to warn their humans; one of my god-daughters, who is Nepali, tells me of the earthquake in Nepal in 2015 when their dog, who was outside the house, began whining and scratching at the door and window. He wouldn't come into the house but was desperately trying to get the family out.

'One should pay attention to even the smallest crawling creature, for these too may have a valuable lesson to teach us, and even the smallest ant may wish to communicate with a man,' commented Black Elk, medicine man of the Oglala Lakota. *Even the smallest ant.* Before a bushfire, some ants will cover their nest-hills with tiny pieces of sparkling quartz which reflect heat and so protect the nest, and if people read the sign, they can see it as a fire warning. As Chickasaw writer Linda Hogan notes, 'The action of ants saves human lives.'[37]

The animals are speaking: we have to attend.

Polynesian sailors would pop a pig into their boat when they went on long voyages because the pig could smell land miles out at sea, hours before people could see it, and would give a Tell, pointing their snout towards it.[38] Sailors have traditionally known to watch animals for both guidance and weather forecasting. If they see no birds except the storm petrel, they take it as a warning: the storm petrel is known to be the last bird out on the oceans before a tempest arrives.

In 2014, golden-winged warblers arrived in their regular breeding grounds in Tennessee, having flown 3,000 miles from South Africa; all being normal, they would have stayed, recovered from the flight, and begun mating, but they didn't. Instead, they suddenly took off in what is called an evacuation migration and flew 400 miles away. Just after they left, eighty tornadoes struck the area, killing thirty-five people. At the point when the birds took wing, the twisters were 250 miles away but it seems the birds knew: it is thought that the birds were responding to the strong infrasound from severe storms. A public health alert, put out by the birds. Had humans noticed them raising the alarm, they could have been prepared.

The senses of animals are often more acute than ours. They may alert us to danger and we would be wise to listen. In Britain during the Second World War, dogs could alert people when a bombing raid was imminent, giving warnings by whining, barking, hiding or leading the way to an air-raid shelter. Cats and birds in Germany also gave warnings of British air-raid attacks, with one German-speaking parrot saying, *Da oben!* (Up there!)[39]

I have a friend, Fran, who is an organic farmer in Mid Wales. She is also a listener. She has the quietest presence and the steadiest gaze. Soft in her voice and movements, she attends to the voices around her, listening gently enough that animals come to her. When she was a teenager, she would go and sit for hours at a stretch on a bank of badger setts, watching them. After some weeks, they became so accustomed to her in her stillness that the badger cubs would play, sometimes so close that they would run over her legs. Animals trust her not to harm them, and perhaps that trust is a result of her patience, time and gentleness. If you listen, animals may well speak.

Fran tells me she can tell the health of her farm by listening to its sound: thriving, birdsung and humming with insects. She has a bird-friend, a male swallow, who would perch on a stone in her bedroom and sing. He did this for three years, and in the fourth year he brought a mate back with him and they nested in her bedroom, six feet above her toes when she is in bed. The female was at first nervous but found Fran so calming that in the end the birds produced two broods of chicks in one year.

When the swallow wakes, he sings for half an hour in her bedroom, a madrigal that is a medicine of joy. 'You get lost in the intensity of awe,' she says. She listens, and the bird's song 'eclipses worry and stress' and puts life into perspective, reorienting her to connect with everything. A musical medic, he guides her heart and her mind, for when he leaves at the end of the summer, she follows him in her thoughts, considering the route of his migration, with the inevitable fear that he may not make it back another year, his life in jeopardy because of the impact of the climate crisis and the loss of insects for him to feed on.

The birds are guiding us like doctors, warning us of risks so frightening that we have to pay attention. In Mi'kmaq culture (of Canada's Atlantic province) 'bird medicine' includes the art of interpreting bird language and behaviour, in order to understand their guidance.[40] We need that guidance now.

In 2021, the Indigenous Totonac people of Mexico wanted to send an urgent communiqué to humanity. They created a huge totem pole of a hummingbird – in Totonac culture, hummingbirds are messengers – and sent it from Mexico to Glasgow in time for COP26. The pole, fifteen feet tall, had presence and beauty. Brightly painted in blues, reds and yellows, the bird's wooden feathers sung like wind chimes. It was carved by Jun Tiburcio, whose first name means 'hummingbird' in the Totonac language. On its journey, while the totem was at the Port of Veracruz, the area was battered by Hurricane Grace and Jun Tiburcio's home was largely destroyed. The climate itself, he felt, had spoken, 'letting us feel its rage'.[41]

~

We humans would mostly be gone from the world within a few months without . . .

Without what? Without money? Without mobile phones? Without the Internet, space exploration or toilet paper? Without doctors? Without education? Without sacred places and the prayers to fill them? Without love?

None of the above.

Without insects.

As E. O. Wilson, biologist and naturalist, said in 2007: 'If we were to wipe out insects alone, just that group alone, on this planet – which we are trying hard to do – the rest of life and humanity with it would mostly disappear from the land. And within a few months.'[42]

Of all the animals, insects are the most necessary to our very survival. Many animals have saved our individual lives but it is insects that actually give us life: daily, hourly, they keep us alive. They are our sustainers, our very life-support system, a flight of angel paramedics in constant attendance to us and other living things. Insects pollinate three-quarters of our food crops and 80 per cent of wild flowering plants and keep the soil healthy, recycling nutrients.

Some societies cherish insects, and in Costa Rica a suburb of San José has given citizenship to every bee, bat, hummingbird and butterfly. The oldest continuously surviving human cultures – Indigenous Australian civilizations – respect and honour the tiniest creatures in a kind of ecodeistic reverence. In central Australia, honeybees feature in totems, rock art and creation stories: in the beginning was the bee. Across Australia, insects are honoured in songs and feature in mythology, place names and personal names. Insects are part of rituals, including the 'increase ceremonies' once widely held to promote the abundance of particular species.

Insecticides perform decrease ceremonies to promote the destruction of insects. Every litre of insecticide doled out is a deadly ritual of killing. In place of creation stories that put insects at the heart of life, every advert for insecticides is an annihilation story. An insecticide-sprayed field poses as food; it is actually starvation. It pretends to be profit; it is actually loss. It pretends to have only killed the insects; it actually threatens the lives of our grandchildren.

Insects are the most despised of all creatures, the ones killed in the largest numbers, and the weaponry used against them has multiplied in lethality in the post-war years. It isn't only chemical warfare. Light pollution contributes to the ritual of decrease because when insects such as moths flock to artificial light, a third of them will be dead by morning. They will either be predated upon or simply die of exhaustion.

Insects are thought to have been alive on Earth 480 million years ago. That's 1,524 times longer than us, as *Homo sapiens* has only been here some 315,000 years. Insects, who were here so long before us, and have been cherished by humans for thousands of years, could all but vanish within a century, a whole world quietly disappearing.[43]

Some insects are on the increase, including locusts, cockroaches and horseflies, but the insects most badly affected include bees, butterflies, moths, beetles, dragonflies and damselflies.

I swim in lakes near me in Wales, summer and winter, and I have done so for decades. I used to see swifts streaming in arabesques of flight, catching insects in large numbers, soaring above my head as I swam, or swooping down to water level and catching them right in front of my eyes. Every year I've seen fewer. Yesterday, a warm summer morning, I saw barely six. According to the British Trust for Ornithology, swifts in Wales have declined by 72 per cent since 1995. The reason is obvious. I barely see any insects, in an area that should be a birds' banquet. As the swallow guided Fran's thoughts across the deserts, and as the swifts speak to me in their relentless declining, the birds are guides as certainly as storm petrels, telling us of storms to come.

The swifts are singing through their songlessness, a silence that speaks of their migration routes as ordeals across deserts, not only natural deserts but over vast deserts of industrial agriculture, for without insects to feed on, the birds risk death at every wingbeat through the starving skies.

How is it possible for modernity to have so much knowledge and yet so little wisdom? How is it possible to chronicle so carefully our death foretold and yet fail to take the actions necessary to avert it? With the noise of shouty human messages, modernity has deafened itself to the healing truths of bird calls and bird silence that signal what we most need to hear: a public health alert of the gravest importance.

If we would listen to the advice of the swift clinicians and be guided now by their eloquent silence, we would be able to read our own story in these emptying skies: the loss and hunger, the silencing of all our songs, all our loves, all our lives.

And we would transform ourselves, changing direction mid-flight, as elegantly and certainly and fleetly as a swift's wing turns.

8

Midwives for the Dying

'The art of living well and the art of dying well are one'
— Epicurus

'I lost my beloved mother last summer to a sudden, fierce and rapid illness,' the artist Amy Shelton tells me. 'It took her from enjoying the early spring promise of her garden to her burial on a sparkling day in early September.' Her mother, Daphne Shelton, was a keen gardener, 'so rooted and real in life', says Amy. Her mother had no religious faith but had 'a capacity to find the beauty and meaning in living an ordinary life that was one of her most inspiring characteristics'.

In the last few days of her life, Daphne became preoccupied with bees: she said the bees were coming to visit her, that she must decode what the bees were trying to communicate to her, and that she had 'ordered a death from a bee'.

Although her mother was in no way a bee expert, Amy's artwork reflects a deep and ongoing interest in bees, and she says that might have been why her mother ('who was also my great friend,' says Amy) focused on bees. And yet during those last days, Amy was startled by how her mother seemed to be experiencing a direct discovery which was both revelatory and intriguing. She wasn't referring to an idea already known to anyone but rather expressing a novel and personal realization of something previously undetected: 'She was giving the information as a new and extraordinary thing.'

Over the days of her active dying, Daphne said she had to concentrate hard to 'go with the bees', who were trying to show her the way in order to be able to undertake the journey of death. Repeatedly, she said that a solitary bee was coming to guide her and that it was stopping off in a hedgerow, expecting her to follow it, but she didn't know how.

Her mother's extraordinary preoccupation with the bees was a consolation to Amy, it 'suffused the atmosphere of those incomprehensibly sad days as I began to lose the person I so loved'. Daphne repeatedly spoke of there being a misunderstanding over how to die, and that she 'had to follow the bee and understand its messages in order to be able to die'. She kept telling Amy that people had been failing to understand the significance of bees in life, and that they were actually the guides between this world and another realm, between the living and the dead.

Amy had talked to her mother about bees on and off, but her mother's dying experience was not in the category of exterior knowledge or research: it was coming to her as intuition and revelation. 'She wasn't asking for any context or information; it was beyond history or discussion. She only wanted to describe the scenes she encountered. For me, it was heart-stopping.'

Her vivid visions of the bees were, says Amy, 'gentle, unlike the illness. Having ordered her death from the bee, she described the next steps as both alluring and elusive. There were guidelines she needed to follow that the bee was trying to communicate, and she was working hard to understand.'

The bee death she encountered was 'remarkable, something of great amazement' to her mother, who, as she stepped closer to death, described a transition both utterly beautiful and highly complex.

'What a lovely way to go – to go with the bees,' her mother said, convinced that they were guiding her 'up into the sky'.

When she woke up she was disappointed – 'Am I still here then?' – and was noticeably frustrated. 'Amy, I didn't get to my bee bed, why can't I have a Death Day?'

A little later, she slept and woke again and Amy saw what she calls 'a lightness in her whole being'. The scene is etched in Amy's memory.

'How marvellous,' said her mother. 'I was alive and now I'm not.'

Amy, startled, took her hand. 'You are alive, Mum.'

'No, not in the same way, Amy. I ordered a death from a bee and I got one. Before I just didn't understand it, it's very complicated – one single tiny bee has done it for me.'

From that moment, Amy says, her mother 'never really returned. I believe that this moment she so lucidly described was when her consciousness shifted and it truly felt like her soul had been displaced, that she had departed.'

~

When Queen Elizabeth died, the royal beekeeper, John Chapple, went to the bees at Buckingham Palace and Clarence House and tied black ribbons around their hives, thick black sashes that wrapped the boxy hives like sad gifts. In the middle of life there is death, looping its black ribbons through it all. Then he told the bees of her passing and spoke to them of the immediate royal thread of succession – 'The queen is dead: long live the king!' – in that phrasing where death is a pause no longer than the colon of punctuation.

According to an ancient and widespread European tradition, bees need to be told about deaths and births because they ferry souls into life and out of it, tiny stevedores loading and unloading cargoes of souls. Honey has been reported in funerals from the *Iliad* and the *Odyssey* onwards, healing the psychological wound of bereavement. Honey literally heals the rupture of wounds, as the bees metaphorically mend the rupture of death.

The idea that animals aid our dying is both ancient and perennial, a constant in the human mind. In considering that there is a world of the living and a world of the dead, the human mind seems to agree that the hard part is the transition between them and that the animals are our helpers on this shrouded and troubling journey.

At the funeral of Queen Elizabeth II, her cortège was driven up the Long Walk to Windsor Castle where her Fell pony Emma was standing to one side, waiting. Tacked up but still. Saddled but riderless. To me, this is one of the most poignant expressions of death, the emptiness of the place where someone used to be. Looked at through the lens of myth, the horse stood ready to carry her rider's spirit on the daunting ride it must undertake. In myth, animals often perform this role, the formal title of which is *psychopomp*, from the Greek *psukhe*, meaning 'soul', and *pompos*, 'guide' or 'conductor'.

At the castle, as if to greet the monarch at the end of her longest journey, were her corgis, Muick and Sandy, two of a lineage of beloved dogs that had accompanied her all her life. As her pony had physically carried her, so her dogs had emotionally carried her across difficult stretches of her life, and when Prince Philip died in the forsaken time of the pandemic, her family gave her more corgis to help heal the wounded months.

Only a few months before her death, the queen 'met' Paddington Bear during her Platinum Jubilee celebrations. A short film was made of them having tea together at Buckingham Palace, each revealing they always kept a sandwich stashed away for safety, a marmalade sandwich in his hat, a jam sandwich in her bag. After her death, among the valedictory floral tributes were many little Paddingtons.

When she died, the state declared ten long grey days of national mourning, heavy as clay. The BBC, tasked with expressing and guiding the national mood, knew that it had to carry the public over the border between the days of extraordinary mourning and *normal service resumed*. The jarring transition needed special reconciling, a kind of honey to mend the rupture, and the BBC, with perfect pitch, chose to screen *Paddington 2*. While not everyone is a royalist (I'm not, as I don't believe any living creature should be kept in a zoo), everyone loves Paddington Bear. I doubt the commissioners at the BBC would have known this, but they were walking an ancient path in choosing a bear. Bears have often been given a crucial role in death, and among the Ojibwe, for instance, the bear was traditionally a guiding spirit, leading people during their lives and showing them their way in death.[1]

Paddington is a quintessential teddy bear, an ur-*ursus*. Teddy bears offer security for children holding them in the dark bed of sleep, and indeed they comfort adults too in that deeper darkness that is the bed of the grave. I want to be buried with my teddy, and I'm not alone.

Twenty-seven per cent of British people would want to be buried with their teddy bear, comforting them in the long sleep.

At the queen's funeral, New Zealand prime minister Jacinda Ardern wore a cloak of black feathers, inspired by the Maori *kakahu* worn at times of transition. For the Maori, birds are messengers between the physical world and the spirit realm, and they carry us on their wings. For the Lakota, a spotted eagle comes to a dead body, lifts up the soul and carries it away on its journey.[2] The birds and other animals are conductors, guiding the music of life and death. For ancient Egyptians, the soul was often depicted as a little bird with a human face which would flutter over the coffin of the dead because only the body had died while the spirit had wings, its melody merely transcribed for a different instrument.

In Ojibwe tradition, dead ancestors may become owls who summon the spirit of someone who is about to die. The dying person's soul cannot see in the darkness of death's night, the path occluded, so the owl lends its night vision. The owl is said to *mediate* between life and death.[3] Similarly, in Scottish Gaelic folklore the redshank is called an *intermediary* between the living and the dead.[4] The owl is a bird of time's borders, the dawn and dusk hours, and is associated with the night-time of death. The redshank is also a bird of borders, mostly living between the upper and lower tide limits on the shore and existing symbolically between life's high tide and death's ebb. In Scottish Gaelic tradition, a song based on the redshank's call should be sung to help the dying on their journey, writes Canadian composer Emily Doolittle.[5] (Ah, Doolittle, in lovely nominative determinism, seems named to work on animals in music.) By the notes of a redshank the psyche is guided on the ebbing tide.

Dolphins have been known to create a cortège accompanying the dead. One day in the Bahamas, a dolphin expert, Dr Denise Herzing, had taken her boat out with other passengers to watch dolphins, expecting all the usual playfulness, bow-riding and games. But on this day, everything was different. The dolphins wouldn't come close to the boat and refused to surf the bow wave, inexplicably serious.

Then someone made a sad discovery: one of the people on board, who had apparently stepped down for a short rest in his bunk, had in fact died in his sleep. The humans had not known, but the dolphins seemed to have ascertained it.[6]

As the boat headed back to harbour, the dolphins approached the boat but maintained a fifty-foot distance, and began paralleling it in what Dr Herzing called an 'aquatic escort'. It is as if they marked the passing by flanking the boat, acting with distanced reserve and a solemnity quite unlike their normal playfulness, carrying something of the emotional freight like pall-bearers charged with a heavy cargo.

In death, the animals are intermediaries, medics to the spirit, and dogs are widely understood to bring remedies. In Mexico the Xoloitzcuintli, or Xolo for short, is a dog named after the Aztec god of death, and the one most associated with the Day of the Dead. This was the breed beloved by Frida Kahlo, who kept them, painted them, and cradled them for consolation. As dogs guide us in life, they are said to guide us in death when, in an image I find very tender, they carry the soul of their owner in their mouth.

Dogs guard the doorways of houses in life, and they are said to guard the doors of heaven in death. In Zoroastrian belief, the Bridge to Heaven is guarded by dogs, and a gaze from a dog can release the spirit into heaven (the bliss of oxytocin is, after all, paradisiacal). A Zoroastrian funeral ceremony called Sagdid (meaning 'dog sight') involves a dog being brought in to inspect the dead body. Done for spiritual reasons, the origin is pragmatic: a dog may be able to detect the most infinitesimal signs of life that we humans might miss. A 'four-eyed' dog (with two eye-spots on the forehead) is said to be best for this, magnifying its vision.

In Hindu myth, Yama, god of death, has two watchdogs with four eyes who guard the gates of death. In Nepal, every November, the Hindu festival of Kukur Tihar takes place where dogs are worshipped and every dog has its day, even police dogs and strays. They are fed meat and eggs. Incense is lit for them. They are garlanded with streamers of marigolds while a vermilion tika, the tiny holy dot, is put on their foreheads. It is done to cherish the living dogs who protect homes in this life, but it is also done to befriend the dogs who guard those other doors and who, properly treated now, will allow people to enter heaven.

When death forms its grey and greasy patina, the animals guide us to the knowledge that the rivers of life will never run dry. In the Amazon, the Shipibo-Konibo people believe that the life force is a giant anaconda which vitalizes waters, forests and all the animals, and if that power died, everything would die with it. For Indigenous Australians, the Rainbow Serpent gave birth to the Animal Ancestors who live forever, and she represents the infinite green ribbon of life that only momentarily turns black at death, and always sprouts up again with the brightness of rebirth, wet with iridescent life.

~

Death gobbles up everyone eventually. Death has a repulsive appetite, perpetually hungry. With its skeletal body, it snacks on a child like a plum or gorges on a man for breakfast. Death has some really nasty habits: spreading germs and bacteria, smirking as it goes, death breeds death. Death stalks across a field of potatoes causing blight and with a withering glance can turn buds to arid husks as a wintering chill announces the callous cold that freezes the heart's warmth. Death feasts on the frozen, licking its ice-cold lollipop lips, and nothing – at first sight – seems to feed on death.

But then, far above, in an enormous wingspan of severe mercy, the death-eaters gather, wheeling in the sky. They flock together: they become a team, the purification crew, the hygiene attendants, cleaners armed with detergent, deterring death. They swoop down to a corpse, put a quick hood up over a dead body and move in to clean it up. Their beaks are surgical scissors, their gaze is astringent as witch hazel. Keen, clean and necessary, they are brisk at their work, in claw and sweep, the vultures.

Vultures in Tibet will swoop down on a body that has been put out in a sky burial, and this carries more significance than simply being a way for nature to process a corpse, for the birds are seen by Tibetan Buddhists as spirits carrying the soul across to a new incarnation.

Considered a tradition of the East (Mongolia, Nepal and Bhutan as well as Tibet), sky burials are thought to have taken place far more widely, including in Orkney, Scotland, with Neolithic peoples believing the spirit of a dead person lived on in the majestic and totemic sea eagle who ingested their flesh.[7]

Vultures can digest and eliminate the bacteria that cause anthrax, cholera, tuberculosis, botulism and rabies, all without becoming ill themselves. Vultures make ecosystems healthy and are venerated in cultures which are grateful for their feeding on carrion. In ancient Egypt, Nekhbet was a goddess with the head of a vulture, worshipped for her association with the bird. At the world's oldest known temple, Göbekli Tepe in Turkey, founded in about 9500 BCE, there is a depiction of a vulture, the bird as psychopomp guiding the spirit into the great beyond, the vulture turning death into wings.

The American poet Robinson Jeffers related lying still on a bare hill watching a vulture who was watching him; the poet imagines being eaten and becoming the bird, being its wings and eyes in a rapturous end: 'what an enskyment'.[8]

Crows compel the attention. Complex and curious, they strut and bob and glint as if their intelligence catapults them into examining everything around them: there's mind behind those bright eyes. They may also, say crow experts, feel passionately for each other, and 'crow funerals' have been observed where crows gather around a dead crow. They arrive, squawking, calling and cawing, sometimes in their hundreds, and hold a fierce ritual of noise for about a quarter of an hour, until they gradually fall silent. After a time, they quietly leave. The dead individual's closest companions seem to express grief at these funerals, although the majority of the crows are there gathering information about the cause of death, any possible threats to other crows and also to negotiate how their society might be affected by the death of this one specific member.[9]

If a magpie dies, her friends and relations may lay grass beside the body and stand vigil by it together before, one by one, flying away.[10] Rabbits can grieve a death to the extent of becoming seriously depressed and, losing their appetite, may starve themselves to death.[11] Donkeys may hold wakes for their friends: after the death of one donkey, others who knew her were seen standing by her grave braying for hours into the night.[12] Female chimps and gorillas whose babies have died carry the dead child with them for days, and they behave as if they are in emotional agony, sitting alone, sometimes whimpering, sometimes crying inconsolably.[13] Orca mothers may feel utterly devastated by the death of one of their calves and in one instance Tahlequah, a Pacific Northwest orca, was seen bearing her dead child, lifting him into the air as if to help him breathe, continuing thus for seventeen days. Having carried the calf inside her for seventeen months, she was grief-stricken and in her mourning she carried him a thousand miles. A few years ago, game wardens went to a small lake in Minnesota and, apparently just for fun, planted explosives and blew up a beaver dam. A sound recordist happened to be there and stayed long after the wardens had left. He recorded the heart-rending sounds of the male, whose mate and young kits had been killed in the explosion. He had survived physically but was left heartbroken, crying forlornly, swimming slowly, stunned and bereft.[14]

Elephants are known to mourn a death among them as a grievous loss. They bury the body, kicking up the ground, digging up dirt and putting the earth over the body while some break off branches and leaves and place them on the corpse. They then stand vigil. If at any time on the trail elephants find the skeleton of a dead elephant, they stop, growing quiet and tense, reaching their trunks to the body, smelling it, lifting the bones and feeling the skull, seeking to recognize individuals they knew.[15]

At a safari ranch in Zimbabwe, three black rhinos were kept with elephants and they befriended each other, strolling together often, and two of them, one elephant and one rhino, were both pregnant at the same time. One night, poachers killed the rhinos in a brutal attack to hack off their horns. The elephants would have heard their screams and the gunshots. The ranch workers buried the rhinos and, honouring the friendship, took the elephants to the grave. They responded with tears running down their faces, while the pregnant elephant screamed and shrieked in grief and dug a yard down to try to reach the pregnant rhino's dead body, supported, physically and emotionally, in her anguish by the other two elephants.[16]

How do these stories help us? How can the evidence of animals mourning a death give us humans any consolation? When an individual human is bereaved, they almost always seek out others in an instinct to share the grief, to know they are not abandoned. Through the animals we can see that as a species we are not the only ones to feel bereft in the grief of death. We are comprehended and consoled in a wider circle of creatures. We are not alone.

When the heart breaks, it breaks as if it were made of brittle bone. We need the apothecary of animals, the comfrey or knitbone of a cat's purring to comfort us (and which does, literally, aid the mending of bones).[17] When the soul is wounded, it is ruptured like ripped flesh. We need the stitchwort of the bees (and stitchwort has a medicinal use in mending wounds), whose honey stitches the psyche back together when it has been sundered by death.

The animals give us a gently amended version of bereavement, showing us how our story is part of a larger narrative, a story of hurt but ultimately not of harm, a wrench that may make us collapse with loss but also lets us know that when we fall, the wordless others may give us wings sufficient to fly.

~

Animals can be midwives for the dying, as they may bring their natural medicine into the noxious sterility of a hospital death.

Dr Stephanie Hodgkinson was a palliative-care consultant in southern England during the late 1990s and early 2000s. So, in a way, was Straws, a female black cat with golden eyes. Dr Hodgkinson told me the hospice hadn't chosen to have a pet but Straws 'just sort of magicked her way in'.[18] She lived on the wards and ate in the communal area and was considered part of the core staff.

Straws seemed to feel a duty of care, to attend the dying by simply accompanying them. Her special skill was knowing when one of the patients was very close to death – something that became invaluable to the staff as they could ensure the patient's family had some advance warning. 'She would pick it up before we did,' said Dr Hodgkinson. Straws used to go deliberately to people at their end and, as one nurse said, 'Straws was always right. When someone was about to die, she would go into people's rooms and jump on to the bed and stay there.' One night three people were very near to dying, and Straws paced all night from one to another, 'not wanting to leave one out'. Dr David Dosa, an expert in geriatric care, reported a similar phenomenon with a cat at a nursing home in Rhode Island who correctly predicted imminent deaths; Dr Dosa reported it first in the *New England Journal of Medicine* and later in book form.[19]

If, Dr Hodgkinson told me, the staff thought a patient might be very close to the end, they would consult Straws for a second opinion and would take the lead from her. If the cat wasn't there, the patient was not as close to death as the staff thought. Often, after that initial staff–cat consultation, Straws would go to that patient the following day, correctly judging it was *now* that they were in their last hours.

Straws had the right personality for the work. She was 'a companionable and self-effacing cat, not demanding attention', but was 'a quiet presence', says Dr Hodgkinson. 'She was not invasive, she would curl up at the bottom of the bed and just be there.' *Comfort* is a word Dr Hodgkinson returns to: 'Her presence gave comfort to many families. We would always ask whether the family wanted her there, and they usually did. Her being there meant that for someone dying it was a much quieter, comforting and secure environment where you would feel at peace.' Straws stayed at the hospital until her own death aged about fourteen.

'In hospital, people don't get a lot of touching,' says Dr Hodgkinson. A cat can offer that. Also, her quiet companionship made the situation 'less clinical and reduced the formality'. With an animal body tucked up next to our animal body, there is a gentle reassurance that in spite of the clinical setting, death is as natural as the setting sun and the ebbing tide and we are conducted by an animal walking the mythic path of the psychopomp, leading us to a healing-dying where all is, finally, well.

In a hospital in Calais, Dr Peyo comforts terminally ill cancer patients and has supported more than a thousand people in their last moments. He is a beautiful chestnut horse who works with his handler, Hassen Bouchakour, who says that Peyo demonstrated his vocation, a calling of care, when they did dressage shows. When the shows were over, the horse would pay attention to the people in the crowd, observing specific individuals and staying near them. It transpired that each time, the person the horse picked out had some sickness, either mental or physical. 'When he decides, I cannot hold him back, it's a need, it's visceral, it is in him, he needs to go and cling on to the specific person he has chosen,' says Bouchakour.[20]

The hospital staff nicknamed him 'Dr' Peyo when they saw that his presence brought their terminally ill cancer patients joy and peace. In some cases, due to his influence, the pain the patients suffer from is so significantly reduced they no longer need strong drugs. One patient, Roger, is sixty-four and refers to Peyo as his 'favourite doctor', and his wife notes that Roger sleeps well the night after seeing the horse. Daniel, sixty-seven, was a former equestrian himself, and Peyo visited him when he was diagnosed with terminal cancer. His son remarks: 'As soon as we speak to Dad about Peyo, he cries, he has stars in his eyes.' With Peyo, says his handler, 'we try to recreate life at the end of life.' When Daniel died, at his family's request Peyo accompanied the coffin at the funeral.

Life. Stars. Sweet sleep. There is something Elysian about this. Something as utterly unexpected as a paradise meadow with cowslips, ragged robin, buttercups and clover in a sterile hospital in the middle of Calais. Death is now lit not with the bright white lights of the operating theatre but with the glow of a beeswax candle. The animals seem to guide people towards a dying that is as easy as a breath, the softest breeze that shifts the lightest curtain.

One thing about Peyo puzzles the veterinary scientists who have studied him. Sometimes when a patient is dying he seems to move into the role of a guard, barring others from entering the room. Strangely, another animal has been reported behaving in exactly the same way.

A parrot.

Joanna Burger is a behavioural ecologist and owner of an Amazon parrot called Tiko. Burger's mother-in-law moved in with her family in the final year of her life, and in the woman's last few weeks Tiko became highly protective of her, preventing the visiting hospice staff from touching the woman and even attacking them, until he had to be moved out of her room when they visited. In the last week of her life, Tiko sat by her head, guarding her. On the night she died, when her body was removed Tiko began screaming and screaming. He had never before, said Burger, made so much as a peep at night.[21]

Dogs may know that someone is dying – for the Koyukon people of Alaska, dogs were considered to have a sixth sense for illness, able to tell when someone is close to death and alerting people by barking breathily[22] – and people may long for the comfort of dogs as they pass. On her deathbed, Queen Victoria, grey-voiced and weak, asked that Turi, her beloved Pomeranian pet dog, be brought to her. Queen Elizabeth's two corgis were with her when she died. Frederick the Great of Prussia requested he be laid to rest in a grave where his beloved greyhounds had been buried.

'I *need* to see a dog. I *need* a wagging tail.' This was Michelle Rivera's mother's dying imperative. In her book *On Dogs and Dying*, Rivera describes how the family acquired a puppy who 'helped to send my mother off, not in an anxiety-ridden and tragic environment, but in an atmosphere of peace'.[23] Another woman, Maria, had been very upset when visiting her dying mother, but began stroking a therapy dog in the hospice and commented to Rivera: 'I wonder why I was so scared before?' This, says Rivera, is why dogs come to the hospice: 'to take away the fear'.[24]

Animals may be a hospice for the heart, care-giving right at the hour of death. Celeste Goschen runs a farm in Suffolk with alpacas who provide a healing service for guests. When she knew she was dying, one woman, Vanessa, spent much of her time sitting with the alpacas because they made her feel less frightened. Close to death, Vanessa had a living funeral to which animals were invited: two alpacas, two guinea pigs and a rabbit. Celeste comments: 'In this poky clinical space, a remarkable metamorphosis happened: all ordinary boundaries disappeared, the ordinary transcended into the extraordinary.'

A hospital is at war with death. Weapons of medicine are loaded with ammunition to fight death as the ultimate foe; monitors are like radars picking up the encroachment of enemy activity. Animals may be wiser doctors in the art of dying, guarding the wards and corridors of the spirit, quelling fear and offering peace.

Animals, so much closer to a natural state, may reconcile us to death as part of nature's processes. The dying so often want to die 'at home' and animals remind us that perhaps we'd be most consoled if we truly died at home, in the profound home that is the natural world of flowers, insects and birds. I know I could die more easily out on the earth, hearing the birds, while I would rage against an indoors death. At death, animals may be quiet witnesses to a peace accord, helping us to make a truce with death's beautiful truth, that we rejoin the great caravanserai of Everything, a dissolution of the mono-stories into the one, great and universal story, and that in burial we are carried by the insect recyclers, the myriad tiny pall-bearers.

~

In Oklahoma on 15 July 2014, with the temperature at 100 degrees, a homeless man died. His dog, a bull terrier, had no food or water and the extreme heat affected him badly, but when animal welfare officers tried to take the dog away he kept pulling back towards his owner's dead body. When he was finally removed to a shelter, the dog showed all the signs of acute grief: he wouldn't eat or sleep and would barely even lift his head. This is what heartbreak looks like.

There are many examples of dogs refusing to leave their dead human companions. Joseph Tagg was born in north Derbyshire, England, in 1868. He became a shepherd and a famous sheepdog breeder, a founder member of the annual sheepdog trials. He lived his later years with his niece and his dog Tip, and became known as Old Joe, shepherd and gentleman. On Saturday, 12 December 1953, aged eighty-five, Old Joe took Tip, aged eleven, to tend sheep in the Upper Derwent Valley.

They didn't come back.

Search parties, including other shepherds, gamekeepers, ramblers and an RAF mountain rescue team, went looking for the old man and his dog but found no trace. Days passed, then weeks. That winter was one of the harshest ever known, with deep snowfalls. On Saturday, 27 March 1954, two men were rounding up sheep and saw Old Joe's dead body with – they thought – a shaggy old coat nearby. It was Tip. She was alive, if only just. Emaciated and dazed, after standing vigil for a hundred and five days and nights, she had felt that dogged need to stay with her owner. The shepherds tried to draw her away but she was unwilling to leave Old Joe and eventually had to be carried away in their arms.[25]

Tip wasn't lost. She knew the territory and also knew people she could have gone to. But she remained. Why a dog might stay with the dead body of their human is unknowable. Perhaps an instinct was struck on the anvil of grief, the fierce desire to protect and to guard unto death and then beyond it. Perhaps it is the devastated howl of a broken-hearted dog or perhaps it is a loyalty that refuses to let their human be alone in facing death.

In Japan, a puppy born in 1923 and named Hachikō was adopted by Eisaburo Enyo, a university professor. Every morning, the professor would catch a train to work, always at the same time, and would be on the train home in the evening, again at the same time each day. The dog would go with him in the morning, see the man off at the station and return home. In the evening, the dog, skilled as many are at timekeeping, would trot off to the station to meet his friend. In 1925, though, Mr Enyo caught the morning train but never returned – he had died quite suddenly at his office. Hachikō went to meet him as usual, waiting and waiting. For ten years the dog would go every evening to the station, at the same time, to wait for the man he loved, until he too died, in 1935.[26]

Greyfriars Bobby is a famous dog of devotion, the little Skye terrier who lived and patrolled alongside a nightwatchman, John Gray, in Edinburgh in the mid nineteenth century. The story goes that when John Gray died in February 1858 and was buried in Greyfriars Kirkyard, the dog then refused to leave his master's grave for fourteen years, until his own death. But it seems that there were two Bobbys, the first happily hunting rats in the kirkyard and fed by locals because visitors would tip them generously to retell his sweet story. When Bobby the First died, the locals wanted to keep visitor numbers up, so the dog was replaced with a near-identical Bobby the Second. The council knew of it, but kept quiet, as did the kirk.[27]

Whatever the facts, this story speaks of the human need to believe in dogs demonstrating heroic devotion, entire and forever. That is a soul-medicine of profound consolation, telling us that there is one thing stronger than death, and it is love.

~

There is a widespread perception that the dead may return in the form of animals. The Indigenous Australian Wurundjeri people traditionally believed that the spirits of their dead would become dolphins, and imagining that the beloved may become that core charisma of the oceans seems comfort enough, but there's more: these dolphins would, from their ocean home, help and guide family members on the land,[28] a belief that would have sustained and strengthened the living.

Some of the reincarnations surprise me: for the Evenki people, spiders may be the spirits of the ancestors; and among the Kaingang people of southern Brazil, mosquitoes or ants may be spirits of the dead.[29] Some are less surprising: there is a near-universal belief that the dead become winged creatures, suggesting the necessary flight through death. Although gulls are not birds with much of a spiritual association, in the West Highlands of Scotland, according to traditional belief, the dead may become seagulls. King Arthur is said to have become a fire crow after death. For the Bororo people of Brazil, when a person dies their spirit enters a new, living body, the best of which, they say, would be a red macaw. The Aztecs believed that the souls of the dead might return as hummingbirds.[30]

In a tender memory, a Canadian Mi'kmaq woman called White Wolf spoke of her mother's funeral. A small bird flitted to the headstone as the minister was speaking, cocked its head and appeared to listen. As the coffin was lowered into the grave, the bird watched and then, at the end of the funeral, chirped and flew off. For White Wolf, it was her mother's spirit who entered the bird and was bidding them goodbye.[31]

For the bereaved, there can be profound consolation in feeling they have had a glimpse of their beloved in the quick of life just in a different form. This is how Liz Jensen saw her son Raphaël, aka Iggy Fox, an environmental activist who died entirely unexpectedly at the age of twenty-five. He often appears to her in the form of birds, which is a comfort and, sometimes, a joke. In her profoundly moving memoir of her son, *Your Wild and Precious Life*, she writes:

> A bird theme is emerging in Raphaël's visits. First the dancing red-tailed bird, my daily visits from the brown pigeon, and now – the day after I asked for a sign – the musvit [a great tit]. It's as if Raphaël knows what I need, and he's doing what he can. Many cultures believe that birds are spiritual beings, capable of acting as messengers between the living and the dead. Perhaps they are right to. For the next few days, I feel a lightness round me.[32]

In an email, she tells me more: 'The more-than-human world has always been a natural messaging service, sending and receiving signals in a million ways, every micro-second.' The messages come to her like a 'familiar epiphany', giving her a 'feeling of delight and grace. To call it healing is an understatement.' She has often seen Raphaël in the form of a bird 'getting unnaturally close and giving out sudden, very loud and persistent squawks. It's hilarious, and there's no mistaking it. It always makes me laugh.'[33]

These appearances offer her a defence against death's finality, 'of life not dissolving into nothingness but transmuting into another form'.[34] She finds a liberation in it. As she writes in her memoir, 'There's a melancholy sweetness in knowing that he can go anywhere and be anything he wants to. He can be a gingko leaf, a stingray, a bat, a tiger, a spider, a sea-turtle, a viper, a jellyfish, a droplet of water in a cloud, a bed of moss, a bacteria, an elephant, a dragonfly.'[35]

Her son was profoundly sensitive to the world of animals and committed to their protection, and Jensen has dedicated herself newly to all that he knew to be precious beyond price. She tells me that for her the animals, seeming to appear for her son, are also a prompt: 'It's a radicalizing, energizing understanding that reminds me daily of the duty I have – the duty we *all* have – to protect the life that in turn protects us.'[36]

~

As I was writing this book, I was doing some gardening one day and I could see from the corner of my eye that I had something in my hair. A fallen leaf, I imagined, and swept my hand to my head without thinking. What fell out were two scarlet tiger moths mating, glued together in a devotion so bonded that even the fall did not uncouple them. I gasped.

The moths have scarlet hindwings with black dots, hidden under black forewings with white and yellow polka dots, and the petticoats can be glimpsed under the overskirts. The full silk skirt, swept sideways, unveils a flourish of colour. They are luxuriously, sumptuously, recklessly beautiful. 'Do I deserve this?' I found myself thinking. How can anyone ever earn this cascade of colours, these wings on wings that put a shimmer in my psyche. Even motionless, they were a flamenco in my hair. It hallowed everything, the garden and the day.

For many cultures, the symbol of the soul is the butterfly. At the ancient settlement of Çatalhöyük in southern Turkey, which flourished around 7000 BCE, there are frescoes that depict a butterfly coming to bright life from the darkness of its chrysalis shroud, a phenomenon that has comforted the human imagination across the world. The ancient Greek goddess Psyche, meaning 'soul', finds her form in the butterfly, and Celtic mythology too sees the butterfly as the symbol of the soul. Butterflies were the emblem for the 1.5 million children who were murdered in the Holocaust, and at the Majdanek concentration camp in

Poland, hundreds of butterflies were drawn and scratched on the walls, symbols of the soul breaking free, demonstrating life after death, as butterflies transmute through the stages of dying and being reborn in flutterby alchemy.

We do, of course, shapeshift into others after death, as our buried bodies or scattered ashes rejoin life's continuance. Obliquely and unknowably, our light is scattered but not extinguished. We are dispersed, diffuse, in the most intimate mediation of the soil where death itself shapeshifts into life. But it is the *animals* we yearn to become, not dust or bacteria. We want to recast the souls of our dead as bees or turn a death into a dolphin or redshank, that shorebird on the edge of land and sea. We seek to transform a bereavement into a butterfly, who has already undergone a death and knows that we may be dying into beauty.

In Mexico, an Indigenous leader once told me the butterfly was the 'soul of nature', but now the butterflies are losing their colours, according to Brazilian photojournalist Lilo Clareto, who spoke just before his death of how butterflies in the Amazon are turning grey, in a devastated mimicry of the incinerated forests. The butterfly, soul of nature, is revealing the true colours of this age, a grave warning to the soul of humanity, because the colour of world-sickness is grey: grey like the bleached coral and the burnt forests and now, ashen-winged, grey like the butterflies.[37]

Black Elk, medicine man of the Oglala Lakota, was given the ability to understand butterflies in a vision of grief, as a cloud of butterflies of all colours filled his sight so he could see nothing else. A spotted eagle spoke to him, saying, 'Behold these! They are your people. They are in great difficulty and you shall help them.' The butterflies were 'all making a pitiful, whimpering noise as though they too were weeping'.[38] What grief would attend him now if he could see those beautiful butterflies of all colours fading to grey and if he could hear the one sound worse than the whimper of butterflies: their silence, as their voices, together with their colours, dim and fade and are gone.

And with them, finally, we will know Absolute Death.

PART THREE

How Animals Heal the Body Politic

This section explores the concept of health further by considering what makes societies healthy. Harmony has long been deemed necessary to well-being, in a figurative way and also literally, and we will look at how the music, song and sounds of the animal world are healing. Societies need a strong sense of ethics in order to be healthy, and there is a good argument for saying that we humans learned our ethics from wolves. Justice and fairness make human societies healthy, and some animals have a lot to teach us in this regard. They can also demonstrate a sense of politics that is necessary for social health.

PART THREE

How Animals Feed the Body Feline

9

Key Signatures for a Sound World

'I am the concert from the mouth of every creature singing with the myriad chorus' – Hafiz

A tiny, furry, holy thing is cupped in my palm. It tickles me with its delicate feet while its mind is awash with the entire Northern Lights.

On this the world rests.

The biomass on Earth, the weight of all life, is about 550 billion tonnes and much of it is brought into being and kept alive directly or indirectly by the bee, who has lifted away from my hand and is now hovering by a laburnum blossom's purchase of gold.

This fragile Atlas. On his shoulders, legs, breeches and pouches, everything we humans value depends, this bumblebee that weighs only a little bit more than the petal he has now landed on. The world is bee-borne.

It is the sweetest – honeyest – paradox on Earth that such power may be almost weightless, and that this utterly necessary creature is so little. So much goodness in something the size of a thumbnail, tender and diligent in all his hours in service to the All.

Bees have been declared the most important living beings on the planet. Honeybees are the world's most significant species of pollinator – and a third of the world's food production and 90 per cent of its wild flora depend on pollinators.[1]

The bees wrap up almost all life on Earth and tuck it into their pockets for safekeeping. They are a synaesthesia of warm, well life, and they sound like they look and they look like they feel in the buzz of their fur while their baggy pollen pouches are as sweet as honey tastes. Honeybees sleep up to eight hours a day, sometimes in flowers. They like to sleep with other bees, sometimes holding each other's feet.[2]

So vital are they for human health that we can say without the bee, the most precious ordinary, we wouldn't be. In Islamic belief, the fate of bees and humans is inseparable: we die as they die. The Albanian language has two verbs for dying. One, *ngordh*, is used when any animal dies but another verb, *vdes*, is used only for the death of a human being or a bee, so close is the association between the sweet bee and human life. In Bosnian-Serbian-Croatian, similarly, the bees 'die' like humans, with the word *umiru* applying to both bee and us, while other animals and insects 'perish', *uginu, crknu*,[3] as if language itself knows their flourishing and ours are inextricably intertwined.

In Mayan tradition, god is a bee, working across all dimensions, shifting energy from flower to honey via the elusive metaphysics of the hive. The flowers need the bees and the bees need the flowers, who offer them their intricate scent-lines on the breeze. The European honeybee is *Apis mellifera*, the 'bringer of sweetness'. A bee lives for an average of forty days and forty nights and one worker bee's life makes less than one teaspoon of honey. Like tiny deities, they can see what is invisible to us, knowing the world in ultraviolet as if while we see a cloudy evening sky, they can see the Northern Lights in the flowers. The bodies of bees have a positive electric charge while the flowers have a slightly negative one. As a result of this miniature electrical effect, the pollen jumps up to meet the bee even while it is still in flight.

If you want to really see the colours of flowers, be a bee. In their eyes, colours come psychedelic, like a rainbow intersecting with a diamond. The eyes of bees and other insects have trichromacy, a three-coloured gift of green, blue and ultraviolet, and this trichromacy evolved in insects hundreds of millions of years before the first flowers, so the ability to see came before the object of their vision.

Being able to see the flowers' special effects, the bees and others selected and pollinated certain flowers, and because the bees chose for nectar and pollen, those flowers lived. In effect, the bees were creative artists — radiant impressionists — and the miraculous was there in the eye of the creator bee. It is as if the bees' eyes were lonely in a less lustrous world and, by being there, by existing and being willing, they invited the flowers into existence, conjuring the colours into being, as the potential of the flower existed first deep in the sight-mind of the bee; and then the flowers, when they knew they would be seen, arrived with their petals of vermilion and coral and gold. (There is a psychological analogy here, for when we feel someone cannot 'see' or acknowledge us, we feel diminished, but when someone sees us, we bloom for them and flourish in their eyes.)

Human society would last barely a handful of years without bees, our health dependent on theirs. The artist Amy Shelton, whose mother had such a poignant and profound feeling for the bees as she died, has created a project illustrating the connectedness of bee health, human health and environment. She calls her project 'Honeyscribe' because in ancient Egypt honey scribes recorded the productivity of the hives. The bees themselves could be said to be scribes, writing in their hives with the honey of their lives, documenting the health of their near worlds. In *Melissographia*, the poet John Burnside has written poems to accompany Shelton's pollen maps, and in sweet, gold words, Burnside sings up the bees, as the hive is literally home for them and metaphorically home for us as a healing place, heard in the bees whose hum, Burnside writes, could have been mistaken for love. An ancient Egyptian marriage vow included a promise to give the bride twelve jars of honey every year: honey the symbol of love at home.

And yet we swap their honey for poison and the bees must now inscribe insecticides, play clerk to chemical pollution and be secretaries to the state of extreme weather events. Colony collapse disorder is widely thought to be a result of neonicotinoids, which damage the neurological functions of bees, and one result is that they cannot find their way home to the hive. That bees — of all — cannot find their way home is heartbreaking when — of all — their humming home is the sound of a sound world.

~

There are bees in the bluebells in my garden now, each bell ringing its assent as the bee gently makes touchdown. It is May and after a cold, wet spring, the sunshine is warm honey pouring through the days and the flowers are flourishing, everything blooming at once: apple blossom, wisteria, wild garlic, lobelia, forget-me-nots, buttercups and irises. The garden has remembered its summersong, and the laburnum is purring with bees.

The words *heal*, *health* and *whole* are all derived from the Old English *hal*, meaning 'whole' or 'sound' in the sense of 'well'. To be healthy is also to be part of the whole: health is not a solo state of wellness for one but is inextricably linked to the health of all. When William Blake wrote his piercing truth 'For every thing that lives is holy,' the key words are *every thing*. The word *holy* is also etymologically related to 'heal' and 'whole', and in order that all shall be well, the bee must be well, this holy thing. Every part of livingkind is implicate with and dependent on the health of other species and the wider environment, co-flourishing.

For the Ojibwe, health is centred on connection and integration, founded on relationships with the animals.[4] In the Ojibwe language there is a profound term, *mino-bimaadiziwin*, that conveys a healthy way of being in the world, living life fully and free from illness, while it can also mean 'a good life' or 'the right way to live'. It is impossible to achieve without the animals, who are crucial to human health and considered as therapeutic allies.

Seeing human health as intrinsically related to the health of animals is a widespread concept in Indigenous cultures. Medicine is not a specific category, something kept separate in a medicine cabinet, but is everywhere around us. Chickasaw author Linda Hogan defines *susto* as a sickness of the soul caused by disconnection from nature, and the cure for this sickness is the healing power of the whole of the natural world, from rivers to forests and animals. For one living being to be healthy, everything it depends on must be healthy and the string that ties them together must be well woven and strong.

Mitakuye oyasin is the Lakota phrase meaning 'all my relations' embedded in a philosophy that finds it inconceivable to limit kinship and relatedness to solely human family. To come to a diagnosis, a practitioner in conventional Western medicine might ask about the health of close family members, perhaps checking if there is a history of diabetes or heart disease, while a practitioner of Native American healing would include the environment, asking for example, 'Are the salmon in your rivers ill?'[5] Because how can your right hand be well if your organs are failing? How can the worms be well if the soil is not?

'From the Native American perspective, medicine belongs more to the realm of healing than curing. These two concepts are not identical,' writes Kenneth Cohen in his decades-long study of Native American healing. 'Physicians aim to cure disease, to vanquish it, to make it go away. Traditional indigenous healers emphasize healing, in the sense of "making whole" by establishing, enhancing, or restoring well-being and harmony . . . Native American healing emphasizes harmony with the Earth as an essential ingredient in personal health.'[6]

For the !Kung of the Kalahari, the distinction is the same, so healing is, in the words of anthropologist Richard Katz, 'more than curing, more than the application of medicine. Healing seeks to establish health and growth on physical, psychological, social, and spiritual levels; it involves work on the individual, the group, and the surrounding environment and cosmos.'[7] One cannot be whole if the whole is not healed.

Philosophy here is like honeysuckle with the nectar of health at its heart.

~

The founding constitution of the World Health Organization (WHO) gave its definition of health as 'a state of complete physical, mental and social well-being and not merely the absence of disease and infirmity'. Recently the WHO has gone further, adding its voice to supporting 'One Health' – a concept initiated in Africa which argues that human health *is* animal health and neither we nor they can be healthy except in flourishing ecologies from oceans to mountains to forests.

A clear example of the principle of One Health is the danger of zoonotic diseases (ones that can be transmitted from animals to humans), including bird flu, SARS, Ebola and Covid, which all demonstrate how the health of animals is inextricably linked to the health of humans. Worldwide, nearly 75 per cent of all emerging human infectious diseases in the past thirty years originated in animals.[8] Zoonotic diseases result from increasing human encroachment into animal habitats and depredations for the wildlife trade. Our health as a species depends on the flourishing health of all the animals, and their losses are ours: their diminishment is our dimming as their sicknesses become our own.

If disease can be contagious, wellness too can be catching and health is a transmissible state. The hilum between pea and pod is a tiny livewire, a filament of thriving, and health sings through it as it sings through the birds, calls through the whales, connecting us all.

The definition of that Ojibwe term *mino-bimaadiziwin* includes 'a life of harmony'. In traditional Navajo culture, medicine men are the 'Singers', illustrating how healing means restoring harmony to the individual and to society. Being well includes maintaining good relationships, so for each being there is a proper way of living in harmony with everything. Human suffering and disease show disharmony, where someone has fallen out of harmony with the world.[9]

Paracelsus (1493–1541), a Swiss physician whose philosophy aligned with that of Indigenous cultures, argued that for an individual to be healthy, they must be in harmony with their environment because the human was a microcosm of macrocosmic nature. Nature, to him, was 'the One Life', a living organism brimful of healing power; the universe in its entirety (including humans) was 'God' and divinely healing. In this intricate and infinite harmony, none of us is a dislocated, separate note, a metallic click of one, but a soft tone in the hum of the hive.

The Qur'an speaks of six revelations given by Allah to creation, in which the first revelation is to the prophets, the second to the Earth, the third to the sky and the fourth to the honeybee: 'And thy Lord has inspired the bee.' This revelation is a sign, says the Qur'an, 'for those who give thought', teaching people to care for communities and to embody the traits of bees.

In the mountains of north-eastern Bosnia, something subtle,

beautiful and wise is happening. In a project titled *Beekeeping in the End Times*, two sisters, anthropologist Larisa Jašarević and her sister Azra, a film-maker, care for bees, recording how the health of the hives is chiming with wider ecological health and how the bees metaphysically rhyme with Sufi lore of the 'End Times'.

In the local Muslim ecology, says Larisa Jašarević, 'there is no world without bees.' Bees act as the conscience of a locality as they are the first to notice and report negative changes. They are affected by all that goes on, and need the best and most ecologically wise decisions in land management, or indeed simply wildness. Bees are considered 'divinely inspired', and their hive products cannot be reproduced in any laboratory.[10]

In Christian tradition, many monks were beekeepers and held bees in high regard for their ethical qualities, working hard for the good of all. There is a mosque in Indonesia known as the Sarang Lebah (Honeycomb) or An-Nahl (Bee) Mosque, because the architecture is based on the hexagonal designs of honeycomb, and the mosque promotes the healthy and harmonious idea of life lived in service, where no bee exists alone. A ḥadith attributed to the Prophet of Islam says: 'Your remedies are two, honey and the Qur'an.'

~

The sound of bees buzzing makes something in my spirit feel calm, reassured and also gently tingly. I felt that it was a healing sound before I learned its factual truth. Bees buzz from about 10 to 1,000 hertz (Hz) and these sound frequencies resonate with organic tissues that promote healing in humans: the sound stimulates the cerebrospinal fluid in our brain and spine, causing it to resonate and aiding the immune system, circulating nutrients and filtering the blood. The bees' sound frequencies also affect our pineal and pituitary glands, the hypothalamus and the amygdala.[11]

The ancient Egyptian physician Imhotep is most likely the first person to have discovered cerebrospinal fluid, around 3000 BCE,[12] and whether or not the ancient Egyptians intuited the healing of the bees, they had a tradition of 'Bee Teachings' in which the humming of bees was understood to stimulate the release of the Elixirs of Metamorphosis, an exquisite phrase for conjuring the soft thrill of good vibrations in the buzzing of bees.

My garden is incomplete if it is silent. It needs bees in order to flower aurally, with that sweet susurrus sounding the blossom in its blessing-song, humming all is well and all shall be well. The bee is a sweet alchemist, turning pollen into honey and hertz into healing.

In Slovenia, a country rich with beehives, there is a tradition of using the sound of bees for healing, involving people lying down in a room with thousands of bees. Firefighters and others with stressful jobs use this as a technique for relaxation and recuperation after traumatic call-outs, noting that the sound and also the smell of the bees – beeswax, earth and honey – is healing. One firefighter comments that he recorded the sound of the bees and, if he has difficulty sleeping, he will 'turn on the bees and float away'.

Many schools in Slovenia have beehives on the premises and at least one primary school holds meetings at the hives, where a psychologist, teachers and parents will gather for a perhaps difficult conversation eased by bees. In those schools, it is common for pupils who are restless and upset to be sent to the bees to be cared for, and the child lies in a net like a large hammock near the hive and the presence of the bees calms the child. The well-being of an individual is linked, in a web of healing, to the co-flourishing of everything in the compass of bees.[13]

The humming of bees is the sound closest to the human *ẓikr*, or invocation, a Sufi tells Larisa Jašarević.[14] Another beekeeper in Slovenia follows the example of her grandmother (and indeed many other grandmothers) in making a bed near the bees where people can rest in the day or sleep at night, describing their buzzing in a tone of glad amazement: 'It's as if I'm lying underneath a waterfall.' A Ukrainian friend of mine tells me that in Ukraine, people sleep above beehives to feel well.

As Indigenous cultures know, health means harmony, which is usually understood as a metaphor but is also literal because the music and song of animals is healing. Whale song has been used for decades to help humans relax and meditate and sleep, as birdsong, insect song and frog song have for longer. A sound world heals: it makes us sound.

If I wake with my cat in bed with me and if it is very early and if my throat is not yet attuned to the human day and if I linger in those misty moments between sleeping and waking, then I may wake to the sound of two purrs. One his. One mine. Cats' purring is regular and rhythmic, their breath, body and spirit so beautifully aligned that we can align with it. Try it. (But don't try too hard: it depends on being exquisitely relaxed.)

The sound of a cat's purr is thought to be healing for humans as well as for cats themselves. Domestic cats typically purr within the range of 20 to 27 Hz but can reach 150 Hz. When treated with frequencies of around 20 to 50 Hz, bone strength can be improved by up to 20 per cent, the bones hardening in response to the pressure, suggesting that the cat's purr could help osteoporosis. The purr-frequencies of cats correspond to vibrational frequencies used to treat oedema, muscle strain, joint flexibility, shortness of breath and wounds. Healing in tendons and ligaments can be treated with higher frequencies, closer to 120 Hz. The range of a cat's purr is known to relieve both chronic and acute pain. Further, a cat vibrates when it purrs, vibrating you if the cat is in contact with you, and vibrational stimulation improves circulation and oxygenation.[15] Old women with their cats on their laps maybe intuit healing properties, unconsciously treating osteoporosis and providing themselves with the furriest and warmest kind of pain management.

Tony Bassett, a sound engineer, has suggested that dolphins may pulse frequencies of around 6 Hz that attune human brainwaves to a theta state and arguably, in this meditative state, bodily healing can take place.[16] Bassett has found that frequencies in the region of 2,000 Hz appear to trigger the production of endorphins in humans, with healing consequences, and dolphins do emit sound in this range, which could be why humans who spend time with dolphins report such powerful healing responses, to the point of euphoria.

Some months ago, David Rothenberg, in his pursuit of animal music, made a recording of insects in a pond and sent it over to me. Listening to this underwater insect chorus with a variety of species crackling, ticking and chirping flooded me with a sense of wellness. It sounds full to the brim, both complete and diverse like a perfect gathering. Beneath the surface of the pond, the insects are an orchestra in an accord of sounds in neat tucked tidiness, intimate and close. It has the same effect on me as ASMR, the autonomous sensory meridian response, where certain sounds make you feel both thrilled and soothed, ecstatic and serene at the same time.

I can't help resonating with insects: they give me good vibrations and I'm not alone. Amazonian people say the song of the insects, humming and buzzing, makes a strong impact on people and is associated with powerful transformation and the fertility of nature.[17] When the Lakota chief Lame Deer described the perfect soundscape for a holy man, he noted the preference for a place with 'no sound but the humming of insects'.[18] Composer David Dunn spent years listening to pond life, writing that 'these sounds are an emergent property of the pond: something that speaks as a collective voice for a mind that is beyond my grasp . . . Now when I see a pond, I think of the water's surface as a membrane enclosing something deep in thought.'[19]

In 2014, there was a competition to find the 'most beautiful sound in the world'. The winner was 'Dusk by the Frog Pond', recorded in Borneo by Marc Anderson. Listening to it, intense waves of sound pour over me, with cicadas, other insects and frogs pulsing their music, as if taking turns to come to the sonic stage, a jazz extemporized by different species at different pitches.

In evolutionary terms, of course, the animal musicians were there before us, squeaking, whistling, singing, calling, carolling, hooting, howling, drumming, lowing and humming. Each is swept up, entranced, into the whole, and we are made whole in the healing wellness of all. The sound of animals creates a sonic diversity as if the very air is a net, a hammock of wild melodies that we can rest in, like a child given to the care of the bees.

Birdsong is the quintessential healing sound of nature. In myth, the Irish goddess Clíodhna cared for three magic birds with songs so sweet they cured every illness. In Welsh myth, the birds of Rhiannon sang so exquisitely that their music banished sadness and, listening to them, eighty years would slip by as if it were a day, and there was no memory of sorrow. In beech woods in southern England recently I was sitting by a campfire with Benny Wenda, West Papua's leader in exile, as he told me about birdsong in his land. 'Traditionally,' he says, 'if you're upset about something, people would go to the forest and listen to the Bird of Paradise. Its song makes you happy.' He smiles wistfully as he speaks, half hearing the bird of his youth.

For Ojibwe people, birdsong enlivens the air, as one Elder remarks: 'The songs are alive, more alive than us.'[20] Owl hoots, for the Ojibwe, can give comfort in distress, reassuring and transforming people.[21] There was a poignant collective love for birdsong in the early days of the Covid pandemic in spring 2020, when the soaring liveliness of their music lifted people's spirits. Birds embody the very quick of things, the life force, and their song is the very quick of music, the poignant nerves of sound running swift through the nerves of the body until the soul is touched.

In Berlin in times gone by, people said, if someone was sick or near to death they would ask to be carried out into the streets at night to hear a nightingale sing for them.[22] Berlin, today, is the capital city of nightingales, home to more of the birds than almost any other European city. The nightingale sings in the dark and makes the spirit radiant, and the word *nightingale* means 'night-singer', for *gale* is from the Old English *galan*, 'to sing', related to words for spell or enchantment.

When Hans Christian Andersen wanted to write of the healing power of animals, he chose the medicine of the nightingale's song. In his story, an emperor of China was suffering from many kinds of sickness, including the moral sickness of being preoccupied with riches and prestige, becoming so obsessed with his porcelain palace and fawning court that he had not realized that the finest treasure of his empire was a little brown bird in the woods. The nightingale healed him with its medicine containing the active ingredients of birdsong: truth, gratitude and tears.

In the words of the Prague-born poet Rainer Maria Rilke, 'A birdsong can even, for a moment, make the whole world into a sky within us, because we feel that the bird does not distinguish between its heart and the world's.' What poets have intuited, studies have demonstrated. Researchers from King's College London have shown that seeing or hearing birds improves mental well-being and helps to lift depression, and the healing effect lasts beyond the time that people actually spend with the birds.[23] Another study shows that hearing birdsong improves people's mental well-being for up to eight hours.[24] Areas with a lower bird diversity have more hospitalizations for mental health crises than areas with a higher bird diversity and, says the lead author, the study also suggests that declining biodiversity may be intricately connected with anxiety.[25]

Having a diversity of species around us is richly medicinal as humans feel well and whole when we see, and hear sounds from, a wide variety of animals, birds and insects,[26] the full harmonies of the living world which Henry David Thoreau called in *On Walden Pond* 'a vibration of the universal lyre'.

For the French composer and ornithologist Olivier Messiaen (1908–92), birds were soul-healers. The meadowlark is 'alleluia-like' while the wood thrush's song is 'full of sunlight, almost sacramental'. He was no stranger to sadness, writing, 'In my hours of gloom, when I am suddenly aware of my own futility . . . what is left for me but to seek out the true, lost face of music somewhere off in the forest, in the fields, in the mountains or on the seashore, among the birds.'[27]

The premiere of Messiaen's 'Quartet for the End of Time', a bird-sung work with the violin like a nightingale and the clarinet singing like a blackbird, took place on 15 January 1941. It was during the dark days of the Second World War, and it was cold – so cold that some of the piano keys became stuck: soundless, these notes were missing from the full keyboard. The musicians were shivering with cold and the cello had lost a string. It was Silesia, Stalag VIIIA, a German prisoner-of-war camp where Messiaen, a prisoner, was playing with his fellow inmates on the only four types of instrument in the camp. Against the hideous ground bass of this ugly, cruel war and in conditions of internment, Messiaen set the freedom and beauty of the birds, and the healing of their song, writing: 'The birds are the opposite of time. They represent our longing for light, for stars, for rainbows, and for jubilant song.'[28]

Between 1967 and 2007, the number of nightingales in the UK fell by 91 per cent. Insecticides can cause the shells of songbirds' eggs to thin and crack in their nests, killing the chicks and killing the music. In extinctions there is silence. One by one, a note from the piano keyboard is lost. The piano keys, as in Messiaen's premiere of 'Quartet for the End of Time', stuck, one by one, frozen in death, and an entire songline ended. Unravel the music. Unhandel it. Take B out of being. Then G. The D, the F sharp too. Music will be very thin now. All the music has missing notes, just dull thuds, gaps, spaces and silences.

~

Who first created music? Who first invented the sounds that make us sound, whole and healed? Insects, says David Rothenberg, were 'the first drummers. For millions of years before humanity, these myriad tiny creatures evolved a world of complex rhythms to further their kind. Human music emerged in forest and veldt, figuring out beats and cries in the midst of a long-standing thrumming insect world.'[29] Frogs, eagles, ravens and lions gave music to the Luiseño people of California, according to their lore, and Tuvan people of Siberia say: 'Our music all began from imitating the sounds of animals.' In early Chinese culture, animal songs and rhythms were said to be the origins of music, while in Christian lore, a dove was said to have dictated plainchant to St Gregory.

For the Suyá people of Mato Grosso, Brazil, music is at the heart of life. Men or women said to be 'without spirits' have a particular gift because although (or perhaps because) they have lost their spirits, they can hear songs from animals, plants and insects. They listen to the music of the forest, the 'true music' that is sung by the animals, and they teach it to others.[30]

The chorus of the Earth is within us all, and we are as much part of it as the blackbird who is, right now, singing for sheer glory at the top of the laburnum, a black note in the bright yellow against the blue, blue sky. We are all makers of the music of this sphere, and the world is a turning song, always and forever playing, and joy rises through us all as air is translated into song.

Bernie Krause is a musician and soundscape ecologist. The sound of animals has been personally healing for him, as he used to suffer the effects of undiagnosed ADHD and anxiety dominated his life. But then, one moment in a forest in Northern California, he experienced for the first time the power of forest sounds, which brought him, he says, 'an overwhelming sense of relief both physically and emotionally. It was a safe remedy I would rely on for the rest of my life.'[31]

For decades, Krause recorded natural sounds, concentrating not so much on an individual creature's performance but on the whole acoustic world of an environment, listening to everything from insects and frogs to birds and mammals. He terms the collective chorus the 'Great Animal Orchestra', where creatures inhabit a sonic niche, a particular place in the soundscape of their precise ecology. Krause was recording in the Masai Mara, Kenya, in the 1980s when he most powerfully heard animals as a myriad of different musicians who yet, collectively, create an entire musical performance.

He had been working hard all that day and, exhausted, had gone to bed. Cocooned in his sleeping bag, he had an epiphany. For the first time, he experienced the sound not as separate voices but rather as 'a cohesive sonic event'. Insects 'set the stage for every other sound', some by continuous whirrs, and some by establishing rhythms. Every bird species would 'mark out its own acoustic turf' while mammals, reptiles and amphibians would fill other niches in the soundscape.[32] What had seemed to him an anarchy of sound now appeared to have a structure. It was, he said, 'a highly orchestrated acoustic arrangement of insects, spotted hyenas, eagle-owls, African wood-owls, elephants, tree hyrax, distant lions, and several knots of tree frogs and toads. Every distant voice seemed to fit within its own acoustic bandwidth – each one so carefully placed that it reminded me of Mozart's elegantly structured Symphony no. 41 in C Major.'[33]

Key Signatures for a Sound World

The world of animal sound is always moving – drifting, ebbing and flowing – but forming an intense and aesthetic concert in various ecologies. At the top, higher than human hearing and far above the top notes of a piano keyboard, are the ultrasonic calls of bats. Down a little are the cicadas and insects. A little further down, the bright screech of the swift. Then, down through the piano's top octaves, the other birds, down to cats, monkeys and human voices. The sloth is said to sing at night, in the musical intervals of a human scale. Bear cubs in the den hum as they suckle, a sing-song swung up and down a scale.[34] Gibbons sing for sunrise in glissando phrases (and in Indonesia their songs are considered so beautiful that Dayak myth says the sun rises in answer).[35] Chimpanzees hoot, in rising and falling cadences, for storms and for dawn. Further down the keyboard is the sea lion's roaring call, and then below the lowest notes of the keyboard is the subsonic humming of giraffes, and the basso profundo of elephants and whales in their infrasonic lowings.

And the bee? The bee is right at the centre of it all. When bees are flower-buzzing, they hum a half-note above middle C, at the core of the keyboard, right where they belong, in the sweet heart of everything. The music of the animals vouchsafes us, leaving us calmed and invigorated at the same time, sung into the eternal present as life is ceaselessly sung into being, sounds swelling, filling, resounding, flourishing and making whole.

~

The Babenzele, also called Ba'Aka or Bayaka or BaYaka (pronounced *bye-jacka*), are a Pygmy people related to the Southern African San Bushmen. They live in the Dzanga-Sangha rainforest in the Central African Republic. The forest shimmers with the music of insects, songbirds, monkeys, gorillas, okapi, elephants, the African golden cat, crocodiles, hippos, antelope, mice, shrews, bats, canaries, pelicans and storks. Beetles buzz, parrots whistle and screech, monkeys scream out, gorillas call and beat rhythmically on their chests.

The Babenzele co-compose music with their forests, with rich harmonies, bright tones and entirely unexpected calls and pitches. It is one of the most beautiful things I've ever heard. It is polyrhythmic, using many rhythms at once, and polyphonous, with different voices singing different melodies at the same time – as indeed does the forest, with different creatures at different times calling louder or more quietly, on shrew rhythm or stork timing, canary song or insect hum. The Babenzele echo the structures of the forest song and its healing sounds, and songs are given to the Babenzele in their dreams, particularly to the women, who, in ceremonies to entice spirits to bless a hunt, sing interwoven webs of sound, created by different threads of different songs from different singers.

Anthropologist Jerome Lewis writes: 'What they are really interested in are synergies: technologies of enchantment, where you lose your sense of self and become aware of a greater community.' Then a sense of both calm and euphoria floods a person, 'a blissful state in which you have forgotten yourself completely and are lost in the beauty of sound'.[36] When I listen to this music it has a particular perfection, as if nothing could be added and nothing subtracted from the wholeness of its sound, as a forest is whole.

In 1984, Louis Sarno, an American musical-anthropologist from New Jersey, heard the Babenzele people's music on a radio programme and it transformed his life, as he described in *Song from the Forest*. Selling everything he had, he bought a one-way ticket to the Central African Republic to find this rhapsody of sound. He never looked back, devoting his life to recording their music, sending collections to the Pitt Rivers Museum in Oxford, among others, and working for decades with Bernie Krause, who, in *The Power of Tranquility in a Very Noisy World*, describes how the healing of the forests assumed particular importance when the Babenzele faced an entirely new crisis.

In the last decades of the twentieth century, the Babenzele suffered a devastating invasion as extractive industries began to encroach on their territory to steal the riches of their forests. Starting from the small towns on the edges, the loggers felled trees, including precious ebony. The fringes of the forest went first. The land was ripped up for diamonds and oil, and elephants were killed for their ivory, for jewellery and trinkets. The vulnerable and precarious way of life of forest people depends on thriving nature, but it was being destroyed, the ebony and ivory stolen, robbing the land of its soul, and all kinds of harmonies that the Babenzele had known were damaged. They couldn't feed their families from the forest any longer, so men from their communities took cash-jobs, hunting bushmeat and elephants, while women were forced into prostitution. The Babenzele people were in an emotional and physical crisis; many became seriously ill and died. It felt like the end of times for them.

So they did what they had always done when they faced catastrophe: they disappeared together, in a moment, into the deep forest, to the heart of their medicine, and stayed there, sometimes for months. There, they could escape the noise of the industries, and find the healing voices of the forest in secret places where it was still intact.[37] They filled themselves with forest music as medicine, and could heal themselves.

But there was only enough of the forest left to sustain them temporarily. When they felt restored, healthy and strong again, they had to come back out to the fringes, returning to the world of extractive colonialism until, again, they couldn't take it any more and would retreat into the healing of animals.

~

Meanwhile, the beekeeping sisters in the Bosnian mountains, as honey scribes for their bees, note all that surrounds them and all that alters. The air is laden with sage and fig while the scent of the hives – honey and wax – mixes with the nectar of flowers. In the 1990s, these lands ricocheted with shells and bullets in the Yugoslav Wars, when neighbour killed neighbour in the bitterest toxicity of civil war until the very air was poisoned. With bees, the beekeepers are hoping to heal the land of blood and ghosts and transform it into a honeyed world. Now, at the former frontline, among landmines and abandoned villages, flowers, herbs and trees blossom with linden and thyme and Jerusalem thorn.

During and after the war, many people were drawn to beekeeping as a remedy to conflict and a cure for nightmarish memories. But the land now suffers something more insidious: the collapse of the stability of its climate, as the seasons buckle and crack. Honey scribes are among the first to notice the ecological disasters appearing in 'the loaded, uneasy moment', as Larisa Jašarević writes, 'while the End is not just yet'. For now, the beekeepers of the Bosnian mountains continue, with their tiny orchestra of bees, to play the music of life's continuance, as Messiaen did with his 'Quartet for the End of Time', in that earlier war.

When the bees are healthy in a healthy world, their presence is healing and they are the signature of harmony, with flowers and bees appearing for each other at the right time. But honey is vanishing now, and it foreshadows a wider waning. Honey, long known to be physical medicine, was a metaphysical assurance, writes Jašarević, a gift from God, inspired by God. On this holiness we depend wholly.[38]

10

Wolves at the Core of Ethics

'Animals are generally really nice' – Eva Meijer

The toughest male wolf ever known in Yellowstone National Park was Wolf 21. He was magnificent – brave enough to take on a gang of eight wolves from a different pack, running out ahead of his own pack with his tail streaming like a pennant behind him. He was also ethical: first victorious in his fights, he would then be magnanimous, seeing off an enemy but never killing them. With pups, he was tender, affectionate and playful, wrestling, sparring and pretending an ambush, letting the little ones beat him in a play-fight but protecting them with his life if needed. He was a very parfit gentil knight.

In a demonstration of his chivalry, Wolf 21 brought down an elk calf one day in early spring. There was still snow on the higher peaks of this boreal forest, and the canyon rivers were brilliant with icy water. Wolf 21 was hungry after a long, lean winter and through the resin of lodgepole pines and the sagebrush curling through the air, he had smelled the young calf, seen it and made the kill. But he didn't eat. There were two female wolves nearby, part of his pack, so he held back and let them eat first because they were both nursing mothers and needed the meat more than he did. He was canny too. Once when he killed an elk the carcass was taken over by a grizzly bear. Wolf 21 and his family hungrily surrounded the bear, but it was dangerous for them so Wolf 21 sneaked up and bit the bear on the backside, provoking the bear to chase him while his family ran in and fed.

Researchers in Yellowstone gave Wolf 21 and other wolves their names, including his mate, Wolf 42. They were devoted to each other, affectionately licking each other's faces, nuzzling, playing and bedding down together when they could. Born in 1995, he was a wolf of presence and charisma, and she was a kind, intelligent and cooperative character, who had learned (from years of being bullied by her sister) that a wiser way to lead a pack was to work together and to support each other. Their pack, the Druid pack, numbered thirty-eight wolves at its height in 2001, and was one of the largest packs ever observed, with most comprising between six and ten wolves. It was so strong because the pair brought a strong ethos of mutual aid and care to the pack. Elegant in ethics, they were beautiful, good wolves.

According to wolf ethics, the pack usually lets the hungriest wolf eat first (to each according to their need). The whole pack will usually share babysitting duties for the young, making sure the pups don't wander off too far from the den and checking for predators. Older wolves will care for and feed the pups, who are born blind and defenceless and cannot hunt for themselves until they are about ten months old. Wolves operate a kind of welfare state, taking care of the sick and injured, sharing food with those too old to hunt.

More than anything, wolves radiate fealty, the grace of allegiance, in a fine balance between the call of the individual and the call of the pack, as if they are ethically twice-seers, seeing once as an individual and then, self-transcending, seeing through pack eyes. The individual needs to be strong for the pack to be strong, and the pack needs to be strong for the individual to be strong.

While many creatures don't have the idea or ethic of friendship, rather working at a more biological level of direct kin, the wolf pack may include not only related wolves but also those who are unrelated but welcome. Friendship is crucial. Wolves hunted in groups with friends as well as direct kin while early humans probably did not, judging by the lack of same-sex but non-kin friendships in other primates.[1]

So vital is friendship that Brian Hare, professor in evolutionary anthropology, notes it as key to the very survival of humans.[2] The development of friendship enabled people to cooperate in hunting large animals in groups rather than hunting small animals alone. Early humans watched wolves and learned from them, say Australian anthropologists. Indigenous Australians put it pithily: Dogs make us human.[3]

Wolves were practising the ethics of cooperation and care millions of years before humans did. The grey wolf ethos is the closest to a human ethos in all of nature, and they were doing it first. In what has been called the lupification of humanity,[4] the effect of wolf ethics on human society is arguably even greater than the more famous impact that humans had in turning some wolves into dogs.

Rick McIntyre, wolf expert at Yellowstone, is the biographer of Wolf 21. He describes being in a potentially dangerous situation, with an aggressive man and a vulnerable woman and a child, and feeling an immense need to emulate Wolf 21. In the moment of decision, he asked himself: *What would Wolf 21 do?* And he protected the woman and child, as the wolf would have done.[5]

'Hear me, Great Spirit! I wish to be like the wolf' is a Native American prayer.[6]

Among the Nootka people on the Pacific Northwest coast, there is a myth that a pack of wolves kidnapped a young man and tried to kill him but found they could not. Instead, they befriended him, taught him wolf culture, and sent him back to his tribe to teach their ethos to humans. It was necessary, the young man told his people, that they should be like wolves.[7]

We were shapeshifted into our better nature.

A Sioux story tells of a woman who had been badly treated by her husband. She ran away through snow and ice and found a cave to sleep in. When she woke, wolves came to her, curling up with her and keeping her warm, going out hunting and bringing back food to share with her. When she was in a state of distress and fury about how her husband had treated her, one of the wolves came to her and stood by her, comforting her. She lived with them for a long time, learning their language and finding her pain eased.[8]

This story, and reading about Wolf 21, makes me think

transformatively about werewolves. Usually represented as creatures of fangs, bloody maws and terrifying claws killing children, I wonder if the truth might be the reverse. Perhaps the idea of werewolves began not in the nightmares of men but in the dreams of women, wishing their husbands were gentler, took more care of the kids, brought more food to the den, were more playful and affectionate and also fiercely protective. Perhaps women dreamed of someone who would be a better man if only he could be more *wolf*.

Animals may often be considered teachers of ethics. Animal behaviourist Marc Bekoff considers a bear to be his ethical role model and he writes heartbreakingly of Jasper, a moon bear, a species so called for the yellow crescent on their chest. Jasper had been held captive for fifteen years in a crush-cage in rural China, physically crushed to extract bile from his gall bladder via a rusty catheter for use in the name of traditional Chinese medicine. Rescued from this torture by Animal Asia's Moon Bear Rescue Centre, Jasper began welcoming newly arrived, traumatized bears into the sanctuary. Bekoff writes, 'When I first met Jasper I could feel his gentle kindness. He is the spokes-bear for forgiveness,' who teaches lessons in 'generosity, dignity, peace, trust and love. I try to practise what he preaches.'[9]

'I take as my code silverback ethics and a sense of gorilla responsibility,' wrote Dawn Prince-Hughes, who held the gorilla Congo to be her ethics supervisor. Gorillas, she says, are teachers of 'gentle care, fierce protectiveness, love, and acceptance'.[10] Congo once intervened on behalf of a human when, on the far side of the glass of his enclosure, some boys were bullying a small girl, shoving her around. Congo noticed. He pursed his lips and then began pounding on the viewing glass furiously until the boys stopped.[11]

In the Amazon, twenty years ago, a shaman gave me feather earrings and a feather necklace he had made for me because he had dreamed that he should. In another community, an old woman gave me a feather headdress which had long red feathers of macaws and other parrots standing proud and tall at the front, with a semicircle of smaller feathers at the sides, brilliant in yellow, green and azure. My immediate response has lasted unchanged through all these years. *Do I deserve these?* I asked myself, exactly as I had felt when the scarlet tiger moths fell out of my hair. *Can I live up to them? How can I become more bird-feather worthy?*

The earrings and necklace I wear only very occasionally. The headdress, never. It rests on a high shelf in my study, never more than eight feet away from me whenever I write. I cherish the feathers, but I feel I must work to merit them. Can I earn them according to vibrant forest ethics, signalled in a flash of turquoise conscience? I must honour what they represent by living up to the gift not only of the human gift-givers but the lasting owners of the feathers, the birds themselves. But I never understood my own reaction until I read with astonishment a precise description of my own feelings.

Indigenous people of the Amazon often wear ornaments made from the feathers of toucans, macaws, caciques, orioles, egrets, hummingbirds, harpy eagles and others. In their view, writes anthropologist Gerardo Reichel-Dolmatoff, the birds retain ownership of the feathers and have merely loaned the feathers to people. As the true owners, the birds watch the wearers and will criticize their behaviour if necessary; the voices of the birds may accuse a person of being morally unworthy of the feathers.[12] Through the language of feathers and birdsong, people are held to a higher ethical standard.

Indigenous cultures are adamant that animals taught ethics to humans. In a rural Indigenous community in Saskatchewan, animals are said to teach humans values such as love, respect, truth, humility, and the vital importance of protecting the young.[13] Robin Wall Kimmerer, Potawatomi author and scientist, comments on the frequency with which Indigenous or Native world views see humans as the younger brothers of the animals. 'We say that humans have the least experience with how to live and thus the most to learn – we must look to our teachers among the other species for guidance. Their wisdom is apparent in the way that they live. They teach us by example.'[14]

Wolf 21 was generous in gift-giving, usually with meat, or perhaps elk antlers as a toy for the kids to play tug-of-war. Wolves are providers, as wolf kills are eaten not only by wolves but by coyotes, foxes and birds. This is why wolves are a medicine that reaches everything in a landscape, and why they were reintroduced to Yellowstone in 1995 to make it healthy. Following the example of the wolf, a man from the Hidatsa people (from North Dakota) named Bear in the Flat took as one of his sacred medicine songs the Invitation Howl that a wolf uses to call other creatures to a feast, a wild howl for an ethic of generosity.

Among chimpanzees there are sanctions for meanness, so those who won't share are less generously treated in return. Worse, a truly mean chimp may be ostracized, which in all social creatures can be a death sentence.[15] In an Ojibwe story, a man catches a fish but he is stingy and unwilling to share it. The owl steps in, calling him out on it, hooting at him and frightening him until he is so scared he runs away, dropping the fish in his haste. The owl's response is an ethical corrector.[16] Meanness is widely seen as simply obnoxious, as in the traditional Cree belief (around Canada's Lake Superior) that if humans don't share meat properly among those in need, the animals will be offended.[17]

Listen well to the animals for guidance. On the north-east coast of Alaska is a place called Naalagiagvik. It means, in the local Iñupiaq language, 'the place where you go to listen'.[18] It is so called because a shaman used to go there to listen to the voices of animals and of her ancestors, and from these she amassed the stories of ethical teaching that steered her people, guided them and protected them.

Humans came late to the stage, and we stepped into a world that was already ethical. Of course ethics are species-specific, but among many animals, ethics are comprehensible and similar. Be nice. Be (reasonably) truthful. Be generous. Say sorry when you need to. Don't be violent except where necessary. Don't be rude. Don't be greedy. Look after the littlest and be worthy of your chance to live in this animated heaven.

The animals are often considered the conscience of the world, its moral arbiters. Ethics is everywhere, both intricate and discoverable, a lattice of interwoven rules that makes a safety net for the good of all.

~

In a study of rhesus monkeys, a hungry monkey was given an ethical test. If the monkey took food when it was offered, another monkey would be subjected to an electric shock. Would the hungry monkey do it? They would not.[19] Other studies show that rats will sacrifice something they want, if their getting it means another rat will be caused pain.[20]

Brian Keenan, who in 1986 was taken hostage and imprisoned in Lebanon for four and a half years, found that his ethical teachers were ants. One particular ant was injured, and he watched a group of ants save it, taking it away to be with other ants, and the incident became a symbol for him. 'We cannot abandon the injured or the maimed, thinking to ensure our own safety and sanity. We must reclaim them, as they are part of ourselves.'[21] Ants do indeed save their wounded. Injured ants release pheromones, calling for help, and when the ant-paramedics arrive, the injured ones tuck their legs in so they can be carried more easily back to the nest, where the ants care for the casualties and clean their wounds.[22]

Wolf 21 was considerate to the sick and injured. He was as good at kindness as he was at hunting. When one of his sons had been injured, his paw having been trapped in a snare, Wolf 21 would lick the injured paw at exactly the point the snare's teeth had bitten, long after the wound ceased to be obvious. He had seen, remembered, and acted on his knowledge in order to comfort his son, and would check on him, bringing him food. On another occasion, he noticed that one of the pups seemed ill and was lying apart from the others, so he went to be with him. A different time, one of the yearlings had been bullied by the others, so Wolf 21 went to the distressed youngster, licked him and then led him to food. As Rick McIntyre says, Wolf 21 'watched over the younger wolves in the pack and gave special attention to ones that were having a hard time, like a human father would to a son or daughter'.[23]

Wolf 21's beloved, Wolf 42, died in the winter of 2003, and for six months afterwards Wolf 21 was seen searching and heard howling for her in vain. On 11 June 2004, he was seen for the last time. Other members of his pack had gone off chasing elk but Wolf 21 took a different direction, climbing to a high meadow overlooking the valley that had been his territory and his world. It would have been a hard climb for a dying wolf. When he reached the wildflower meadow, he lay down in the shade of one lone tree. All around him were forget-me-nots.[24] Wolf 21 and his mate would have bedded down there often over the years, watching their pups eddying around in the meadowgrass, and they would have both marked this one tree many times. On this last day of his life, he couldn't find her but he could trace her image in scent, and in the far horizons of his memory she was unforgotten. He curled up then, this fine, fine wolf, unforgetting and unforgettable, and fell asleep for the final time in the field full of forget-me-nots.

~

The early evening air is warm and heavy, the summer syrup of London, sticky with sycamore and sweat, beer and hot asphalt, coffee, geraniums and car exhaust. I have wine and chocolate in my bag and I'm on my way to meet Mariam Motamedi-Fraser and Monk.

I'm pretty sure Mariam and I will get on – we've been introduced by a mutual friend – and even if we don't, there will be fountains of words for us to play in, but I am a bit nervous of meeting Monk. No words will deflect his judgement: it's the bare self and the naked pheromones that he will note.

It is Monk who answers the door, although of course it is Mariam who opens it. In a split second, both Monk and I are down in a play bow, me grinning on the top step, him just inside the hall. Then he gets up and looks at me to assess me seriously. Monk doesn't suffer fools, I feel, and I want to live up to his standards. He is, after all, a teacher of ethics at Goldsmith's College in London, with his own staff card.

When I met him, he had a page on the website for the Department of Sociology where he had been working since 2017. The module on 'The Ethics and Politics of Animals' listed the teachers as Mariam Motamedi-Fraser and Monk. The staff page detailed Motamedi-Fraser's academic background and then moved on to introduce Monk thus: 'Monk is a gentle, somewhat aloof, black Labrador . . .'

He checks me out before he offers his friendship and it feels like a test. It isn't to do with my mood or my personality – rather that I feel an anxiety about whether I will be good enough for him. Will I be worthy of his time and attention? It feels like an appraisal by someone who will let me know in no uncertain terms what they make of me. Animals (particularly dogs) may have that effect on people.

He can be said to teach ethics through his character, as he is gentle, aware, observant and sober in his mature years. He physically accompanies Mariam when she is teaching and she tells me that for the students, 'the sheer presence of Monk in the classroom transforms their understanding of that space.' Simply being there, the animal reveals how the university is 'premised on the idea of human exceptionalism, for example'. His attendance naturally provokes discussions on the complex ethical and political questions that are raised by domestication, she says, and the 'agencies, opinions, preferences and desires of animals'. Students with a dog in their class will begin to explore the 'connection between prejudices against animals, and prejudices against other humans'.

Mariam did not consciously name him after a literary dog but she had possibly lodged in the back of her mind that the name of Dorothea's dog in *Middlemarch*, a protective, watchful and dignified St Bernard, is also Monk.

He has very good manners, says Mariam, and is very polite. This is important for animals, including us. Otter is courteous in communicating whether or not he wants to be petted. He usually does like being stroked but if he doesn't, he will first start switching his tail. *Nah, sorry, I'm busy*. If that is ignored, he will air-snap a fake bite. *I mean it*. If that is ignored, he will hiss. *Fuck off*. And if a hiss is ignored, he will take a swipe, claws out. He has never been so rude as to attack out of the blue. Whether or not they know Otter, the clarity of his communication means that very few humans go beyond his second warning.

Monk teaches people good manners, particularly on that issue of consent. If a student doesn't have his consent to touch him, they mustn't, and Mariam requires her students to watch a video on how to gain consent from a dog. Let the dog approach you. If the dog doesn't come to you, they are already saying no by keeping their distance. If the dog does approach, watch their body language. If they look fearful, aggressive or worried (with a stiff body, pinned-back ears, lower tucked tail, furrowed brow), then don't pet them. If, though, the dog is wriggly and tail-waggy, then offer a hand towards the dog and pet them briefly, then stop and withdraw your hand. After that brief pet, watch for the dog's answer. 'No' includes turning away, moving away, shifting their weight away from the hand or indeed responding with indifference. By contrast, a dog who is saying yes will actively solicit touch, moving or wiggling up closer to the person or nudging their nose under someone's hand each time petting stops.

This is a difficult ethics lesson, because Monk's friendship cannot be bought and the students have to learn that it is up to Monk whether or not they can have any relationship with him. Mariam comments, 'It's a story about relationships and politeness, about respect and effort – and therefore sometimes also being disappointed.'

The psychotherapist Dr Aubrey Fine, working with young people in Pomona, California, used animals to teach manners, telling his clients to pay attention to whether they gave or withheld consent, so if an animal was not consenting, they must respect that and not try to touch them. The kids also learned to act gently and speak softly, because if they were shouting at the birds, for example, they would startle and fly off. He reported good progress because from the outset of each session it was the birds who, according to Dr Marty Becker, handled 'conduct and deportment'.[25]

Washoe, the chimpanzee who learned sign language, was good at teaching people manners. She was 'especially good at fingering anyone who acted arrogant or bossy', according to her trainer Roger Fouts. The chimps were part of the selection process for human volunteers at the Institute of Primate Studies, and Washoe had 'the right to fire anyone she didn't like, which she usually did by spitting on them'.[26] Sometimes, Fouts recalls, graduate recruits arrived with an attitude of superiority towards Washoe, acting as if they were going to teach her sign language, ignoring the fact that she knew sign language better than they did. 'Washoe was pretty good at humbling these uppity types. She would walk right up to them and begin signing in an extremely methodical and exaggerated fashion, like someone talking English very slowly and loudly to a foreigner.'[27]

At Arnhem Zoo in the Netherlands, the chimpanzees had learned the zookeepers' rule that no one would eat until everyone – all the chimps – was present. One day, two adolescent female chimps were playing outside and wouldn't come in for hours, meaning the other chimps got hungry. This was rude, in chimp terms, and they beat the adolescents for it. The next evening, those two were the first to show up for dinner.[28]

There is etiquette here (literally 'little ethics'). Good manners are not a trivial thing: they illustrate consideration for one's group, something that keeps the body politic healthy. The chimps in Arnhem Zoo showed that rudeness was not okay and that the youngsters needed to be polite if they wanted to belong.

Among dwarf mongooses, someone must stand sentinel while the others go foraging. The watch-mongoose has to be trustworthy and sound the alarm if there is a predator, but must also avoid raising a false alarm. They take turns to be on guard duty and towards evening they gather and groom each other. Those who have done more sentinel duty get more grooming and if, for example, one mongoose has been unkind during the day, perhaps barging another away from food, the mongooses remember and groom that one less.[29] Mind your manners.

One aspect of ethical behaviour is appreciating how important an apology can be. If, Mariam says, someone Monk knows accidentally steps on his paw and apologizes, he'll come to them, pressing his head into them, as if he is reassuring them that he knows it was a mistake.

Jane Goodall, pioneering zoologist and primatologist, wrote of her childhood dog, Rusty, 'If I reprimanded him for something he had learned that was not permitted, he apologized, but if, in his books, he had done nothing wrong, he sulked, facing the wall. Not until I knelt beside him and apologized to him did he cheer up.'[30]

And what about times when an animal considers that they themselves have done something wrong? They may, like us, reproach themselves. The animal behaviourist Konrad Lorenz had a dog named Bully who bit Lorenz once by mistake. Knowing it was an accident, Lorenz immediately tried to reassure the dog but from Bully's own point of view he had broken a fundamental rule: never bite a dominant pack-member. The dog fell into a state of despair in which he couldn't eat, didn't leave his place on a rug, and would sigh occasionally but profoundly, an enactment that looked to Lorenz like remorse. Primatologist Frans de Waal commented on this case: 'We seem to be getting close here to an internalized rule, the violation of which may lead to profound emotional and physical misery that is probably not far removed from guilt.'[31]

Koko, the gorilla who learned more than two thousand words and a thousand American Sign Language signs, was filled with remorse after she had bitten her trainer, Penny. Three days after the incident, she saw the bite mark on Penny's arm and signed 'SORRY', then 'WRONG BITE'. 'WHY BITE?' Penny signed. 'BECAUSE MAD' Koko answered. 'WHY MAD?' Penny asked. 'DON'T KNOW' said Koko. She knew she had been wrong, and an apology would be an emollient.[32] Guilt, the second cousin of remorse.

Roger Fouts notes an incident when his daughter Rachel had handed an apple to Tatu, a chimpanzee. 'Tatu grabbed her hand just long enough to show dominance and scare her. I rushed over to scold Tatu, signing "MY BABY CRYING". Tatu was so taken aback that she looked genuinely remorseful as she signed "SORRY SORRY" to Rachel.'[33]

~

Monk is not the only canine teacher of ethics I came across. Dogs in classrooms in South Carolina are teaching social ethics to kids with enormous success. The background to this programme includes the high rate of violent crime and murder in America, with acts of violence and aggression prevalent through all school ages. *Send in the hounds!* The programme, called Healing Species, takes rescued shelter dogs into schools and, crucially, the dogs are the teachers. In eleven weekly lessons, the dogs teach the kids how to practise prosocial behaviour and how to be empathic by considering the feelings of the dogs and others. The dogs 'convey principles of kindness, empathy and cooperation', according to a study that finds that this programme positively affects the students' expectations about the norms of aggression and increases their levels of empathy.[34]

When Wolf 21 was just a small pup, his father died and he was adopted by an alpha male who mentored him, teaching him the leadership skills of cooperation and audacious kindness that Wolf 21 practised all his life.[35] Myths relate how animals may take pity on the young and adopt them. An earlier chapter has examined the reality of animals adopting human infants, but myths have a different way of exploring the idea.

Intriguingly, several myths say that infants, having been fostered by the creatures of wilderness, grew up to be founders of *cities*. Semiramis, who was fostered by birds in Assyrian myth, became the founder of Babylon. In Roman myth, the baby twins Romulus and Remus were abandoned in the wilds by humans, and suckled by a wolf who adopted them. Romulus went on to found Rome. Remus had two sons, one of whom founded Siena.

This detail fascinates me because cities are culturally understood as a key part of civilized behaviour, the words and the history intertwining, as *civitas* in Latin means 'city' and is related to 'civilized', and 'civil'. In a striking piece of symbolism, these legends tell how humans had treated the infants in a cruel, manifestly 'uncivilized' way while the wild animals rectified it, being more 'civilized' than the humans. Myths make the point twice, first in showing that wild animals may adopt infants, and secondly that their destiny lies in creating cities, where humans learn to live together in huge packs in some kind of harmony. In cities, they learn to be civil to each other, to show good manners and to police good behaviour in the polis and the metropolis. It is wolves who made civil life possible, the legend of Romulus and Remus says. The body politic depends on the wolf. They civilized us.

Myths of wild animals adopting human infants perhaps intuited a truth. Although each tale focuses on an individual, this is arguably what happened to humans universally, in evolutionary terms. We were savage little creatures, scruffy and rude. We didn't have any manners or any friends. We were dirty, foul-mouthed, nasty little starvelings who were unkind even to our own pups. Wolf couldn't help herself: keyed into her nature was a need to care and to teach the young the ethics of how to be. *We* were the young. Wolf stepped in, adopted us and taught us good behaviour.

If in our prehistory wolves gave our ancestors ethical guidelines, some of their dog-descendants are laying down the law today. In the USA, writer and dog-trainer Vicki Hearne reported that a police officer, Philip Beem, was working with a police dog, Fritz, a Dobermann pinscher. One night Officer Beem stopped a young black woman for jaywalking and attacked her. Witnesses saw him clubbing her 'for the sheer fun of it as near as anyone could make out', says Hearne. Fritz was not having it. He attacked Officer Beem, his own handler, and emphatically took away Beem's club. Fritz, says Hearne, 'had his own command of the law in a wide sense'.[36]

Who guards the guardians? Who polices the police? A good dog can.

In March 2022, from Panama City Beach in Florida, footage emerged of a dog upholding the ethics that a healthy society needs. Scene: a parking lot. Glorious sunshine of early spring. A burly, thick-set cop appears. He ticks all the power boxes: physically strong, male, a uniformed police officer, armed and accompanied by his K9 (canine) police dog. The cop is also white. He has an altercation with a young Latinx woman wearing only a bikini, her hair long and loose. He is yelling at her. The power imbalance is acutely unsettling. She walks away but the cop is venting fury and directing the dog at her. Just then, a young black guy, slightly built and looking perhaps between thirteen and fifteen years old, wearing a baseball cap, T-shirt and shorts, clearly tries to defuse the situation, looking protectively towards the woman, but he cannot calm the officer so he walks away, his hands in the air. The officer grabs the kid by the neck and hurls him to the ground. Onlookers are screaming, 'He didn't do anything!' The dog agrees and attacks the officer, sinking his teeth into his arm.

Online comments flooded in: 'Good dog. He knew who was in the wrong'; 'The dog has better morals.'

As a newscaster commented, 'The [canine] sees no colour: the K9 does not see white or black. The K9 is trained to attack the aggressor. The K9 determined that the cop was the criminal. There's some cops that could take a lesson from their K9.'[37]

The ancient Greeks considered the crane to be a police-bird who cautioned people for bad behaviour. In a story from the sixth century BCE, cranes came to the aid of a poet who had been attacked by a thief and left for dead. The poet called to cranes for help, and they followed the thief, hovering over him until he was shamed into confession.

Many Indigenous cultures have understood that good policing is good medicine for society. For the Ojibwe, medicine and policing are overtly woven together in the idea of the Sky Bear, an archetype of the actual animal, born in a Sky den, and living in Sky lodges from where he cares for the Earth. The bear teaches humans the ethical dimension of life and demonstrates the consequences of actions, the positive results of generosity and the negative results of greed.[38] Within Ojibwe human society, Bear Clan people are both the police force and the medics, tying together those two strands of healing, for just as herbs are remedies for the individual, so wise policing is a social remedy for the body politic.

Animals are used to articulate ethical behaviour, invoked as models for the right way of acting. Many cultures have attributed to animals the authority to police human morals. There is a widespread Indigenous idea of the Master, Mistress or Owner of the Animals, an eternal archetype who carefully notes human ethics. It works like a personification of the animal police.

For many Native peoples of northern Canada and North America, the archetypal bear is often called the 'Bear Master', who polices how people hunt. On ethical grounds, people must not take more than they need, nor disrespect the hunted animal. If they do, the Bear Master's goodwill is lost and people's well-being suffers.

For the Naskapi people, of northern Quebec and Labrador, traditionally reliant on reindeer, the Animal Master is, similarly, a powerful spirit who is sensitive to wrong, and who judges whether or not a person is worthy of the life of an individual animal. If yes, he gives the reindeer to the hunter, but if not, he withholds it.[39] He will judge someone unworthy if the person fails to treat animals with respect, or insults them with rudeness, arrogance or ridicule. After a life has been given, the Animal Master requires that everything is eaten and nothing wasted. Violating these rules will make the animals disappear, resulting in starvation and death across the society.

These ethics are remarkably similar across the world, interpreted by ritual specialists or shamans, who negotiate with the Animal Master. Koyukon people consider that spirit animals (like the animal archetype) pay attention to human actions and are offended by disrespectful, irreverent, insulting or wasteful behaviour towards living things.[40]

In the Amazon, there is a widespread concept of the Master of the Animals, whose consent must be sought in hunting and who protects species and ecosystems from overhunting or deforestation. He is a guardian and protector, a powerful figure.[41] The figure of the Master of Animals is a projection of a person's conscience, so if someone sees him or feels his presence in any way, they know they have violated some fundamental norm.[42] The Greek god Pan, a caretaking god of the animals, has an uncanny resemblance to the Master of Animals, and they both seem to activate the human conscience in much the same way. As people fear violating the law of the Master of Animals, just so, perceiving Pan made people feel apprehension, fear and even *panic*, that emotion specifically named for Pan.

The Master of Animals may appear to someone in their dreams, or a person may catch a glimpse of the Master in the forests. The first warning is cautionary, like Otter switching his tail. The dreamer, troubled, is likely to talk it over with a shaman who audibly voices an ethical caution, underlining the warning to the dreamer – Otter's air-snap. If that warning is disregarded, the Master of Animals may then make the animals scarce – Otter hissing – and then withdraw the animals completely. That's it. Enough. You've taken enough. Three strikes and the claws are out.

For Inuit people, dependent on the creatures of the sea, Sedna is the ethics police. Sedna is Mother or Mistress of the Sea, often visualized as part woman and part seal, mother of marine life, with long hair flowing like the waves. One version of her legend says that she was born a woman and grew up disliking the human suitors her father presented to her, choosing to marry a dog instead. Omnipresent as the water itself, Sedna watches over her creatures, jealous in guarding not just their lives but their dignity. If a hunter disrespects her creatures, she becomes angry and will gather the animals towards her, entangling them in her hair, which becomes knotted like bunches of seaweed so the creatures are hidden in her thick locks. The hunt will fail. The shaman must go to her, and wash and comb her long hair softly until she is calm, her hair smooth as lakewater on a windless day, at which point she releases her animals again.[43]

Myth and traditional Indigenous wisdom align with demonstrable facts about animals showing ethical behaviour. Researching this, finding out about animals from wolves to bears and gorillas, chimpanzees and rhesus monkeys, ants, dwarf mongooses and dogs, has left me breathtaken and dazzled. There is not just intelligence surrounding us but morality and a sense of rightness. I had had no idea.

It was as amazing to me as if I'd found out that the moon apologized when it eclipsed the sun. That Jupiter would make sure its babymoons ate before it did. That lightning would make a point of being fair. That chlorophyll would go on sentry duty for other chlorophyll atoms. That the sun might deliberately dim itself so as not to cause a drought. That sand forgave the sandstorm. That snow crystals gave gifts to each other. That a cloud would slow down so that injured clouds could keep up, and a lake would make friends with a puddle and defend it to the death.

11

The Fair Play of Justice

I will never have not kissed a whale, I thought. I hugged my godson, who was with me in the boat. 'And you will never have not kissed a whale,' I said, 'you'll have this moment inside you always.' We wept an astonishment of tears. My head was soaked in seawater, my lips salted and touched with the cool smooth skin of the grey whale. My skin was drenched in the fish and ocean breath of this whale, who had come many times to the boat, rising to our lips. I never want to wash again, I thought. Not ever. If I can't get in with her, I want to take her smell with me wherever I go, into all the rest of my life.

When Gabi Mann was four years old, she was a food-spiller. The local crows, living near her family home in Seattle, noticed, and when they saw her they would scoot in for biscuit crumbs or bits of cheese. From the age of six, Gabi began to share food with them intentionally, often giving away much of her packed lunch, feeding them peanuts in her garden and refilling the bird bath with clean water.

The crows began to bring her bright tokens of regard in turn, including a blue paper clip, a silver ball, a yellow bead, a piece of beer-coloured glass ground smooth, and a pearly heart, leaving these shiny tchotchkes on the bird tray. The crows made the friendship fair in this back-and-forth gift-giving. One present they brought was a little gleaming piece of metal from a necklace that said 'BEST', and Gabi relishes the fact that there would be, somewhere, the matching other half to balance it that said 'FRIEND' and it would be only fair in the scales of friendship if the crows had it.[1]

The Fair Play of Justice

Gabi's crows, notes wildlife biologist John Marzluff at the University of Washington in Seattle, must be planning to bring the presents for her, anticipating ongoing rewards, and in doing so they demonstrate they understand the benefit of reciprocation.[2]

Other creatures also appreciate mutual exchange. Dawn Prince-Hughes reports a moving interaction with Congo the gorilla. She was trying to give him an apple but he wouldn't take it until she first accepted a piece of hay he was offering. 'He thought it was fair that I should have something. Hay was all he had.' It was, she realized, because 'he valued me and cared about my feelings' and the exchange was 'the fine and sacred sentiment woven in all such acts, whether they be between gorillas, human people, or one of each'.[3]

A bit of hay for an apple, or a blue paper clip for a nut. This is not a mercantile relationship, nor a performed trick for a promised treat, but a freely given relationship in gift culture. Mercantilism says, 'I value this.' Gift culture says, 'I value you,' ounce for ounce in the scales of fair friendship.

This chapter explores how animals model fairness and other aspects of justice, including mercy and forgiveness. It notes how justice may be served through sanctions and, in some cases, revenge. Some animals, alert to a sense of balance, express a form of thank you.

It isn't always possible to give a gift for a gift, but 'thank you' is a kind of gift, rebalancing the scales of a relationship, rewarding the giver with warmth. When I put a plate of food down for my cat Otter he will, even if he is very hungry, pause a moment before eating, turning towards me, nudging my hand and giving a quick little happy mew before eating. Nicoletta, my vet friend who has lived with us, also noted it. 'He's saying thanks,' she said. 'No doubt about it.'

Gabi's mother, Lisa, set up a birdcam so the family could watch the crows. One day, Lisa was out in her locality photographing a bald eagle when she realized she had lost her lens cap in an alley. Walking back, she found the lens cap was already at home, left perched on the rim of the bird bath. Reviewing the birdcam's footage, she saw that a crow had not only picked up the lens cap but known it was wanted and by whom, and had flown it back. More: the crow had also rinsed it in the bird bath, flipped it and checked it. It was a present gift-wrapped in cleanness.

Chimps can say thank you. A researcher at a primate research facility in the Canary Islands in the early twentieth century found one day that two of the chimps had been accidentally shut out of their shelter and got stuck in a downpour, something chimps hate. They were soaked, miserable, and shivering with cold. The researcher opened the door for them and, eager though they were to get into the warm, dry shelter, they stopped first to give him a massive hug in gratitude.[4]

Whales can say thank you too. Mick Menago runs nature trips in the ocean near San Francisco and one day, several years ago, he found a whale who had become entangled with 2,000 pounds of crab traps and ropes which were tied around her tail, pulling her down, and meshing around her mouth and head, right across her eyes. She was struggling to breathe. They worked on cutting her out of the lines, which were all so tightly knotted that in one spot a diver knew he'd have to cut right into the whale's body to get a knife under the rope. She let him do it. Finally she was released and free. She swam away and the divers were high-fiving and whooping when she suddenly returned, swimming back to one diver, gazing at him, nudging him gently in the chest, then pausing, and repeating the gesture. She then greeted each diver in turn with the same series of movements, gazing and gently nudging them all.

'I felt this whale was really thanking us,' said one of the divers, and another remarked: 'This fifty-ton mammal was literally saying thanks. Thanks for helping me out.' It was as if she was balancing their gift with her gratitude.[5]

~

Dogs shake paws for the sheer fun of it, many times in a row, with no treat necessary, just because it's a bit of a laugh. Until it isn't. A 2012 study showed that when a second dog was given food rewards for shaking paws while the first wasn't, the first dog refused to play any more, and showed signs of stress, leading researchers to infer a sense of fairness and unfairness in dogs.[6] Researchers have also demonstrated that crows and ravens dislike it if another bird is rewarded for a task but they are not.[7]

Frans de Waal and reciprocity expert Sarah Brosnan conducted a famous fairness experiment with capuchin monkeys where the monkeys are engaged in an apparently simple task-reward situation with a human. Each monkey has pebbles in their cage and is asked to pass a pebble to the human and, in return, the human gives each monkey a slice of cucumber. If you are a capuchin, you sort of like cucumber. But only sort of. You *really* like grapes. Each monkey hands over a pebble and is given a cucumber slice which each is quite happy to eat. So far so good. But then the experimenter gives one of the monkeys a grape in return for the pebble, but continues to give the other monkey a mere cucumber slice. The latter monkey hates it, hurls the cucumber at the human and shakes the cage, agitated and upset. The monkey, says Frans de Waal, 'seeks to equalize outcomes, which is the only way to keep cooperation flowing'.[8] The monkey acts as if it has been wronged, injured by injustice, and wants the situation righted, because things are not only what they are (a slice of cucumber) but also what they represent.

Chimpanzees may object not only when they get less than another, but also when they are given more, and this, says de Waal, 'brings us close to the human sense of fairness'.[9] He notes a bonobo called Panbanisha who was being tested in a cognition laboratory and who was getting a large amount of milk and raisins as rewards, while her friends and family (who could see what was going on) were not getting anything. Panbanisha began to refuse the rewards, staring at the experimenter and gesturing to the others. Only when they were included would she enjoy her food.[10]

Fairness matters to parrots. African grey parrots, given the choice between food just for them, or food to share with a human, will choose the 'share' option if they trust that the human will be fair and will reciprocate a gift in turn.[11] Irene Pepperberg, animal cognition scientist, writes of Alex, the famous African grey parrot who she taught letters of the alphabet, and who performed his knowledge to observers. When he did so, she rewarded him: nuts for letters, fair's fair. On one occasion, though, she was short of time and failed to perform her half of the bargain. Alex got irritated: it wasn't fair. Then, says Pepperberg, Alex 'gets very slitty-eyed and he looks at me and states, *Want a nut. Nnn, uh, tuh.*'[12] N-U-T. He'd spelled it out for her.

~

The opposite of a gift is not theft but unfairness. If gift-culture says, 'You are valued,' unfairness says, 'You are of no value, you are lesser and diminished.' Unfairness causes emotional harm: irritation in the parrot, stress in the dog, anger in the capuchin. It's unhealthy.

Countries with the most equal income distribution, including Norway, have healthier populations than countries such as the USA which are more unequal. Epidemiologist Richard Wilkinson argues that inequality causes social stress that leads to ill health.[13] When people feel unfairly treated, particularly over the long term, there is a damaging impact: painful conditions worsen[14] while the risk of heart disease is greater.[15] Injustice creates stress that can lead to mental illness too, undermining psychological functioning.[16] Unfairness is bad for the health.

But when injustice stings, go to the animals. Crows are a jury who will find in your favour as Dog is your judge. Capuchins agree with you all the way. Take heart, for the animals, who are so much older than us in evolutionary history, are on your side: guides to justice, doctors to the health of society.

Marc Bekoff hit on a line of enquiry into fairness that is elegant and yet simple, both outwardly demonstrable and innerly known: fair play.[17] How does play relate to fairness? What are the rules of the game? What happens to those who cheat and deceive? What are the health consequences?

Bekoff elucidates the four rules of play ethics for dogs.

Rule 1. Communicate clearly. If you want to play, say so by making a play bow. If you want to fight or have sex, say so. Be honest and don't mix your messages.

The Fair Play of Justice

Rule 2. Mind your manners. Play fair by creating equality, self-restraining: rein yourself in if you are bigger, older, faster or more powerful. Let everyone take a turn at winning.

Rule 3. Admit it if you make a mistake. Bekoff notes that animals show surprise and stop playing if a playmate gets aggressive or tries to mate. There needs to be an apology, by gestures such as a renewed play bow.[18] The apology, between dogs as between humans, shows you care about the other's feelings. (For pigs, by the way, the equivalent of the play bow is bouncy running and head-squiggling.)

Rule 4. Be honest. The apology, like the invitation to play, must be sincere. If an animal lies about play, signalling 'let's play' but then attacking for real, there are sanctions. Coyotes who lie are ostracized from other games and find it hard to get playmates and this in turn increases the likelihood that they will leave the pack,[19] which is a risky and dangerous situation, almost trebling their risk of mortality over seven years.[20] A dog who cheats may be shamed and avoided by others.[21] Fair play matters for pack well-being.

It matters for us too, and we can perhaps thank the animals for this. 'The origins of virtue, egalitarianism, and morality are more ancient than our own species,' Bekoff writes. 'While fair play in animals may be a rudimentary form of social morality, it still could be a forerunner of more complex and more sophisticated human moral systems.'[22]

Darwin in 'Notebook M' wrote that 'any animal whatever endowed with well-marked social instincts would inevitably acquire a moral sense or conscience.' There are many humans who could learn from the parrots, primates and dogs. Only saying.

Animals who are most sensitive to inequity, says Frans de Waal, include chimps, capuchins and canids, who 'hunt in groups and share meat'[23] like us. Those animals whose societies are most like ours set us an example of social health through justice, ancient, enormous and everywhere, that doesn't need courtrooms because the Law is within us, old as mammal memory and close as your breath.

~

Fair means both beautiful and just. *Kalon*, in ancient Greek, means both beautiful and good. *Ewa*, in the Yoruba language, is both outer beauty and a moral quality.

There is an aesthetic of morality going on. Fairness, kindness and honesty are beautiful. Unfairness, nastiness and deceit are ugly. Part of the aesthetic includes the widespread understanding of virtue as a quality of light, a radiance of goodness, unashamed and shining. Cheating and dishonesty are underhand, covert and hidden from light. Part of the aesthetic is to do with harmony, because justice creates the harmonious ethos of a healthy society while injustice jangles and throws things out of tune. Part of the aesthetic concerns form. It's 'bad form', the English language says, suggesting that bad behaviour is warped in shape and twisted out of true. Virtue, by contrast, is associated with good form, the visual fairness of beauty, in a symmetry and balance which is aesthetically pleasing. Balance is at the heart of both beauty and justice.

Lady Justice is not only fair (beautiful) and fair (just), she is also the emblem of balance. Her statue at London's Old Bailey shows her in perfect bodily equipoise. She has a pair of scales in her left hand and the two dishes are also in balance, smoothly level.

Frans de Waal wrote of two juvenile chimps quarrelling over a leafy branch. A female, a little older, played the role of Lady Justice in what de Waal called 'second-order fairness', which involves caring about others being treated equally. She took the stick, broke it in half and gave each one a piece.[24] Dispute settled. Scales balanced.

~

In Croatia once, I visited the Old Pharmacy in Dubrovnik, founded in 1317. Among the ancient illustrated medical books and the vials and bottles was a set of gilded scales and tiny measures, for finding the finest balance, weighing out precise doses of medicine in scrupulous measures. The word *medicine* derives from Proto-Indo-European *med*, the concept of measure. That same root, *med*, gives us *remedy* and *remedial*. At the heart of medicine and at the heart of justice is the measure of the scales.

The Fair Play of Justice

The links between medicine and justice are everywhere. A remedy can be a medical remedy or a legal remedy. We speak of an illness as a *complaint*, just as in legal terms we speak of a *complainant* or *plaintiff*. Social well-being is closely related to societal justice.

Some animals demonstrate one particular aspect of justice: being able to give discerning judgement.

James Anderson and his colleagues at Kyoto University examined animals for their responses to watching a human behaving unfairly. In one experiment, capuchins watched two people, Actor A and Actor B. Each actor had three balls. Actor A made it clear that they wanted balls from Actor B, who would play a generous role, giving all three balls when asked. But would the gift be reciprocated? And more to the point, would the capuchins care? Actor B then asked for balls from Actor A. Actor A might balance the situation, giving back three balls, or might play dirty and refuse, keeping all six to themselves. And then both actors would offer the monkeys a reward.

The capuchins, like a jury of wise monkeys, made moral judgements. If Actor A had played fair, equalizing the situation, the monkeys didn't mind taking a reward from either actor, in other words happy to maintain social relations with both. But if Actor A had not returned the balls, the monkeys would specifically choose to accept a reward from the victim of the unfairness, allying themselves to them, and would refuse a reward from the other, cutting a social tie with the unjust one.

The same Kyoto team wanted to see how the capuchin jury would judge unhelpfulness. The monkeys watched someone struggling to open a plastic container, then approaching another person to ask for help, which the second person willingly gave. But when the same situation was replayed, a different person was asked for help and they refused to give it. The monkeys would not have anything to do with the unhelpful one, not accepting food from them, as the uncooperative meanness was clear to them and they disliked it.[25]

In the 1980s, Kenya's Amboseli National Park had a problem with tourists mistreating the local elephants. The holidaymakers shouted at them, threw things, hit them and laughed at them. One elephant,

Tania, had issued the little hooligans with a series of cautions, tossing her head and sometimes making a charge at the tourists, who would run screaming back towards their lodge. One day, though, Tania was really angered and made a charge at a woman who tried to flee but fell to the ground. Tania could have trampled her, or killed her with one sweep of her trunk, but she didn't. Instead, she skidded to a halt to avoid hurting her – there were deep marks of her braking sharply, ruts in the earth. Then she backed up, turned away and walked back to her family.[26] This could be interpreted, says Carl Safina, as forbearance.[27] In terms of justice, this is mercy, as socially necessary as fairness.

~

I would subpoena Lady Justice herself and find she moonlights – perhaps as a capuchin monkey, with her scales holding pebbles and grapes; perhaps as a coyote, cutting off a cheating coyote from the pack. In her right hand Lady Justice lifts the sword of justice, representing the sanctions of law, its revenge. Perhaps Lady Justice is now moonlighting as a crow, wolf, elephant or tiger, whose claws are drawn swords for revenge.

Just as human courts of law are able to impose punishment as retribution on behalf of society, similarly some animals demonstrate ethical revenge, something that is, writes Marc Bekoff, 'a complex cognitive reaction, involving memory, self-awareness, logic, hurt, justice, blame, and more'.[28]

Take the crow, Lady Justice in her black robes, adept at balancing gifts in the scales of friendship for Gabi in Seattle. She may also use the avenging sword. John Marzluff has captured many crows for his research, measuring them and banding them. The crows hate it and exact their revenge. Whenever he and his colleagues are on campus, the birds pick them out of some forty thousand people and harass them, scolding and dive-bombing, alerting other unbanded crows, teaching them which humans to avoid; those crows seem to get the message, uttering what Marzluff describes as 'a call that sounds to us like vocal disgust'.[29]

A good justice system defends the victim and allies itself against a perpetrator, and there are flashes of this in animal behaviour. Wolf 42 in Yellowstone had been bullied for years by her sister, who frequently attacked for no reason, injuring her and likely killing her pups. That same sister also bullied many others and eventually the pack turned on her and killed her, meting out punishment. This word *mete* (to allot, to give out appropriately) is also from that root *med*, and the pack meted out a tough remedy for the sake of their collective health.

Animals may focus a gaze as severe as a judge on a criminal and target precisely people who have been cruel. In Morocco, in the early twentieth century, a camel was being badly treated by a fourteen-year-old camel driver. The animal was repeatedly beaten, but didn't respond, biding their time until no one else was close enough to intervene. Then the revenge. The camel seized the boy's head in their mouth, lifting him into the air then flinging him to the ground, until part of his skull tore off and his brains were scattered on the earth. It was reported by Edward Westermarck, a Finnish anthropologist and sociologist, who interpreted it as retribution that was, in his view, part of the suite of behaviours that animals – including us – need as an aspect of morality, necessary to societal health.[30]

African bush elephants used to roam in huge herds over the tip of Southern Africa but were ruthlessly hunted by Europeans. By 1919, the remnants of one herd had gathered in the Addo area of the Eastern Cape, a forested wilderness where they seemed relatively safe. On the contested grounds that the elephants were damaging nearby farms, Major P. J. Pretorius was sent to exterminate them. 'He was not a hunter. He was an executioner,' said a local farmer.

From June 1919 to August 1920, Pretorius shot about 120 elephants in what was called the 'Pretorius Massacre' reducing them from about 130 to 16. He then went back to get the last ones. The remaining elephants singled him out, hunting him and forcing him to flee to save his own life.[31]

In 2005, researchers described widespread 'elephant breakdown' across Africa as elephants suffered serious psychological injury after witnessing the killing of their family members. Trampling homes and gardens, blocking roads and showing aggression to humans, as *New Scientist* reports, a number of scientists said elephants were en masse 'taking revenge on humans for years of abuse'.[32]

A young male chimpanzee called Franz was captive in the Yerkes Laboratory of Primate Biology in the 1960s and 1970s. He would habitually throw faeces at particular people he disliked, including a man called Larry. Passing Franz's cage one time, Larry saw it had been cleaned. Franz had no ammunition, so the man teased the chimpanzee: 'You can't get me – *na na na na na.*' Franz stared at Larry, waiting for the man to finish his taunts. Then Franz regurgitated partially digested food and threw it at the man in revenge, splattering him, and performed a victory dance.[33]

In the 1960s, chimpanzees were held captive at the Institute for Primate Studies in Oklahoma under the director Dr William Lemmon, a clinical psychologist. He not only imprisoned them but controlled them and intimidated them, using chains, cattle prods, pellet guns, electric fences and Dobermann pinschers. When two chimpanzees managed to escape (from their quarters, not from the institute) they acted with eloquence, making for Dr Lemmon's own house and going right to his bedroom, where one of them pointedly took a shit in the man's bed.[34]

In human justice systems there may be a long delay between a crime and subsequent trial and sentencing. Animal justice may also operate with delayed retaliation if necessary. On a mountain road between Mecca and Taif in Saudi Arabia in 2000, a baboon was hit and killed by a car driver. The rest of the troop gathered in grief and anger and they waited. Other cars passed, and the baboons did nothing. But they watched. Night and day they waited at the roadside at the exact spot where their friend had been killed. Then, on the third day, one of the baboons saw the driver and car that had caused the death and screamed out an alert to the rest of the troop. They grouped and picked up rocks and stones, hurling them at the car in a frenzy of fury. The driver was forced to stop, the baboons climbed on to the car and ripped out the windscreen as the driver fled.[35]

The animal most famous for revenge, however, is the tiger.

Christmas Day 2007, San Francisco Zoo. Shortly after closing time, three young men approached a four-and-a-half-year-old Siberian tiger called Tatiana, yelling obscenities, taunting her, gesturing in postures of violence and throwing sticks at her. They felt safe because Tatiana was behind a twelve-foot-high wall. But fury can send our muscles into overdrive. Tatiana climbed the wall and went for the young men, killing one immediately with blunt-force injuries and a severed jugular vein. The other two (who were brothers) escaped and she began searching for them, roaming the zoo, hunting them but not attacking anyone else. This wasn't a blind response, it was targeted revenge. It was about righting a wrong, rebalancing the scales of justice.

Tatiana prowled, looking and sniffing for the brothers, finally hunting them down near a cafe where they were trying to hide. She got to them, injuring them severely with deep bites and clawings – and then she was shot and killed by police, her blood pooling with theirs.[36]

Around the world, from the Amazon to India and Siberia, the tiger or jaguar is the quintessential exemplar of ethical revenge, the most severe advocate for justice. Tigers of wrath, targeting their fury against those who cause harm. Sahil Nijhawan, anthropologist and expert on relations between tigers and people, comments that among the Idu Mishmi, in Nagaland, India, it is dangerous to kill a tiger because 'the tiger is vengeful and a keeper of justice. Tigers are so important in maintaining human social order because they are *moral* predators.'[37] They reorder society with tooth and claw in a fierce restoration of justice. They have a sense of law and are willing to implement it.

In the Russian Far East, Siberian tigers (also called Amur tigers) used to live in wary harmony with humans. The Indigenous people of the land had worshipped and lived among tigers for centuries, even sharing kills from their hunting with the animals, and they believed that if someone killed a tiger without just cause, they would be killed in turn. But things changed in the early 1990s, when a quarter of the tiger population was killed by non-Indigenous poachers who slaughtered them for their organs, their blood and their bones, to be used in the name of traditional Chinese medicine. Tigers fought back.

In John Vaillant's book *The Tiger: A True Story of Vengeance and Survival*, the author speaks to one expert on tiger attacks in the Amur district, who tells him: 'If a hunter fired a shot at a tiger, that tiger would track him down, even if it took him two or three months.' The tigers are, say hunters, 'very powerful, very smart, and very vengeful'.[38]

Late in 1997, Vladimir Markov, from Sobolonye in the Amur district, had gone missing. He was known to hunt tigers and was believed to have killed a tiger cub recently and even, some said, to have wiped out an entire tiger family. It was also possible that he had stolen food from a tiger. What was certain was that he had shot and injured one in particular. That tiger tracked Markov back to his cabin and lay in wait for days, very close to the shack. The tiger was not hunting just anyone, he was hunting Markov. It was personal. It was revenge.

When he finally caught the man, he killed him in a rage. 'A hand without an arm and a head without a face,' reports Vaillant of the scene, 'the boots, luminous stubs of broken bone protruding from the tops.' One of the government's anti-poaching team had never seen a human 'so thoroughly and gruesomely annihilated'.[39] The fury extended to Markov's possessions. Everything that smelled of him had been examined by the tiger and much destroyed, his water dipper savagely chewed, a steel saucepan scratched and dented, his axe handle gnawed to bits.

When the anti-poaching team found the body, they were shocked and also terrified. The tiger was still in the vicinity and they were themselves at risk: when they saw the tiger, they shot him dead. That was when they understood what the tiger had suffered. Over the years, he had been shot countless times, his body bearing witness, with dozens of bullets, balls and birdshot: 'This tiger had absorbed bullets the way Moby-Dick absorbed harpoons.'[40]

Melville's *Moby-Dick* is said to have been inspired by a true-life story of a whale's revenge. It was 20 November 1820, and whale hunters had set off from Nantucket. They had harpooned three whales, causing

The Fair Play of Justice

pain and terrible suffering. Suddenly, as the first mate Owen Chase reported, another whale came at them from the pod where the hunters had struck. The whale tore into the ship, ramming it repeatedly 'as if fired with revenge for their suffering'. The hull splintered and the ship sank, and the whalers piled into three small boats, endangered in the open ocean and so slow in their passage home that the men starved and, reports say, turned to cannibalism.[41]

Tilikum was born in 1981, captured as a two-year-old infant in Iceland, sent to north America and held in captivity for life, dying in 2017. In an undisguised irony, as they robbed this orca of his family and whale nation, those who imprisoned him gave him his name, which means in the Chinook language of the Pacific Northwest, 'friends, relations, tribe, common people'. Orcas in the wild rarely attack people and are never known to have killed. Captive whales, though, including Tilikum, seem to exact revenge for their unjust imprisonment. Tilikum was involved in the deaths of three people, two of whom were his trainers. On 20 February 1991, at Sealand in Victoria, British Columbia, a trainer slipped and fell into the whale pool. Tilikum and two other orcas dragged her down deep into the water. When people tried to reach her with a pole and flotation ring, the whales prevented her from reaching them, pulling her under repeatedly until she eventually drowned. On 24 February 2010, at SeaWorld in Orlando, Florida, Tilikum grabbed the trainer Dawn Brancheau and pulled her into the water. He scalped her, according to the autopsy report, bit off her arm and kept her down until she drowned.

That is what revenge looks like when creatures feel so wronged. But if whales can be moved by revenge, they may also be motivated in an entirely different way.

~

My godson Euan and I were camping at Punta Piedra, on the shores of Laguna San Ignacio, a sixteen-mile-long lagoon deep in Baja California, at the invitation of poet, author and whale-lover Steven Nightingale. Each day, we would go out on the small boats called pangas, which sit low in the water, longing to see the grey whales that come here in January and February to give birth and nurse their calves for about three months. It is a sweet, playful time in the whale year. The calves nuzzle and rub their mothers, who lift their babies up and let them slide down their bodies and then create a jacuzzi effect, blowing bubble bombs that the babies play in.[42] The mothers use this time to socialize their young, introducing them to family members and giving them a nursery education.

Going out on the boats to find the whales feels at first like gazing at a blank night sky, hoping for a shooting star. Breath held, eyes searching. The boat engine is hunched at the back of the panga like a heron praying for fish. One of the guides, Ramina, working with the ecotourism company Baja Discovery, tells me the whales may be drawn by the purring sound of the motor – *purr* is *ronronneo* in Spanish – and she adds that the whales, too, can purr, mostly the mothers to their babies.

The whales swim on average at about three to four miles per hour. Some boats from various whale-watching companies approach the whales three times faster, which disturbs me as no one can see where the whales are underwater and the boats could injure them and certainly frighten them. I ask Ramina about this, and she sighs heavily. 'I try and try and try to tell them this,' she says flatly. But all the boats, when they know they are near whales, cut their engines. It means the whales can decide whether or not to come close.

Look! Just there! A whale breaches right ahead of me where the horizon meets the sky. Another, and another. Each time I see a whale breach, I want to applaud its strength and exuberance, as they thrust themselves up near vertically into the air, making of their bodies a living cathedral, cascading waterfalls down their flanks.

I'd hoped for a shooting star but was given a meteor shower. As they dive, their tail flukes arc sideways at a perfect right angle to the tailstock, the tail's centre, a sculpture of wings. The tail fluke is the very last thing you see after a whale breaches, as it sinks back into the water, an elegant kinetic farewelling in a quarter turn of a flowing S, the gentlest and most enormous calligraphy, written on the axis of a helix. It leaves a pool of flat water, a footprint like a giant water lily.

A grey whale may be the size of ten elephants, and their heart weighs about as much as a whole human being. They are giants and they play giantly. They blow bubbles under our boat, then pitch up, gazing at us, breaching and tail-slapping, the exuberance of an inexhaustible ocean of spirit, and then suddenly they are everywhere, churning the water – almost certainly mating, say the guides – rubbing, twisting, splashing, swerving, diving, rolling, plunging, and all the sea is whale.

When whales breathe, they first need to exhale, and grey whales blow a heart shape because they have two blowholes, with each 'nostril' making one side of a heart. A mother will blow, then her baby puffs a little breath, mama-spout and spoutlet, and the sunshine makes rainbows in their spray, a big rainbow and a little one. From the shore, their breathing is like a sea-hymn, the ocean's breathing life. When the whales have exhaled, they suck air in and seal their blowholes, and the whole breath, out-and-in, lasts about three seconds. Three seconds is also the interval between two waves breaking on a shore, and the time it takes to gasp with delight; three seconds is the average length of a hug or a goodbye wave or a musical phrase or an infant's bout of babbling. For humans and many other animals it is considered, physiologically, to be the length of the present moment.[43]

In breathing, they leave their eternity in the water for that one precious moment in the air – the moment that gives them the breath of life but which in the past was the moment that killed them, for whalers would watch for the spout and then pursue. Whaling is thought to have begun with Basque people, who started whaling in about 1,050 CE, approaching a millennial milestone now. As technology improved, slaughter accelerated, and during the course of the twentieth century some three million whales were killed around the world.

This lagoon and others nearby were once scenes of mass murder, as the whales were hunted in vast numbers, the waters red with the blood of the harpooned mothers, their orphaned calves left in deep distress, first circling the whaling ships then starving to death. In fury and anguish, the whales would try to defend themselves and their babies, smashing up ships, injuring and killing the sailors. The men referred to the whales as 'hard-headed devil fish'. I imagine the whales described humans in similar terms.

When grey whales were critically endangered, a ban on hunting them was declared in 1949 by the International Whaling Commission. In 1979, the Laguna San Ignacio became an officially protected whale refuge, now part of a wider area that has been protected as a biosphere reserve since 1988.[44]

Since the 1970s, the whales here have enacted something that seems miraculous, given the history. The whales seem to befriend humans, deliberately and consistently. A fisherman, Pachico Mayoral, was out in Laguna San Ignacio one day in 1972, when one whale came close. He was frightened, as their reputation was fearsome. But when this whale came towards the boat, as Steven Nightingale tells it, Pachico responded in a way that others had not. 'Slowly, tentatively, quietly, he did just what no one does, he made the straightforward, strange, simplest gesture: he put forth his hand and touched the whale.'[45] Over the next few years, more whales began to approach the boats, including, in January 1977, a friendly whale nicknamed Amazing Grace who would come to a boat and lift it out of the water enough to let it slide down her body. She'd sometimes swim beneath the boat, exhaling a huge burst of bubbles, and then would lie beside the boat where people could rub her body.[46]

It became a more frequent occurrence, but never seems less than miraculous considering that the parents and grandparents of these whales were speared and cut to ribbons here. At the time when they first tried to befriend humans, there were likely to be whales for whom the slaughter was in living memory, as whales often live up to sixty. (One, killed in the 1960s, was estimated to be eighty years old – and pregnant.)[47] Some of the mothers, wrote journalist Charles Siebert in the *New York Times* in 2009, still bore harpoon scars and yet would seek out the boats and gently shepherd their calves towards people. The young are brought up by several generations, including their grandmothers, who would have been able to teach the calves their own anguishing experiences. But as marine mammal behaviourist Toni Frohoff says, 'they've now come to consider us as safe in these areas.'[48]

I felt that perhaps our luck would have run out as, after the mating display, I could hardly hope for more. But there was. The following day, the whales approached the boat repeatedly, often upside down and open-mouthed. It's likely, said the guides, that they see the boats better upside down, while if a whale keeps her mouth open, she can see more by looking through her baleen, because her eyes are positioned so far back in her head. They seemed happy, playful, rolling and turning again through all the sweet sashays that you can do in the fluency of grace – if you happen to be a whale.

One swam right up to our boat, drawing alongside, and I leaned over and stroked her silky cool skin. And then that one whale returned over and over again to our boat, paralleling it, spraying us, being stroked, visiting another boat and returning to ours. She had a calf nearby, but she was leading the interaction. I found myself searching for her eyes, so deep down in her face, so low in her huge head. I loved her. Quite suddenly. Quite absolutely. And then in her easy, slow generosity, she opened her mouth wide, in a gesture that seemed happy, trusting and intimate. She stayed by us, and three times in one hour I was sprayed by whale breath. A whale healing. I was longing for my lips to touch her skin, a caress in the huge simplicity of bodies. And that was when she came so close, right up to my face, and feeling a rapture that washes my spirit and always will, I kissed her. She came to my lips again and again. She was choosing to kiss rather than to kill when she could have done either. It was like kissing the cathedralized soul.

One moment I was leaning so far over that I thought I might fall in. And I didn't care. I wanted to make the same decision that the cetaceans made some fifty million years ago, to go back in. Back to the ocean, the home and heart of it all. Back down low into the swinging tides and profound minds of our common primordial past.

I wanted to slip overboard, off the dry ships of stranded humanity, to swim away with them, dissolving into an ultimate healing of the separation between us and all the others, leaving behind the opposable digit and all the dry technis that we have created.

I wanted to live in the lithe and lovely body of the whale-world, liquid and sinuous and singing in the uninterrupted music of the all, the everything, touched with the song whistling through them, sounding the endless sounds of worlds before ours, the singing bowls of the ocean whose song – for humpbacks – can reach a thousand miles in the saltwater that preserves their perspectives and priorities, these whales, made of marvels by marvels with marvels in honour of the marvellous.

I didn't even realize my face and head were actually underwater until the others in the boat told me.

I am whalestruck.

Whaleswept.

The buoyancy of it. That is when it comes to me that this is forever. I will never have not kissed a whale. Not ever, ever again.

I cry.

Absolute tears. From the heart for the heart of everything. I am crying for the sorriness of my species. Tears are holy. Our tears are our reliquary of the oceans, a lachrymatory and the last left to us by which we know our salt past and the salt truth. Tears acknowledge ocean and grandeur.

Some have suggested that the whales are behaving in this friendly way for no purpose beyond playful curiosity, but most experts feel that may be an insufficient reason. One possibility is that the whales, in their huge nurseries, are behaving as good mothers, educating their children. Perhaps they are not only teaching their calves but teaching *us* how to behave, and have perhaps come to regard us as the 'young' who are in great need of being socialized. Euan, my godson, is struck by the whale mother–child bond we see all around us, a relationship, he says, 'so fast, so secure, so unique, impossible to mistake. And they are the grownups: we are the kids.'

It is a truth of evolutionary history that we are very much the new kids on the block. While whales with such advanced brains have been around almost thirty million years, we have existed for about one-thousandth of that time, says biologist and environmentalist Roger Payne, adding: 'We have a lot to learn from whales. They know how to avoid destroying the world. We don't. What would a lesson like that be worth? A trillion dollars? More? All the money that was ever minted?'[49]

Are the whales perhaps simply showing us their normal behaviour, the stance they would naturally have taken towards us had we not slaughtered them? For thousands of years, says Payne, 'we were as aggressive toward whales as we could manage. Now that we have changed our stance we are finally able to see for the first time what their normal approach to us is.'[50] Peaceable. Tranquil.

Are they, like the crows, making a gift of their friendship, to which we humans seem to respond with profound gratitude? They are neither coerced nor coaxed into interactions with us and where necessity stops, grace begins.

There is another possible explanation. Toni Frohoff has been observing these whales here since the late 1990s. She notes the way they are actively engaging in communication with humans, through eye contact, touch and perhaps also acoustically, and says significantly, 'something like forgiveness is a possibility.'[51]

Frans de Waal comments on forgiveness as the internal aspect of the external reality of reconciliation, observable in many animals. Chimpanzees kiss and hug after a conflict, monkeys groom each other, and bonobos resolve social tensions with sex.[52] He picks out forgiveness, along with revenge and gratitude, as emotions that sustain social relationships and keep a society functioning.[53]

Forgiveness is social medicine, a remedy in purest form, as those wounded beyond measure then give beyond measure. It is an iridescent medicine, the rainbow in the heart-shaped spray of the whale. They have mighty and moral authority as great in its way as their physical size, and Steven Nightingale perceives nobility in these ancient creatures, writing, 'the noble are those who forgive when they are able to avenge.'[54]

Interpreting the phenomenon is different from attempting to interpret the individual motive of a specific whale. No one can be certain that this precise whale forgives us, but in sum their forgiving friendship after such unforgivable slaughter is the narrative of grace, the shape of grace, the geometry of grace. What carries sound better than ocean? What carries goodness better? To forgive is to be the bigger one, and they are indeed the bigger ones, offering a redemption song sung by those with the largest of hearts.

12

Political Animals

A friend of Dalí's once spoke of the artist's pet ocelot, Babou:
'I only saw the ocelot smile once, the day it escaped.'

Loukanikos was runner-up in *Time* magazine's 'Person of the Year' in 2011. He hated austerity measures and corrupt politicians and was, according to Athens' deputy mayor, 'a symbol of freedom'.

In 2008, the Greek government had decided to put 28 billion euros into its banking system while not paying its medicine suppliers, with the clear inference that the health of the banks was more important than human health. That December, there were huge demonstrations in Athens against corruption and against Greece's imbalance of wealth, with the minority living as overlords and the majority as underdogs.

Enter Loukanikos.

He was a fearless golden-tawny street dog who joined the demonstrations of his own volition and often led the protests, right out in front, barking at the heavily armed police. He'd snarl an inch away from the riot shields and stayed with the demonstrators despite water cannons being directed at him, being kicked by police and having tear gas hurled in his face. He was known to protect people by grabbing tear gas canisters and pushing them away and he always sided with the protesters against the state.

By 2011, the anti-austerity movement was growing in strength and Greek unions were on strike. Democracy, one of the purported legacies of ancient Athens to the world, had gone AWOL, people said; one of the slogans of the movement stated: *Error 404, Democracy was not found*. There were protests at Syntagma Square in Athens, and Loukanikos returned. In September of that year, a group of police officers went on strike, marching in the centre of Athens, with ranks of riot police lined up against them, and Loukanikos was confused by the two lines of uniformed police. Which side should he be on? Then the riot police attacked the striking officers and Loukanikos applied his signature politics – always support the underdog. He immediately sided with the officers on strike.

So appealing was his presence and his message of political solidarity that he made headlines around the world. He died, though, in 2014, from the after-effects of the tear gas.

Another denizen of Athens was Aristotle, who argued in *The Politics* that only humans could be political animals because only humans could distinguish between right and wrong; but Aristotle clearly had not met many dogs.

Unlike Diogenes.

Diogenes the Cynic (or Diogenes the Dog) was a fourth century BCE philosopher who, like Loukanikos, protested against corruption in Athens. Here's a portrait of the philosopher as a young dog: he slept in a barrel in the marketplace, farted as openly as a honey badger, pissed wherever he liked, including on people who insulted him, masturbated in public and took a shit in the theatre.

Plato once described Diogenes as 'a Socrates gone mad'. Although Diogenes shared Socrates' ambition to be a doctor of souls, Socrates was not his role model. Instead, Diogenes followed the politics of the Dog party, saying: 'I am Diogenes the dog. I nuzzle the kind, bark at the greedy, and bite scoundrels.' (It is possible that Diogenes was taking an insult and turning it to political advantage.) In a world of greed, he chose poverty, preferring to be the underdog. He lived simply, using that simplicity to political effect. It was part of his philosophy to be as natural as a dog, believing that artifice was unhealthy and caused unhappiness.

Diogenes believed that humans should look to dogs for political healing. His epithet 'Cynic' is from the ancient Greek *kynikos*, meaning 'dog-like', and, *pace* Oscar Wilde, a dog is someone who knows the price of nothing, and the value of everything.

Dogs get my vote.

~

This chapter looks at how animals can offer us political medicine. They may work collectively, forging alliances, operating referendums and making decisions by consensus; they may practise cooperation and resistance.

Fieldfares are birds of the thrush family who are good at collective action. With a blush of gold at their chests, they form a consensus of beauty as they flock and roost with chucking calls. And they have an enemy, the hooded crow, who'll sneak eggs from fieldfare nests. It's horrible to have a hoodie on your tail, but the fieldfares deal with it in a demonstration of political power. Fieldfares are far smaller than the crow and they know they can't fight alone, so they adopt the first principle of political action – find allies. Then, in communal defence, the fieldfares fly together above the hooded crow and do a massive synchronized shit.[1] They bomb the bird. Importantly, they make a consensus decision on the timing, as one poop is no poop but a flock shitting at once can defeat the hoodie, whose plumage gets oily and loses its insulating properties so the crow has to slink off and clean up. Birds of a feather shit together in the turd-world wars. The scientific name for the fieldfare is *Turdus pilaris*.[2]

A shoal of herring acts collectively because they are safer together than scattered. At night, though, they can't see each other too well, so they communicate by deliberately taking a sip of air and farting with it, something like a fish sneeze or a high-pitched raspberry.[3] Red deer too, in their nervous elegance, know their safety is in numbers, so after a period of feeding or resting they also come to a consensus decision as to when they will set off again. They move only when an average of 62 per cent of the adults in the herd are up on their feet, voting with their hooves in a wise referendum where there is no change unless a clear majority wants one.[4] There is no despotic deer-leader, but distributed decision-making power for an uncoerced agreement.

African buffaloes similarly make a group decision about when to leave a site and which direction to take, but it is only the females whose votes count (the converse of Athenian democracy). A female buffalo who wants to set off will stand up, gaze in the direction she wants to go and then lie down again, while each watches the others to note the votes, and when enough of them have signalled their agreement they will set off. However, if they can't all agree, they agree to differ, with some members splitting off and grazing apart before the whole herd joins together again.[5] The collective noun for them is an *obstinacy* of buffalo, which isn't very fair to these animals, who take such amenable account of each other.

A clattering of jackdaws (their collective noun) makes a collective decision for when to take wing. They roost together in their hundreds overnight and in the day they split up into smaller groups, but how do they time their take-off? They create a crescendo of squawks, and when their clattering reaches a particular degree of intensity the birds get behind the decision and they all take flight.[6] Good flock politics.

Geese may take a sensibly collective attitude too, often keeping crèches in which goslings of different parents are looked after together by one pair, allowing many adults to forage and feed, free of childcare duties.

Then there's the hive mind of honeybees (specifically the species *Apis mellifera*). 'One bee is no bee' is the beekeeper's motto and the unofficial maxim of the bees. They need to know as much as possible about their situation and to communicate as truthfully as they can. They share information about pollen and nectar sources, relayed in the waggle dance. When one honeybee has found a good foraging site, she'll return to her hive and tell the others, who will need to know what direction it is in, how far away it is and, crucially, how good it is.

She'll perform the answers. Which direction? It's the angle of her waggle-run relative to the sun. How far? This is expressed in the duration of her dance, where one second represents about a kilometre, so if her dance lasts two seconds, it's roughly two kilometres away, while if it lasts half a second, it's half a kilometre away. How good is the food source – how rich is it? She answers the question by the measure of her passion. The better the quality, the more lively the dance and the more often she performs the circuit, in a sweetly comprehensible way, dancing in italics: 'It's *wonderful*, honestly, it's *gorgeous*!' (Or perhaps, dancing with her enthusiasm checked in brackets like a shrug, 'It's okayish.')

Honeybees swarm when a home hive gets too crowded and about two-thirds need rehousing. They leave the old nest before they have chosen their new one, forming an assembly of about ten thousand (a swarm) that settles and waits. From the swarm, a few hundred older and more experienced females, called scouts, fly off to scope out the territory, looking for protected cavities with south-facing entrances and somewhere snug but roomy enough to store their honey for winter.

The scouts are independent researchers, sent out to investigate, who will return to the other scouts with their findings. Those who don't find anywhere useful stay quiet, no showy posturing, while those who do find somewhere will report their findings truthfully and will do so in the language of dance.

The watching scouts learn from the dance how to find the sites and after a while they fly out to make their independent inspection, like a peer-review process. When they return, if they are also impressed by the site, they too dance for it. From disparate voices and diverse experiences, a parley for a parliament, the choices are gradually, over hours or days, honed down to a honeyed consensus when all the scouts agree. The new nest is chosen when they are all vigorously dancing the same dance.

The bees' skill at making good choices, comments Thomas Seeley, author of *Honeybee Democracy*, 'arises from a truly ingenious balance between interdependence and independence among the debating scout bees'.[7]

For human societies to be healthy, we could use some political medicine from the honeybees. Tell the truth. Don't suppress dissent. Always dance. Listen well to the advice of experts.

Plato's *Republic* proposed that those with the most expertise should govern: the philosopher-kings who would apply knowledge for the good of all. According to legend, swarms of bees surrounded Plato's cradle when he was a baby: bees were seen as the philosophers of the animal world. Bees often represent wisdom, and in ancient Greece the oracle at Delphi was called the 'Delphic Bee', rooted in the idea of the bee nymphs (Melissae) who were divine messengers. 'Go to the bee, thou poet: consider her ways and be wise,' wrote Irish playwright George Bernard Shaw.[8]

Honeybees demonstrate how the hive mind is wise because it is collectively more intelligent than the cleverest individual in it. Honeybees offer a direct model of the consensus-building politics called citizens' assemblies or popular assemblies, which allow autonomous voices to come to cooperative decisions after listening to the advice of experts and deliberating carefully.

Martin Lindauer conducted early research into honeybee communication. He had been drafted into Hitler's army in 1939, and was injured. While recuperating, he learned about bees and it was honey to his damaged soul: he felt he was returning to 'a new world of humanity'.[9] The contrast could not have been starker between the best of politics and the worst.

~

Some animals demonstrate the importance of collaboration, working with other species including humans. The honeyguide is one such.

Honeyguides are small brown birds treasured for their ability to guide humans to honey. There is wild honey in the baobab trees in the Niassa National Reserve in Mozambique, a huge area of woodland, open savannah and dambo wetlands with mountains and towering inselbergs, those island mountains that rise from flat plains like huge cliffs. This area is home to the Yao people, who are often subsistence farmers, living in thatched houses in small sand-swept rural villages. The soundscape is the same as any rural village, with kids playing, cooking noises and human voices in the choir of the everyday, but people listen out for one voice in particular, a sound like *VIC-tor*, *VIC-tor*, where the *VIC* is an upswept note and the *tor* is a slide down the scale.

Quite different from their mating or territory call, this call is from a honeyguide who is hungry and has come to fetch a human helper. Let's say this one is female. Although the honeyguide loves beeswax, she is too small to break open a hive and needs help. The bird's Latin name is *Indicator indicator* and she does what it says on the tin, indicating all the way. First, she indicates that she wants people's attention with her repeated call and then, checking they are following, she indicates the route, flying in short swoops towards the hive, flirting her tailfeathers and alighting frequently on branches so the honey hunters can catch up.

At the honey location, the bird makes a different call – *here, now* – and then she waits as the honey hunter climbs the tree, smokes out the hive, axes open the comb, takes out the honey and leaves the beeswax for their bird guide. Yao honey hunters in turn may summon the bird by making a rolling 'r' sound, *brrrr*, then a hefty exhale, *hhmph*, and the birds understand it so well that a hunter who calls like this is more than twice as likely to attract a bird collaborator than a hunter who makes other calls.[10]

In the Kalahari desert of Southern Africa, humans and bird are joined by the honey badger, who also follows the bird's calling. Arriving at the hive, the badger puts his backside up against the hive's entrance and farts with such potency that the bees are knocked unconscious. (Yes, this is for real.) The San people take honey, giving some to the honey badger but leaving enough honey for the bees and enough wax with bee larvae for the honeyguides. The honeyguide is a guide to the honey, but also a good guide to the political medicine of cooperation.

Dolphins were said to collaborate with Indigenous Australians. The Noonuccal people in Queensland would call to dolphins through sounds and whistles, and the dolphins would drive a shoal of mullet towards the fishermen's nets; the men would then give some of the catch to the dolphins in thanks.[11]

Koyukon people say ravens can help hunters find game because the bird flies over them first then on towards an animal, crying, say the Koyukon, *ggaagga . . . ggaagga* ('animal . . . animal') and the bird will do that to get a share of the meat.[12] Ravens similarly work in alliance with wolves. From the skies, the ravens can spot potential prey and call out to the wolves, who interpret these calls, follow the birds and make the kill. The ravens then feed on the carcass. Wolves are themselves experts in cooperation, hunting in packs with a coordinated dexterity to bring down prey that one wolf could not kill alone. They may also help each other lift and carry things too heavy for one.

So will the burying beetles who need to lay their eggs in a dead body (a mouse is ideal) so that their larvae can eat. A corpse on the ground decays too fast, so they prefer to bury the body, but one beetle alone is not strong enough to bury a mouse, so they put out a call for helpers. Although they are usually quite solitary, they gather in groups of perhaps six to ten to help each other, like a roof-raising or a harvest.[13] There is *opera* in co-*opera*-tion, a concert resulting from concerted effort, a chorus of singers whose voices together lift the burden of a song that is too heavy for one.

Many writers, from the Russian political thinker Peter Kropotkin to Brian Hare, have shown how competition (aka the selfish-gene theory) is not the key component driving evolution, but rather that mutual aid has been a crucial factor. Some animals will take concerted, cooperative action where there seems no immediate benefit but there is actual danger, as, for example, the lapwing and the wagtail, who defend other small birds from aggressive and predatory gulls and hawks.

I love all birds but I have a particular fondness for sparrows. Staying recently in Grenada, in Spain, I would put breadcrumbs out for the birds on the terrace and watch. Magpies would fly in, alone and silent, and snatch all they could for themselves. The sparrows, though, would call out to their pals that there was food to share. A study backs this up: free-living solitary house sparrows first chirrup their invitation, then wait for company before they forage.[14] The sparrow is sacred to Aphrodite, goddess of love and beauty, but to me it is the pin-up bird for mutual aid and friendship.

We need sparrow medicine. The super-rich could learn a lot. The profoundly unhealthy politics of billionaires offends the unionizing spirit of the sparrow. Jeff Bezos, famous union-buster, flies into space in a penis-shaped rocket, the prick in the dick yanking himself off, off and away from the shared and sharing life on Earth. Then there's Elon Musk, that human sick-note, the twat in the tweet, promoting the presidential fart, the twat in the cap, to world domination, that one-man ethical fade sponsoring an assault on political truth-telling that would make the bees weep.

Sorry. Where was I?

Healthy politics not only involves cooperation and community but also a strong sense of autonomy. Here, too, animals are good political role models. When Geoffroy Delorme lived in the forests with the deer, he noted how dependent they were on each other, as every herd or pack needs to be, but he also remarked on their profound independence. 'Each deer is a complete individual, one who makes choices, and the sum total of those individual choices ensures the cohesion of the group.'[15] When author Andy Merrifield spent time with donkeys, he was impressed by their autonomy and their willingness to stand their ground, not so much obstinate as proudly autonomous.

Autonomy is a basic psychological need that is fundamental to well-being. Autonomy enhances life satisfaction, increases happiness, protects against depressiveness, lessens conflict, promotes more trust and has a significant impact on people's sense of engagement and meaningfulness.[16]

Autonomy, from the Greek, means 'self-governance' and is an inherently political state. Many creatures seek autonomy at almost any price, demonstrating that they are, literally, political animals.

The healthy body needs the autonomy of unrestricted movement, stretching when your leg muscles require it, yawning when a yawn encounters your mouth, falling asleep at times of the body's choosing. Without that autonomy we suffer ill health in its miasma-form, never entirely well, tired all the time, when the spirit feels more like cardboard than chlorophyll. The healthy mind needs the autonomy of mental sovereignty, directing its own attention, shining its light where it chooses. The body politic needs autonomy: self-rule in civic health.

Autonomy is a sensibility, a stance, a social attitude perhaps best illustrated in contrast to its enemy – constraint.

Autonomy authors free-handed generosity. Constraint writes a mean little memo.

Only with autonomy do relationships run true, in freely given company or cooperation, in free associations of friendship. Constraint deals in transactional alliance.

Autonomy can aim for honour. Constraint reaches only as far as duty.

Autonomy means freedom of expression and the language of gift. Constraint raises a pro forma invoice.

Autonomy activates the senses, quick to every scent of pine or chicory. Constraint redacts life and hinders the spirit. Without autonomy, the free life of the spirit is diminished, whether it belongs to a human, a hedgehog or a pine marten.

~

Although other animals may get caught in traps, Coyote, they say, never does. Coyotes have been known to dig up traps, turn them over and then urinate on them, making their feelings known.

Animals need freedom. They seize it, fight for it and plan for it with vehemence and determination, escaping with dexterity and subterfuge. Primates are serious about freedom, pursuing it as you or I would seek to get out of prison. One capuchin called Oliver was being held at a zoo in Mississippi in 2007 and picked the lock of his cage to escape, but was caught within a week. The manager said, in an understatement, 'I know he wasn't happy when we caught him.' The zoo put new locks on the cage, but Oliver worked out their mechanisms and let himself out a second time.[17]

Lucy, born in 1964, was a cross-fostered chimpanzee brought up as a human child. She would be locked in her bedroom but would always let herself out, and her human parents could never work out how she did it until one day they found her letting herself out with a key she had 'stolen' and which she hid in her mouth every morning.[18] When Dr Lemmon imprisoned chimpanzees at his Institute for Primate Studies, a group of chimpanzees were devoted to escape, doing so with formidable skill. There was a heavy chain-link fence that kept them in, and one of the chimps would begin to twist an end-thread of the chain until they grew tired and another would take over. They would do this for days, one after another working on it until the chain-link broke, and they would unravel the whole section. They never worked on it when they could see humans about.

It isn't a game. The life of the spirit is on the line for liberty, and in some cases reports show the hatred and fury that humans have engendered in the animals they capture. In the nineteenth century, Carl Hagenbeck, an animal trader, described a raid to seize baboons to be used in research laboratories. Traps were set for the baboons and many were slaughtered while the youngest were taken captive. It's hard to read about the young ones, held down with a forked stick, muzzled, with their hands and feet tied, seeing their parents and other relatives shot dead. Torture. Howls of pain. The grief-shriek.

And then the resistance. Older baboons who had avoided being shot would fight for their friends and family, carrying little baboons away safely if they could. The captive baboons would be taken in long caravans of wheeled cages to a port where they would be sold and transported. On the way, the caravans would often be attacked by other baboons, trying to rescue those trapped. In one case in then-named northern Abyssinia (Ethiopia), a caravan of cages was passing through a valley with captive baboons crying out, when an immense herd of baboons surrounded the caravan, grunting and yelling. Hagenbeck writes, 'they refused to leave us, running along on either side of us, keeping up an incessant conversation with their imprisoned relatives. Now and again one would advance to within twenty paces of the cages, and with violent gesticulation and screaming would seem to be adjuring the captives to break loose and come to join them.'[19] Hagenbeck referred to this as an 'amusing incident'.

Hagenbeck killed and caused untold pain and grief, including causing terrible suffering to an elephant in his circus who then attacked him. 'The monster must be executed,' said the man, and by his order the elephant was hanged. The monster that was Hagenbeck died when a snake bit him.

The animals cry freedom with an adamantine seriousness that *to be* is to be free, and that they cannot live under a life sentence. The soul is a flame, a candle extinguished by prison. The wall, the fence, the chain, the lock, the glass, the moat, the electricity: primates take on everything.

For orangutans, escape becomes an obsession as they learn quickly how to dismantle their cages out of sight of humans. One orangutan named Ken Allen, born in 1971, was imprisoned at San Diego Zoo and dedicated himself to freedom from when he was very young. He would unscrew the bolts of his cage and threw rocks at a TV crew and when he ran out of rocks he threw his own shit. In one attempt at escape, he made a ladder with fallen branches. He once noticed a crowbar left accidentally by keepers, and threw it to a female orangutan called Vicki who immediately put it to good use prying apart glass panels in their enclosure. Ken climbed the walls of a moat, although he hated water, and at the top he got electrocuted. But he watched and waited until one day the electricity was turned off, and he got out. After their escape attempts, he and Vicki were held in solitary confinement, something that splinters the psyche of anyone, a person or a 'person of the forest', the literal translation of *orangutan* in Indonesian.[20] Were these humans, we would have no difficulty in seeing these animals as political prisoners trying to escape in fervent and justified political action.

For animals penned in before slaughter, escape is a matter of immediate life or death. In Britain in 1998, two pigs escaped from a truck that was taking them to slaughter. Nicknamed the Tamworth Two, they nudged their way under a fence, swam across a river and fled into a thicket, winning huge public sympathy: only in their escape were they recognized to have the kind of personhood that is denied by their identity as 'pork' or 'bacon'.

Animals can aid each other, committing themselves to a cause of liberation beyond themselves, escaping generously and helping others to do so if they can. In New Jersey in 2017, dozens of goats and sheep were being held at an auction yard. One goat called Fred escaped but deliberately returned to the auction house and, just after he arrived, about seventy-five animals broke out. The auction house manager said he was almost positive they were aided by Fred headbutting the gate that was penning the animals in. Though the others were recaptured, Fred remained free for a year, spending his time with roaming deer.[21]

A herd of antelope was being held corralled in a boma (an animal enclosure) in Empangeni, in what was then Zululand, but one night a family of eleven elephants approached the boma, circling the perimeter fence. The elephant matriarch, called Nana, approached the gates and began working on the metal latches, undoing them all with her trunk. Then Nana swung the gate open, stood back with the rest of the herd and watched as the antelope ran from the boma and darted off into the night. It was clearly, said conservationist Lawrence Anthony, 'a rescue'.[22]

Freedom is a thing of wings. 'A Robin Red breast in a Cage/Puts all Heaven in a Rage,' wrote William Blake. Seeing a bird imprisoned, often in solitary confinement, breaks my heart and when their cagers say they 'love' their birds, I cannot speak.

~

Humans have looked to animals as moral support in political battles, conjuring the animals' desire for freedom and allying themselves to a shared need for the natural world to be protected.

The bird of paradise is the national bird of West Papua, and understood as the symbol of freedom, although West Papua is far from free. Indonesia instigated a genocidal invasion in 1963, and Papuans have resisted it ever since, dedicated to freedom, for which they are imprisoned, tortured and killed. Visiting a few years back, I was overwhelmed by the beauty of the land and by the shining courage of Papuan people, who believe their political right to freedom is shielded by all the animals, especially the ants and wasps who attack Indonesian soldiers, and the Papuans co-opt the animals as fellow freedom-fighters.

The winter of 1995–6 was perishingly cold in the treehouses of the anti-road protest in Newbury. I visited many times, writing about it first in the *Guardian* and *Observer* and later in a short novel, *Anarchipelago*. One morning in February 1996, film-maker Mark Carroll was filming a huge oak tree being felled on the site and he caught an astonishing moment.[23] It's a cold day, and misty sunrise wreathes the woodland. While birds are singing from the trees, some five hundred security guards and police in high-vis jackets and helmets arrive, the fluorescent ugliness jangling in this place of slaughtered beauty. There are a few scattered protesters and a handful of mounted police officers whose horses are alert but still. The giant oak tree is being chainsawed and the sight and sound of it feel like a torque of cruelty. The land shakes as the tree falls.

Quite suddenly, two black horses appear from nowhere. They are wild horses and this is their territory: they know these trees. I asked equine therapist Louise Reynolds to watch the film and interpret their body language and behaviour for me. The wild horses, she notes, arrive disturbed and anxious, moving urgently with their heads and tails high, lacing right through the line of security guards even when the men attempt to shoo them away. The horses first try to get close to the felled tree, but then they seem to change their minds and approach the police horses instead. One of the wild horses, who Reynolds surmises is a mare from her behaviour, aligns her head with the larger, possibly male, police horse. Forehead to forehead, nose to nose, they remain absolutely motionless like that for a long moment, in poignant communication.

The mare then suddenly pulls away, striking out a leg, not aimed at the horse but into the air, and the police officer pulls his horse away. The wild pair are not aggressive towards the humans but seem bewildered and distressed. 'The horses are trying to understand what's going on, looking for the sense in what is happening,' says Reynolds, and there is, for her, for the protesters, and for me, a sense that the horses are asking, distraught, *What are you doing? Why is this happening?* The protesters felt that the presence of the horses worked a sympathetic political magic. It was profoundly moving, and seemed to underline how this was a senseless act of state violence against the natural world.

In the history of political protest in Britain in the last thirty years, animals are often evoked as an essential benignity and a medicine for the body politic. At a recent trespass for the Right to Roam, in Berkshire,

England, protesters arrived dressed as animals, the creatures of the commons taken as political role models who embody the politics of the commons, each belonging and none owning.

When it comes to an animal uprising, orcas recently swept to fame. Between 2020 and 2024, orcas have attacked almost seven hundred boats in the Straits of Gibraltar, damaging dozens and sinking several. The whales rammed one boat's side and slammed it for an hour and a half, holing it in two places. Coastguards rescued those on-board but the boat, a Swiss yacht called *Champagne*, was scuppered and sank before it reached harbour.

Some experts suggest the whales are playing. Others say it could be revenge for whales being injured in agonizing collisions with boats. Others comment that the orcas seem to want to just drive the boats out of these waters. Interestingly, many people yearned to co-opt the whales into a political context, a protest against the wealthy conducted by the creatures of the sea commons. The Straits of Gibraltar are a playground for deranged millionaires with an unhealthy desire to own more yachtage than any one person can enjoy, and some have expressed the hope that the whales sink Jeff Bezos's $500 million superyacht, which is sometimes seen off the coast of Spain.

Ships create noise that is hideously painful and distressing for whales. Also, over-fishing has badly depleted food that whales depend on in these waters. Perhaps the whales want to put a stop to the boats not because they would recognize the term *Götterdämmerung capitalism* but because it's perfectly possible that they have an equivalent and equally damning term for what we do and how it damages them and their world.

When Walt Whitman wrote the poem 'I think I could turn and live with animals', one of the attractions was their healthy politics: 'not one is demented with the mania of owning things.'

~

Gamekeepers on pheasant enclosures set traps for owls, who are caught by their legs and left terrified and fluttering all night until the gamekeeper kills them in the morning,[24] all to ensure that the wealthy can get their pleasures from killing pheasants. It sickens everyone else.

Animals have rights, for their own sake and, inextricably, ours. The German artist Joseph Beuys created a political party for animals, wanting their voices to be heard. In the Netherlands, similarly, there is a Party for the Animals, whose manifesto explains its motivation being 'to protect the interest of the weakest against the alleged right of the strongest. In all this, the animals are the most vulnerable. After the liberation of slaves and women, and giving rights to children, the next logical step is to take the interests of animals seriously.' In the 2023 general election, they received 2.25 per cent of the votes and the party has seats in the House of Representatives and in the Senate and one seat at the European Parliament.

This sensibility is a new iteration of an ancient politics, the Indigenous idea of 'natural democracy'[25] whereby the whole community implacably includes all creatures, birds, animals, insects and plants as well as humans, each of whom has their rights. 'This concept of life,' wrote Luther Standing Bear, Lakota author and philosopher, is 'sane, normal, and human'.[26]

On 3 January 1889, on the streets of Turin, Italy, Nietzsche reportedly saw a horse being savagely beaten by a carriage driver. He threw himself on the horse's neck to shield the animal from the whip and burst into tears. This was the moment that precipitated his eleven years of insanity: cruelty to animals damages us as well.

For George Orwell, the ill-treatment of a horse was the instigation for *Animal Farm*. The book, he explained, was not only an allegory for human–human politics but a searing depiction of the politics between people and animals, as he wrote in the introduction to the Ukrainian edition.

> I saw a little boy, perhaps ten years old, driving a huge cart-horse along a narrow path, whipping it whenever it tried to turn. It struck me that . . . men exploit animals in much the same way as the rich exploit the proletariat. I proceeded to analyse Marx's theory from the

animals' point of view. To them it was clear that the concept of a class struggle between humans was pure illusion, since whenever it was necessary to exploit animals, all humans united against them: the true struggle is between animals and humans.

Animals are treated cruelly for our entertainment, in fox hunting, circuses, zoos and films. In the making of the Clint Eastwood film *Every Which Way But Loose* and its sequel, *Any Which Way You Can*, orangutans were used as actors. One was trained by being viciously beaten the day before filming, to make him docile. Another was 'caught stealing doughnuts' and was violently attacked with an axe handle in punishment, dying soon after of a cerebral haemorrhage.[27]

Most circus elephants are trained with a bullhook and if they do something 'wrong', they get repeatedly beaten with it or stabbed with the barbed end, to stop them doing it again. In 1988, the San Diego Wild Animal Park was holding captive an African elephant called Dunda. She was continually 'disobedient' and was being 'disciplined' (in the words of the supervisor). Trainers had chained each of her legs and pulled the chains taut. They then went to work on her, beating her around the head with axe handles for four days.[28]

Every animal in captivity, argues animal activist Jason Hribal, knows which behaviours are rewarded and which are punished, through beatings, torture, starvation or solitary confinement. They also know that they can rarely escape and that fighting back is usually both futile and hideous for them.

But still they resist.

Captive elephants repeatedly refuse commands or deliberately injure trainers in spite of the beatings. Some people theorize that elephants respond like this because they are suffering from PTSD. Hribal counters this: yes, they may well be psychologically suffering, but, he says, 'resistance is not a psychological disorder. Indeed it is often a moment of distinct clarity' as, using intelligence and tenacity, they are acting with intent. 'They are choosing to fight back.'[29]

To resist includes making a stand against something, to stop the course of something, or to refuse to comply. Animals fighting back are not reacting in an automatic reflex response but truly resisting, argues Hribal. That difference between responding and resisting is the reason why their actions can be called political.

Animals can protest against ill-treatment, operating slow-downs or refusals. Whales forced to do performances in aquariums will sometimes go on strike, taking swims between routines, using delaying tactics or refusing to perform.[30]

In cows, people have been noticing resistance long enough to name it; the Irish term *bó dhodach*, for example, is used for a cow that purposely spills her milk pail when it is full.[31] Purposely, not accidentally. And *when it is full*: this is what strikes the note of resistance.

The electric cattle prod, high voltage and strong enough to inflict significant pain, is recognized as an instrument of torture when used on humans. Used on cattle, it is naturalized as if it were a normal interaction. This is how dinner is made: first torture someone, then serve them up in a bolognese sauce with spaghetti for tea.

Andrea Arnold's *Cow* is a film like no other. Almost without human voices and entirely without commentary, the film follows the emotional life of one cow, Luma, held in an intensive dairy farm, as she gives birth, and in the brief time she has with her calf. They lick-kiss each other with long and gentle tongues, lowing and loving. When her calf is seized, she goes on hunger strike. Full of milk and love, the grief she feels is evident. She calls for it, lows for it, lowering her head; she looks for it through the legs of other cows and under their udders, at calf-height. And then she sinks her face into another cow's shoulder as if the weight of her grief is too heavy for her to lift her head. Her heart is breaking and she weeps.

In an interview, Arnold says that during the edit, quite involuntarily, she found herself repeatedly saying, 'I'm seeing you, Luma. Don't worry, Luma, we see you.'[32]

Luma has six calves, and they are all stolen from her. She becomes angry and aggressive when she watches another cow being separated from her child and this is a moment of resistance for the sake of someone else, a political rebellion. Over time, her udder becomes so swollen that it almost scrapes the cold concrete floor, filthy with mud and shit, until she can barely walk and is of no more use. She is taken into a barn and shot dead.

'For the animals it is an eternal Treblinka,' wrote Jewish author Isaac Bashevis Singer. 'In relation to them, all people are Nazis.' He wrote this in a collection called *Eternal Treblinka*, with a foreword by Lucy Rosen Kaplan, daughter of Holocaust survivors.

They suffer from our totalitarian politics.

They are also part of the resistance to totalitarianism.

Totalitarianism works by isolating people, as the political theorist Hannah Arendt maintains, noting how all tyrannies base themselves on loneliness, 'on the experience of not belonging to the world at all, which is among the most radical and desperate experiences of men'.

By safeguarding us against loneliness, animals offer us a vaccination against totalitarianism, preventative medicine for the body politic. Animals help us keep our paws on the ground. They lead us into the belonging world where we matter and they matter, where matter matters, where the unashamed physicality of our being is embedded in the true world, shared and alive.

~

Media reports from China say that young chimpanzees have become 'addicted' to mobile phones. Gorillas, say zoo experts, are 'fascinated' by screens, and one teenage gorilla imprisoned in a Chicago zoo became 'very much distracted' by mobile-phone screens.[33]

Nassir is a thirteen-year-old gorilla and a total teenager. He is held at Toronto Zoo, which noted on its website, 'Screen time would dominate his life if he had his way.' Zoo visitors had begun showing Nassir videos on their mobile phones, and the zoo's director of wildlife conservation said that he was 'just so enthralled with gadgets and phones and the videos'.[34] (I'm not surprised, as zoo animals experience excruciating boredom.)

'We just want the gorillas to be able to be gorillas,' said a spokesperson for the Toronto Zoo, noting, 'When our guests come to the zoo, we want them to be able to see gorillas in a very natural state, and [doing] what they would be doing naturally.'[35]

Would she be suggesting the blindingly obvious that it is not natural for primates to be obsessed with phones? Would I be stating the blindingly obvious that it is not natural for primates to be imprisoned in zoos?

Zookeepers plead with visitors not to show screens to the animals, not to let them become as addicted, distracted and fascinated as we are. Attendants put up signs to stop visitors sharing videos with the animals and rope off areas to physically prevent visitors from doing so. Let the apes be animals, natural and untechnological, the zoos are trying to say.

It's a fascinating situation, as the chimps and gorillas reflect our enthralment right back at us and also challenge our perception of what is natural. There is a profound uneasiness here because, of course, many visitors were delighted by the shared-screen interactions but the zoo authorities were voicing something else, the fact that we humans desperately need animals to stay as animals because it comforts us.

While we humans are living in times of flux, technologies sweeping their changes at breakneck speed, making many people feel dizzy, dispossessed and perpetually edgy; while our communities feel unstable and the political world is in upheaval; while jobs are unpredictable and housing precarious; while social ties are weakened or (online) unreal; while behind it all, the true and coming ghast of the climate crisis wreaks blind havoc with the sustaining steadfastness of the living world, we need the animals more than ever.

The combination of all this can lead to a seasick sense of insecurity, a bewildering sense of unpredictability, as if the ground we walk on is not solid. In this fragile world, animals can provide the continuity we need. A cat is a cat is a cat and should be forever so. In 364 CE with St Jerome, in 1564 with Montaigne, in 1964 with Ursula K. Le Guin, in 2064 with your granddaughter. We need the animals to stay animals for our sakes, providing us with a constancy of being, a still point in a spinning world, because our collective health requires it.

PART FOUR

How Animals Heal the Soul Politic

This section looks at how animals are healing for the collective psyche in art, spirituality, dreaming and medicine stories. They are the foundation of our art and it is impossible to imagine human creativity without the influence of animals, from cave paintings to heraldry and language itself. Animals are at the heart of spirituality; primates have spiritual instincts and animals are considered divine in many cultures. Animals dream and the dreams of the soul politic are stored in medicine stories and folk tales which stress that animals are the source of healing for the public mind. The oldest doctors of the world, shamans, have always said that it is the animals who heal, and we examine the role of shapeshifting as a healing power.

13

Pink Pink Stink Nice Drink

'Birds are not like ideas. They are ideas' – Paul Shepard

If the imagination were an animal, it would be the hare. The mercurial hare races quicksilver, like a flash of thought swiftly appearing and instantly gone.

Hare is intuition, that glimpse of insight that hardly seems one's own, leaping as it does from beyond the self, landing on its paws for a fleet moment in the mind, then off in one bound back out into the boundless. Hare is the illuminator as art is, as on a cloudy night a full moon may break through briefly, washing its otherlight over a sleeping world, before eloping with your dreams. Glimpsed at moonrise or moonset, maybe moonstruck or maybe changeable as the moon, Hare is associated with the moon from India to Africa and the Americas. Hare is moonshine, and to swallow the hare means to get very drunk.

Hare, the quickener, springs up with the grasses of springtime and is associated with springs of water and of life. Fecund, they represent the fertility of Oestrous Easter and were beloved of the goddess Eostre, whose lights were carried by hares. Symbol of generation and regeneration in China and Europe and elsewhere, so alive is the hare that the ancient Egyptians used this animal as a hieroglyph for the verb *to be*, and for existence itself. This hieroglyph is a beauty: the animal's body is outlined with the ears running back along the length of the body, and even as a picture the eyes are bright and the whiskers seem to twitch while a wave of water ripples underneath the image. Albrecht Dürer's famous watercolour of a hare seems to come alive if you watch it by candlelight.

Hare is meaningful medicine, and many animals are similarly freighted with meanings that fertilize the collective imagination. Their symbolism provides a common vocabulary for the collective psyche that can speak through the animals and will be understood.

The eagle was the bird of Zeus, supreme deity, and chosen by the Roman Caesars as their symbol of rule. The Hindu king of the birds, Garuda, also has the beak and wings of an eagle. While the eagle represents emperors and kings, in cultures where power was more equally spread, for example among the Vikings, the bird of power was often the raven, and in Celtic myth the king of birds is the wren.[1] The wren! The tiniest and sweetest musician of them all, the bard of the birds, it symbolizes wisdom and divinity precisely because while it is hard to see, its song carries far and inspires the music of the soul.

In Alexandria in the first centuries after Christ, a book called *The Physiologus* ('The Doctor' or 'The Physician') was compiled to demonstrate animals as physic for the collective imagination because they were perceived to show moral virtues. The phoenix, who sacrifices herself in the pyre and rises from the dead, was taken as an image of Christ; while hoopoes, caring for their elderly parents, were a model for the young. The bestiary – a compendium of beasts – became popular in the Middle Ages as a morality dictionary, and animals were enlisted as role models or cautions. Turtle doves, for example, were applauded for 'chastity' as the female dove was understood to be faithful to her mate even after his death, and priests would use this to exhort widows not to remarry. The boar represented the sin of lust but was also a model for fearlessness. The otter symbolized Christ because it was believed to attack crocodiles, who were associated with Satan. Similarly using animals as lessons, the Koyukon people consider the osprey to be a miser, wrote cultural anthropologist Richard Nelson, 'because it can hold slippery fish as it flies, clutching its possessions and refusing to part with them. Koyukon people regard this as a highly disagreeable characteristic.'[2]

Wresting animals into ideological propaganda, bestiaries paved the way for the medieval and Renaissance animal trials across Europe and the Americas, where animals were literally tried in courts of law and could be found 'guilty' of natural animal behaviour and killed in punishment. These trials were not common, but they were remarkable. In 1457, at Savigny-sur-Étang in France, a sow and her six piglets were put on trial for the murder of a young child. The sow was found guilty and sentenced to death by hanging, but the piglets were shown mercy, pardoned because they were young and innocent, and also because their mother was said to have set them a bad example.[3] Rats overran Autun in Burgundy in 1522, destroying the barley crop and the vineyards. The rats were summoned to court by a town crier: they did not appear. A lawyer for the rats argued they couldn't come to court for fear of journeying through the ferocious cats of Autun, and the judge spared them execution but ordered them to vacate the fields within six days.[4]

Animal symbolism floods the collective imagination across the ages. For the ancient Egyptians, the dung beetle represented the eternal cycles of life and resurrection. For St Augustine, 'the truth is like a lion; you don't have to defend it. Let it loose; it will defend itself.' In Kenneth Grahame's *The Wind in the Willows*, the stoats and weasels are creatures of theft and threat, while Toad is a self-indulgent, boasting hedonist, though one whose reckless splendour splashes charisma across every page.

Heraldry uses animals as imaginative aspiration. An animal – lion couchant or badger rampant or boar passant – cues strength, intrepidness or fierceness, and the animals in heraldry are exactly that: heralds, messengers sent ahead to announce who someone is or how they would like to be seen.

A gyrfalcon is fit for a king, a sparrowhawk for a prince, a peregrine falcon for an earl, while a lady's bird is the merlin, according to a 1486 book on heraldry and hawking, *The Book of Saint Albans*. A deer trippant, with delicate ankles and exquisite alertness, dances across the arms of Europe. One heraldic symbol is the 'crane in its vigilance', in which a crane stands holding a stone in its claw, and it is thought to originate in the writing of Pliny the Elder, who noted that a flock of cranes are able to sleep as they choose one to stand sentry holding a stone, and if this bird accidentally falls asleep, the stone is dropped and the bird is woken by its noise.

In canting arms, the name of a family is recalled (incanted) in the name of the creature, so the Bowes-Lyon family features lions and Princess Beatrice of York has three bees (bee, thrice), while many families whose names begin with 'Be . . .' also choose bees: nine bees volant (flying) perhaps, or three bees argent (silvered). The municipal arms for Berlin features a black bear (*Bär*) and the arms for the village of Hensbroek in Holland features a hen in breeches. Heraldry includes species that are not grand, including the mole (moldiwarp), the hedgehog (urcheon), the tortoise, grasshopper and – in the coat of arms of the Pullici family of Verona – the flea, *pulce* meaning 'flea' in Italian.

Heraldry is alive and well and walking among us, in the form of companion animals. Pets are often tellers of who people are or wish to be, or how they want to be perceived. They are sent out as our heralds. Bulldog couchant. Kitten salient. Poodle rampant.

For author Barbara Cartland, a Pekinese. For Queen Elizabeth II, her corgis. For the British rural middle classes, Labradors, spaniels, pointers and golden retrievers are heralds of group identity, while for New Age travellers, traditional poaching dogs such as lurchers are badges of belonging.[5] A study looking at young male immigrants to Germany in the 1990s demonstrated the popularity of the fighting dog, the *Kampfhund*, often given names like Gangster and Rambo.[6] Chosen to express aggression and machismo, the dogs may unwittingly reveal their owners' sense of vulnerability.

The England national football team, the Three Lions, and the basketball team the Chicago Bulls use these animals as aspiration for their spirit of success. Banksy opts for rats: 'If you feel dirty, insignificant or unloved, rats are a good role model. They exist without permission, they have no respect for the hierarchy of society, and they have sex fifty times a day.'[7]

Animal companions are a social shorthand for novelists to amplify characterization. So Charles Dickens gave Bill Sykes, the villain of

Oliver Twist, the bull terrier called Bull's Eye, while George Eliot gave her heroine Dorothea the St Bernard, symbolizing virtue and a seeking nature, to express her pursuit of knowledge and moral goodness in outer animal form.[8]

Jane Eyre opens with the young Jane reading Thomas Bewick's *A History of British Birds*, alerting us to Charlotte Brontë's use of birds to paint the character of Jane (a dove, skylark and linnet) and of Rochester (eagle and cormorant). Using animals this way has timeless eloquence: the linnet was as alive to Brontë as it was to poet Christopher Smart, writing 'Let Linnet, house of Linnet rejoice', or to Yeats in his poem for his daughter's peace, praying that nothing 'tear the linnet from the leaf'.

Italian Renaissance painter Pisanello created portraits on medals and frequently put animals on the verso (the reverse side) of each medal, representing and almost summoning the spirit of the individual portrayed, so Cecilia Gonzaga, for example, a fifteenth-century classical scholar and nun, is portrayed with a unicorn in a moonlit landscape.

In order to create his pen-portraits, Philip Pullman puts animals on the verso of his characters' psyches in his deftly specific daemon-animal motif that is the tutelary genius of his work. Lyra has her pine marten, Lee Scoresby his Arctic hare and Mrs Coulter her golden monkey. Through their daemon, a person both knows and is known. The daemon is the intuition within a character and also the visible form of a person's authentic being. If a person is separated from their daemon they sicken and die, and this, to me, bears a far larger truth, both poignant and tragic, that humanity's psychic survival must be linked to the animal realm and when that link is severed, we die. There is no medicine more necessary for the collective mind.

The full imaginative reach of being human needs the animals. We are made of the snort of a horse, a hedgehog bristle and badger's teeth. We are wren-sung and swallow-built and seahorse-etched, and our imaginations are flecked with turquoise, thanks to the dragonfly. Through the animals we know ourselves, and without them our identity is as threatened as a Pullman character without their daemon.

For the Desana people of Colombia, the human brain can be

pictured in various ways, sometimes as a humming beehive with hexagonal honeycombs, or as a flock of butterflies, as a school of tiny sparkling fish or a trembling mass of frogs of many colours.[9] The collective psyche teems with dazzling animals. Traditional healers of the Seminole people in North America use different birds to bespeak their specific healing practice. A healer who works much like a GP, practising general medicine for many types of disorder with a generalist's wisdom, wears an owl feather in his hat, while a healer who specializes in curing headaches wears the feather of a yellow-flicker because he probes for the problem as the flicker probes for insects.[10]

~

The ancient Greek satirist Aristophanes wanted to make his feelings about warfare widely known, so he invented the idea of Cloud Cuckoo Land. It was a city that men created in the sky, believing that birds rather than gods should rule the world, and offering bird-wisdom over militarism.

The habit of using birds to deliver military meaning has never left us, and people have often used doves and hawks as symbols for those who support peace or war respectively. The terms were widely used in the Vietnam War as polarized positions, while Senator George Aiken said, 'I'm not very keen for doves and hawks. I think we need more owls.' The eagle on the American dollar bill, with an olive branch in one claw and arrows in the other, sends messages to the world that war or peace is on its terms: America rules.

Birds carry our meanings. Sparrows are commoners:[11] cheeky, chirpy and chatty, they are never soloists but love rowdy, beautiful gatherings. The panache of the peacock suggests boastful bravura and represents the gilded wealthy: the collective noun is an ostentation of peacocks. When Belgian artist Francis Alÿs was invited to the opening of the Venice Biennale in 2001, he did not go but sent a living peacock in his stead, in a work titled *The Ambassador*. The peacock preened, belled and flirted his tail feathers. Alÿs knew that we can all speak peacock and understand the bird's preposterously pretentious meaning.

Johnny 'Rooster' Byron is one of the greatest characters to have strutted the stage in my lifetime. Breakfast is milk, vodka, speed and an egg. He is Dionysus on forty-five pints of Guinness, a one-man fugue of fire, Lord of Misrule, a reprobate shaman, debauched and drunk on his own spunk. In the play *Jerusalem* by Jez Butterworth, Mark Rylance plays Rooster, crowing, cockerel-chested, a cock of all roosts. The spirit of Rooster is a force of nature burning through a wan culture to bring on dirty, real, red life. Rylance seems to shapeshift, almost to become a rooster on stage, evoking the animal spirits who are our imaginative fertility.

Advertising and marketing invoke the power of animals. A sheepdog sells Dulux paint, a Labrador puppy sells toilet roll, we have the Peugeot Lion, the Jaguar car, the black horse of Lloyds Bank, and Camel cigarettes. An Edinburgh cafe used cartoons of Peppa Pig to sell bacon sandwiches, which didn't go down very well as parents feared their children might learn the devastating truth that they were half-pint cannibals eating their friends. Red Bull Energy Drink depends on the bull of its name and would hardly sell as well were it named 'Pink Dormouse Energy Juice'. This is sympathetic magic, coined in today's currency.

Animal spirits signpost us to the madlands of alcoholic spirits: Badger ale, Woodpecker cider, and the lion for Singha beer. John Bull, his Union Jack vest stretched over his beer belly, lover of dogs, horses and ale, struts into the national psyche as a personification of England and would have an honorary seat in the corner of the Bull, the pub that is the pumping heart of village life in the fictional village of Ambridge, in the United Kingdom's longest-running radio soap opera, *The Archers*. Pub signs often sluice the juice of animals in the Blue Boar or the White Hart or the Red Lion, but the Bull is paramount.

The bull, with his muscles of iron and weighing 1,500 pounds, ferociously pawing the ground, speaks of supercharged strength and sacks of semen-cargo. Venerated for his thundering power and gigantic size, the bull is colossally libidinous and has been sculpted, painted and invoked for thousands of years. With Wall Street's bronze sculpture *Charging Bull*, New York financiers seek to channel his macho spirit, charging towards aggressive financial trading and charging a bullsack for their services. Capitalism, like shamanism, conjures spirit animals for its own purposes.

~

When I was in Dublin a few years back, I went to see the Book of Kells and I was knocked sideways. It is a manuscript of the four Gospels, believed to have been created in a Columban monastery in Ireland or Scotland about 800 CE. It is illustrated extravagantly with illuminations of gold leaf and pigments of red, yellow ochre, verdigris and indigo. Animals teem through the pages. You'd think the artists have drunk the hare, then let the kittens into the church organ and invited the otters to play havoc in the monastery library, their minds bendy as a baby elephant's trunk, as they listened to a Latin Mass played on a kazoo by kangaroos. They are cartoons of imagination but conjured by real animals. Take the animals out of the Book of Kells, and it loses its soul. Take the animals out of many cartoons, and the brains and intuition are gone. Tintin without Snowy. Charlie Brown without Snoopy. Wallace without Gromit. The lead of Disney's cartoon *Robin Hood* is not a man but a fox, quick-witted and charming.

~

In contemporary society, humans are predominantly interested in the doings of other humans, gazing fascinated at ourselves. Narcissus, staring at his own reflection in the lake, was so self-absorbed he forgot to eat. He didn't notice the animals that surrounded him and who are a jubilant remedy. He didn't see the mother-of-pearl rainbow on a dragonfly wing. Hungry and thirsty, he refused lakewater, drinking only his own image, taking the mythic selfie until he faded, famished, desolate and alone. In a world gradually emptied of animals, the great commons of the human imagination risks becoming narcissistic. Without the Others, human culture is sere and self-regarding, its species-selfie a cracked wing-mirror in an arid desert reflecting on nothing but itself.

Those whose politics and traditions oppose that species-centrism may directly identify themselves with animals, so environmental activists have named themselves after particular creatures, such as Badger and Reed Warbler in Britain, while in the United States they have taken forest names including Thrush, Rabbit, Skunk, Minnow, Sparrow, Earthworm, Magpie, Turtle, Grasshopper and Butterfly.[12]

Native American societies by tradition honoured animals in name-giving. Some of the followers of the old Sioux chief Red Cloud were named Smoking Bear, Eagle Horse and Wolf-on-a-hill, while Luther Standing Bear writes of White Hawk, Swift Bear and Black Crow,[13] and Black Elk names Eagle Wing Stretches, Rattling Hawk and Bear Sings.[14] The mother of Chief Plenty-Coups, of the Absarokee or Crow Nation, was called Otter-woman; his father was called Medicine-bird and one of his grandfathers was Coyote-appears. (His mother's mother was intriguingly named It-might-have-happened.)[15]

Animals are a necessary invigoration in our cultural life. Museums and galleries are usually enclosed and cut off from the animating forces of nature, and the National Portrait Gallery is an exemplar: silent, stony and still portraits of people frozen in time, the sitters ever unalive. The sheer deadness overwhelms me – dead art portraying so many dead people, almost all of whom are enclosed, solipsistically sequestered in a square for one. But over the course of a night in 2004, an extraordinary animation took place: a fox was released in the middle of the night in the gallery, a piece of performance art called *The Nightwatch*, by Francis Alÿs in collaboration with Rafael Ortega and Artangel.

Fox is on the loose with his 'sudden sharp hot stink', in the words of Ted Hughes.[16] Against the pale blue walls, painted like the studied sky of eternity, the fox is rough-red and prowling. By dint of simply being a living animal, the fox (name of Bandit) seizes your attention, sniffing, listening and unpredictable. Bandit is a good name for a fox, being a Trickster animal. Tracked by security cameras, Bandit is first curious and inquisitive, with his ears pricked, until after some time he jumps up on to a bench under a painting, curls up and sleeps.

Take the wolf and watch how it galvanizes culture. The wolf lopes through Jack London's books – his first story collection was titled *The*

Son of the Wolf – he named his dream house 'Wolf House' and loved being called Wolf. The wolf calls to the wildness in us. Hilary Mantel heard the wolf howl in Wolf Hall. The band Wolf Alice took their name from an Angela Carter short story, with the feral, fierce, beautiful wolf within it. A wolf note, a wolf whistle. Wolf will out, creeping into grandmother's clothes or striding out in a suit and tie, like the werewolf of our worst side in *The Wolf of Wall Street*. Wolf provokes a siren shiver, a quiver in our own hackles. It is an utterly unjust portrayal of wolves, but it demonstrates how culture is dynamized by so wild and so unrestrainable a creature. When the Nordic gods tried to chain the death-wolf Fenrir, the only thing that worked was magic: the dwarves devised a 'supple fetter' and a subtle one, made from the footfall of a cat, the breath of fish, spittle of birds, the anguish of the bears and barely existing things.

Animals are the life blood of art, pulsing through time. Dolphins swim in a seascape fresco on the walls of the royal palace at Knossos in Crete and they have been smiling there since about 1600 BCE, thought to have been chosen to decorate the queen's bathroom there. The horses of George Stubbs seem almost alive, as do the dogs of Edwin Landseer, who seem to be playing in front of our eyes. Landseer's lions in Trafalgar Square have presence, power and pride. Wherever you look, animals vitalize art. At Somerset House recently, Chila Kumari Singh Burman installed an ice-cream van decorated in the traditions of the artist's Punjabi heritage, with, on the roof of the van, a neon tiger, and that was the detail which flickered the neon in the audience's mind.

The shamanic German artist Joseph Beuys knew the imaginative power of animals and in 1974 he spent three days in an art gallery in New York with a coyote, in a performance piece called *I Like America and America Likes Me*. On arrival at the airport, he was wrapped in a large cloak of felt, driven to the studio by ambulance and carried in on a stretcher to highlight that this artwork was about collective sickness and the role of animal spirits in healing it.

During those days, the young female coyote is sometimes unnerved, occasionally hostile and often curious. She tugs at the felt robes while

Beuys moves into a kind of symbolic communication, trying to make eye contact with her, throwing his leather gloves for her to catch, holding the coyote in a brief hug, gesturing with his hooked shepherd's crook, all the while making his movements into a kind of ritual.

Copies of the *Wall Street Journal* are brought in for the coyote to piss on, with fresh copies supplied daily: the contempt of the artist for the bulls of Wall Street enacted. (There's something about animal responses that delights us: the redoubtable journalist Amol Rajan got the giggles on BBC Radio 4 when his interviewee told him about urban foxes in London pissing on copies of the *Financial Times*.)[17] Coyote, for many Native Americans, is Trickster, teaching humans survival skills. For Beuys, Coyote was America's spirit animal, holding within itself a history of predation, racism and attempted annihilation. 'You could say that a reckoning has to be made with the coyote, and only then can this trauma be lifted,' Beuys said.

I have in my study a precious Nick Hayes woodcut with a fox playing a clarinet and a hare playing a banjo: every time I look at it, I feel a surge of joy as music and animals are combined. 'Happiness isn't happiness without a violin-playing goat,' says Julia Roberts to Hugh Grant in the film *Notting Hill*. Marc Chagall, whose work both characters love, was a goat-summoned artist. A goat plays a blue violin in one work, while in others there are sky goats. In a 1930 painting, *The Old Man and the Goat*, the man sits in snow while a small goat nuzzles his hand, as if about to suckle on his fingers, and both the goat and the man seem ecstatic because of the love between them. Chagall's imagination is most truly expressed through an animal: he is goat-sung and goat-whispered.

~

Animals not only inspire art but sometimes create art themselves. Bowerbirds famously make bowers with found objects, usually blue, chosen and artfully curated as part of the process of attracting a mate, while the satin bowerbird paints the interior of his bower with pigments made from plants and saliva.

Carl Safina writes of a baby bottlenose dolphin in an aquarium who watched a trainer smoking a cigarette and puffing out the smoke. At this, the dolphin went to her mother, suckled for milk and returned to where she could see the trainer. Then, she puffed out the milk. Safina comments: 'Dolly came up with the idea of using milk to represent smoke. Using one thing to represent something else isn't just mimicking. It is art.'[18]

An elephant, Siri, was born in 1967 and captured in the wilds in Thailand as an infant. Utterly bereft, for some years she was the sole elephant at the Burnet Park Zoo in Syracuse, New York. In the early 1980s, a trainer noticed she had a stick in her mouth and was drawing lines in dirt on the ground. He gave her pens and paper and paint, with which she seemed to create a repeated leitmotif of elephants' trunks. She was, perhaps, recreating her earliest memories of her mother and others, after those searing years of solitude. The artist Willem de Kooning called her a 'damn talented elephant', while Onondaga chief Oren Lyons commented, 'You can't speak for the animal. All you can do is appreciate what she has done – if you dare.'

Koko, the gorilla who learned sign language, also made art. A fledgling Steller's jay was rescued after a storm at the compound where Koko was living, and the bird often visited the gorilla. She painted it as a streak of blue, a flurry of feathers in red, with a yellow splash, and she gave it the title *Bird* in sign language. It doesn't look exactly like a bird, but it goes one better: it looks as alive as the soul of flight. Although she lived in captivity, Koko did have some access to nature, and one of her most famous paintings was a stream in a valley with pink flowers and blue-grey water flowing into white. She titled it *Pink Pink Stink Nice Drink*. (PINK PINK was her sign for 'pink'. STINK was her sign for 'flower'. NICE DRINK was her sign for 'good fresh water'.)

Koko taught Michael (1973–2000), a silverback gorilla, how to sign, and Michael also created art, including a painting done from memory of playing chase with his friend, a black-and-white sheepdog called Apple. Michael signed to humans that he was titling it *Apple Chase* and the picture captures the dog at full pelt in the vivacious energy of play, the flow of animal spirits in the flow of the paint.

~

Poetry is vitalized by animals, and poets are alert to them: as George Mackay Brown wrote, 'poetry should be given on the wind, like a lark or a falcon.'[19] In 905 CE, the poet Ki no Tsurayuki noted how animals were the very genesis of poetry in Japan: 'A nightingale singing among the blossoms, the voice of a pond-dwelling frog – listening to these, what living being would not respond with his own poem.' With baffling concision worthy of Wittgenstein, when Jacques Derrida considered the question 'What is poetry?', his answer is *hedgehog*.

The Irish poet Leanne O'Sullivan found her life devastated in 2013 when her husband, Andrew, became seriously ill. He was diagnosed with encephalitis, an inflammation of the brain, and fell into a coma for three weeks in hospital. Doctors said his survival was not assured and, even if he lived, he was likely to have catastrophic brain damage. In his illness, his brain on fire, Andrew had hallucinations of animals. This is not unusual among people recovering from strokes and brain injury: damage to the mid-brain often results in visions of animals,[20] as if right at the core of the human mind animals are living medicine, and the collective psyche knows it.

It was foxes and cats at first, and Andrew would see them from the corner of his eye. Coming out of his coma, Andrew tried to communicate what he saw. Leanne viewed the animals as a potential link between her and Andrew, a common language they could share. He spoke of seeing wild animals and birds whose voices reawakened a kind of healing knowledge in him, showing him 'how to return' to health. The animals, O'Sullivan says in an interview, were so important that they were almost totemic. 'Some other kind of intelligence [was] at work in his body.'[21] She decided to participate in the animal medicine, letting herself figuratively and emotionally melt into the fox that her husband saw, messenger between the worlds of the ill and the well.

Writer does not know Reader, but we meet in the forests of original thought, the Ur-language, where we *know-together* the turquoise glimpse of kingfisher or the boxy badger's snuffle. Like Leanne O'Sullivan meeting her husband, we too meet in the animalscape of the mind where both of us belong.

~

In the history of writing, early pens were made of feathers whose quills were sharpened into points called 'nebs' (now nibs), a word also used for the beak of a bird, so the writer's hand held the feather of flight and the beak of song.[22] Animals swoop, soar, glide and scamper through world literature, in every culture and every age. They tumble through the Epic of Gilgamesh; they shapeshift in medieval Icelandic literature as animal-warriors and berserker bears. A cock crows with unmitigated boast in Chaucer's Chaunticleer. They inhabit Japanese haikus; African literature is lit with legends where humans have an animal double; Russian literature rumbles with animals.

Children's literature fizzes, pops and squeaks with animals from nursery rhymes onwards. When Little Miss Muffet sat on her tuffet, 'Along came a spider and sat down beside her.' 'Hey diddle, diddle, the cat and the fiddle'; 'Hickory dickory dock, the mouse ran up the clock.' The latter possibly relates to a thirteenth-century astronomical clock at Exeter Cathedral, which was kept in working order by being greased with animal fats. The fats attracted mice. The mice ran up the clock. So from 1305 until 1467 two cats were 'paid' a penny a week to chase the mice, and the ancient door of the cathedral was even fitted with a cat flap, a hole in the door below the clock, to let the cats in to chase the mice.

Beatrix Potter grew up with animals as friends, and her pets included mice, frogs, bats, rabbits and a hedgehog; her work offers back to children the friendship of animals. As a child grows older, there is Pooh Bear and Tigger, the Gruffalo, and Fantastic Mr Fox. Animal stories are the right size and shape for a child's mind, inquisitive about capture, fear, bravery, nests, night and friends. Children's writers give animals voices and lead roles, and Aslan the lion speaks in tones of such strength and assurance that the psyche can be protected for a lifetime. Not many stories are written 'by' animals but there are some, and my favourite is Archy, the cockroach-author grappling with a typewriter, as written by Don Marquis.

Children's literature would be unrecognizable if you removed the animals. What would Alice do in Wonderland without the White Rabbit and dormouse and lobster and hookah-smoking caterpillar? The kitten at the beginning is associated with the mirror which enables Alice to cross over into the looking-glass world where the room has an unheimlich quality. Cats are border-crossers, half tame but never wholly; creatures of the dawn and dusk.

My favourite example of animals in vernacular art is the teddy bear. Medicine for the soul of childhood, a teddy bear helps a child sleep, a soft solace woven around them all through the night, and the teddy is still there at the drowsy fringes of the day when the child crosses back into wakefulness.

The contract between the teddy bear and their child is unconditional. Being loved, a teddy will love their child back. A teddy bear is the objective correlative of a cuddle, the paws outstretched for a hug, and the kindness of their eyes offers constant and tender attention. Guardians of sleep, protectors of the heart, teddies call a child into the warm den where they know themselves cub-beloved and never, ever alone. In the world of teddyhood, a child's soul is healed into the wholeness of the small animals they are.

Is a teddy bear, to a child's mind, alive? The Velveteen Rabbit knows. Stitched out of fabric and stuffed, the Rabbit is loved in the book by Margery Williams, but then abandoned for years. Eventually, though, he comes alive because he is loved a second time.

My childhood teddy was a monkey called Charlie, who I named after Charlie Chaplin. He came with a red collar and lead that I immediately removed, thinking he wanted to be free. He has a hard plastic face, big green eyes, and his head can turn all the way round. I slept with him for decades (yup), he in my right hand, lying across my chest with his left cheek pressing against me. So long was the love, and so repeated was the position, that his plastic face gradually morphed until it is now lopsided.

And was he alive for me? Of course he was. How? He was alive like a guardian angel is alive, because with him, I knew I'd always be okay in the end, and his consolation was a force field around me so my soul was protected and safe. It is no exaggeration to say that as a child and teenager I don't know what I'd have done without Charlie. Growing up, we had very few toys but I was (and remain) adamant that Charlie was not a toy. He was a talisman. Teddies provide comfort for life.[23]

Charlie slept with me until Otter arrived as a kitten when I was in my forties. One day, I was working in my study and heard an appalling fight going on in my bedroom. Otter, who seemed to think Charlie was as alive as I considered him to be, was attacking the little monkey, ripping him open, chewing ferociously at his threadbare legs. Charlie had to be rescued and relocated to a high shelf, and he now lives out his retirement in the most precious place in my study, with my gratitude forever.

~

Animals fertilize the collective mind in language. Someone may be as 'mad as a box of frogs'. Activities can be 'like herding cats' or 'going on a wild goose chase'; a person can be drawn to something 'like a bear to a honeypot' or 'a moth to a candle'.

Language, like an intelligent insect, keeps its antennae up for good expressions. Nervousness is most perfectly somatic when we speak of having 'butterflies in the tummy', while the feeling of being socially awkward is like being 'a fish out of water'. Animals scamper through our vocabularies, pounce into sentences and vivify our verbs: to dovetail, to badger, to fox, to squirrel away, to be a lounge lizard or a snake in the grass, to act kittenish, to be sheepish, dogged, coltish, or bat-shit crazy.

Animals wriggle into language, proliferating and often alliterative, busy as a bee, or stepping out rhyming with ants in your pants. Language is warm with animals, happy as a pig in a puddle, funny as a barrelful of monkeys. To play possum or to be as chipper as a squirrel in autumn. The dog's bollocks. The cat's whiskers. The bee's knees. To be owl-blasted is to be bewitched. We speak of moving like a bat out of hell. We know puppy love and horse sense, the latter meaning 'common sense'. We watch like a hawk, or go at a snail's pace, see someone taking the lion's share, or let sleeping dogs lie. According to Joseph D. Clark, author of *Beastly Folklore*, which compiles thousands of animal-based expressions, no other category of things is found so often in speech.

The presence of animals is written in sky maps. All over the world, cultures have seen animals in the stars. Hare, *lepus* in Latin, who leaps across the mind's sky, in the real sky gives its name to the constellation Lepus. For the Skidi Pawnee (of Nebraska and Kansas), part of the starscape is a herd of antelope,[24] while the people of the Pacific island of Kiribati see Dolphin in a constellation of stars,[25] and in what some call the Bear, the Saami see Elk and the Inuit see Caribou. Indigenous Australians refer to one constellation as 'Emu in the Sky'. The word *zodiac*, from ancient Greek, means a 'circle of little animals'.[26]

~

Art, story and song from Indigenous Australia is replete with animals, right from the beginning of the collective imagination, in the famous mythic concept of the Dreaming, or the Dreamtime. It looks at first sight like the past, an origin story as vast and ancient as the land, but it is more than that. It is a depth of time that surrounds the present, an other-time, ambiguous and diffuse, which envelops the now. The world was created in the Dreamtime by the Ancestors, who walked the land and sang it into being.

The Ancestors were the animals. Mythic beings, they were the combined imagination of collective life, and they made the waterholes, rivers or rocks where they slept, had sex and ate, giving shape, meaning and memory to every aspect. Their actions in the Dreamtime fertilized the now, ceaselessly giving birth to the present. The Emu is always at the Waterfall, and Possum at the Bluff. Indigenous Australian painting cannot but tell of the Dreamtime, and it bursts with animals, Yellow Goanna, Kangaroo Dreaming, and Wallaby Dreaming.

As the Ancestors walked and sang their way, they created paths that are known as Songlines, both music and maps of the land, and indeed also codes of Law and how to live well. Animals guide people walking the Songlines, so, for example, the Pitjantjatjara, living in the vast deserts of central Australia, understood insect maps. Follow the route as long as you can hear green ants singing, they would say, and when their song ends, head towards another voice, and onwards.[27] Take the animals out of Indigenous Australian art and its spirit fails, nothing left but dust and an appalled silence.

There is a bird whose song is a map. The marsh warbler migrates between their breeding habitats in Europe and down to Southern Africa. They mimic European blackbirds, sparrows, linnets, skylarks, stonechats, magpies and willow warblers. As they migrate through Africa, they imitate the birdsong they hear on their way, including the notes of the black-eyed bulbul and the calls of the bush warbler, the blue-cheeked bee-eater and fork-tailed drongo. They add more to their repertoire, collecting tunes from the Boran cisticola and the vinaceous dove. This is, says David Rothenberg, 'the one bird in the world who can recount its migratory path as a kind of songline, where the journey is mapped into the music itself.'

~

It seems appropriate that the Lascaux Cave in south-western France, with its ancient paintings of animals, should be discovered by one – a dog called Robot.

On 12 September 1940, Robot began curiously investigating a hole by an uprooted tree, and his companion, eighteen-year-old Marcel Ravidat, followed the cue of his dog and the astonishing works were found.

The Lascaux art includes a pregnant ibex and a pregnant horse: here, in the deep dark cave of the human imagination, fertility is made incarnate. The drawn animals seem to move, switching their tails, galloping, leaping, sweeping through the mind. They would have seemed almost alive in the flicker of the sandstone lamps the cave artists would have used.

One part of the Lascaux Cave is called the Axial Gallery, and here red aurochs' heads are painted in a circle, as if thought was flowing between their minds, and there are reindeer with antlers branching like creative thinking, each line giving rise to more.

The main chamber is mostly aurochs, literally the ur-ox, the original or first ox. I pause on that because it conjures, in my mind, a sense of absolute ancientness. Ur-ox. There is an ancient bear in the Chauvet Cave in south-eastern France, and the word for *bear* in ancient Greek, *arktos*, contains the root *arkh* ('chief', 'first' or 'primary'), also found in words such as *archangel*, *archaeology*, *archetype* and *archaic*. These caves speak of the ur-life of the mind, the subterranean, primordial and archetypal thinking from archaic time that fertilizes us with the spirits of animals, fluid, fleet and forever.

A lion's tail spirals in the cave art found in Tassili n'Ajjer, in Algeria, which also has images of giraffes, elephants, a sleeping gazelle and a round-nosed, big-eyed baby hippopotamus. In cave paintings, it is animals that are painted. This is so well known that its importance can be overlooked. The earliest art, in other words, was inspired by a thrilled, observant and almost certainly shamanistic entrancement with animals.

When San shamans of Southern Africa painted animals – an eland, for example – they are understood to have touched their essence and found, through the power of the animals, how to enter the spirit world.[28] Half a world away, an Ojibwe spokesperson calls Native American pictographs 'true teaching', 'a map for your mind', 'the path to travel in the spiritual world', and 'painted dreams'.[29]

In the Colombian Amazon, vibrant ochre rock paintings have been discovered, dating back 12,500 years. Indigenous people who accompanied the researchers pointed out the half-human and half-animal figures that they thought were likely to depict transformative states of shamans shapeshifting: the figures include a bird-human, a lizard with a human head, a sloth-human and deer-human.[30]

In most cave art, while the paintings of animals are wonderswept and awestruck, the humans are haphazard little stick people. Are the animals touched with the glory of being gods? Are they a necessary route to the spirit world? Surely yes and yet more.

Animals are foster-parents to thought itself: they are how humans communicate ideas. Conjuring the animals in art or by gesture or mimicry, we could translate thought from one mind to another. We could express 'leap' by evoking the leaper hare, 'prowl' by noting the fox, 'vision' by pointing to the eagle, 'power' by the bull, and 'size' by the auroch. We could indicate the dazzling shapeshifting of the octopus, or the lowing, licking mother-love of cow.

Animals gave us an animate vocabulary and the embodiment of ideas as distinct as feather from fish-scale. Each species vouchsafes an entire and exact thought, uniquely selved and never elsewhere expressed, a way of being that is utterly its own, weighted precisely and freighted exquisitely, which speaks its part out into the world for other species to note, and each species fertilizes the imagination of every other.

'For EARTH which is an intelligence hath a voice and a propensity to speak in all her parts,' wrote Christopher Smart in *Jubilate Agno*. Each creature – including humans – is a thought in the full, complete intelligence of Earth. 'For I will consider my Cat Jeoffry. For he is good to think on, if a man would express himself neatly,' wrote Smart. I wonder if anthropologist Claude Lévi-Strauss had taken advice from Cat Jeoffry when he wrote that certain animals 'are good to think with'?

When Apollo, god of healing, sought guidance to find the right site for an oracle, he chose to transform himself into a dolphin, and the Delphic oracle is dedicated to this animal's wisdom. Dolphin mind was a good way to think. The contemporary American poet Eleanor Wilner writes marvellously of the word *elegy* as a large word 'with a nine foot wingspan'.[31] The bird is good to think on. Without birds we wouldn't know a wing by which to measure the span of thought. Thinking less and less through the animals, modernity is writing itself out of the script, paragraph by paragraph, parakeet by parakeet, worm by worm and word by word.

All species are imaginatively necessary for the human mind, in its myriad variety. When we think with animals, we humans draw on a wider imagination, and one that is stronger and more energetic by being more diverse. We think with animals, and our wild brains are hooting in the treetops, soaring in the skies. The ability to conjure animals as units of thought is necessary to cultural well-being, and the animals gave us the first sense of metaphor, 'as timorous as a mouse', 'as fast as a cheetah', 'as sensitive as an antelope'.

A sparrow flew through the mind of a man in 627 CE. Watching the bird, the man, a chief advisor to King Edwin of Northumberland, considered it as an image for the life of humans on Earth, coming from unknown darkness and after death returning again into a great blackness:

> It seems to me like the swift flight of a single sparrow through the mead-hall where you sit at dinner on a winter's day with your theigns and counsellors. In the midst there is a comforting fire to warm the hall; outside the storms of winter rain or snow are raging. This sparrow flies swiftly in through one door of the hall, and out through another. While he is inside, he is safe from the winter storms; but after a moment of comfort, he vanishes from sight into the wintry world from which he came.

In one moment, in one mead-hall, one sparrow gave wings to a thought so illuminating and profound, the sparrow making comprehensible what was incomprehensibly large in time and space. The story was written down by the Venerable Bede and the venerable bird was made immortal.

The sparrow fostered the metaphor that gave the thought its wings to fly. And it has flown for hundreds of years and into forever, one of the earliest written metaphors in English and still one of the loveliest. This is what the animals do: they offer a tumult of ways by which we can think the world, they make and keep the collective imagination in robust health, and the single voice of the human is interwoven with the songs of all the Others, and we see that sweet and only ever half-abandoned truth that the animals are our Ur-Imagination.

14

Wild Alleluia

'In ancient time, cats were worshipped as gods: they have not forgotten this' – Terry Pratchett

There is a waterfall in a forest, a cascade of silver six times the height of a human, and at the top the water seems to pause a while, then it leaps down in a thousand points of brilliant sunlight. This is the Kakombe waterfall in the Gombe Stream National Park, in Tanzania, where a chimpanzee is engrossed in a 'waterfall dance'. He approaches the falls with bristling hair, a sign of heightened arousal, and as he gets closer the sound of the wind, rustling the wet leaves of this fig forest, is drowned in the roaring falls. Jane Goodall describes it thus:

> His pace quickens, his hair becomes fully erect, and upon reaching the stream he may perform a magnificent display close to the foot of the falls. Standing upright, he sways rhythmically from foot to foot, stamping in the shallow, rushing water, picking up and hurling great rocks. Sometimes he climbs up the slender vines that hang down from the trees high above and swings out into the spray of the falling water.[1]

Chimpanzees normally avoid water, but in these dances, which last ten or fifteen minutes, the chimp is charged up with the power of the falls, throwing rocks which crash as percussion, drumming with the waterfall in uproarious exuberance. Although he has come alone, he does not act as if he is alone: he is dancing with the waterfall, magnifying its force, his godbody on full alleluia.

The chimp is porous to the waterfall's power and as it pours, his spirit surges. He scampers up rock ledges to the top and takes a flying leap over the cliff edge, then grabs a branch, standing on one leg with a vine in one hand, swaying and swinging back and forth, then hopping, elastic with delight. His sheer enthusiasm (from *en-theos*, 'the god within') jubilantly collides with the thundering waterfall and he shakes the branches to rattling, getting everything going, struck by his primordial imperative: *dance*.

Chimps perform rain dances in heavy downpours, and thunder and lightning that make the air electric are often the overture to these displays. It is almost always adults and mainly males who perform these dances, often alone though sometimes in groups,[2] and they seem to choose either places which are most animated – waterfalls – or times that are most alive – thunderstorms at the beginning of the rainy season – saluting them with their own life spirit.

In one rain dance, filmed at the Mahale National Park on the shore of Lake Tanganyika, a jungle storm crackles brief but heavy and a chimp climbs a tree, swinging on a vine with a thumping rhythm. Visiting humans are standing motionless in identical grey cagoules like drenched ghosts, perhaps thinking it might be risky to move in such a charged atmosphere. The chimp climbs up a slender elastic branch until his weight bends it down into an arc to swing on, and he pushes himself forward and back and side to side, then drops to the ground and runs. From a cloudy day in Mid Wales, watching safely online, my mirror neurones go AWOL, totally flipped out by the chimp's stamping swing, and I am swaying side to side on the same vine, with a chimp I've never met, in a place I've never seen. As in the waterfall displays, it feels as if he is rousing the sleeping world to the dynamism of the dance of life, storming encouragement. *Animé! Go for it!* Then he climbs again, sits, curls up and remains still. The rain is slowing and it is all over.

At the end of the waterfall dances, too, the chimp goes very quiet and often sits on a rock right in the stream, his gaze following the falling water in a place – and a mood – of reflection. Jane Goodall writes, 'Is it not possible that these performances are stimulated by feelings akin to wonder and awe? ... Would they worship the falls, the deluge from the sky, the thunder and lightning – the gods of the elements? So all-powerful; so incomprehensible.' As Goodall points out, the chimp's brain is so evidently like ours and they display emotions close to our own, including happiness, sadness, fear and despair, and she asks, 'Why wouldn't they also have feelings of some kind of spirituality, which is really being amazed at things outside yourself? I think chimpanzees are as spiritual as we are.'[3]

Chimpanzees also perform dances for heavy winds,[4] for earthquakes[5] and for wildfires: when savannah chimpanzees at Fongoli, Senegal, encountered a wildfire, an adult male was seen performing a slow, exaggerated display *towards* the fire,[6] and perhaps as the waterfall dance is addressed to the waterfall, so the wildfire dance is directed at the wildfire and, with the wind dances and quake dances, they are elemental rituals for earth, air, fire and water. Perhaps the primates feel the transcendence that dance can offer, the ecstasy of trance-dance, when the spirit is both embodied and ecstatic, known in spiritual traditions from Jesus as the apocryphal Lord of the Dance to the Sufi whirling dervish.

Adult male chimpanzees in the Gombe Stream National Park have been seen climbing alone to the top of a ridge at the end of the day, greeting another chimp at the top who has had the same idea, and holding hands as they sit down together and watch the sun set.[7] Chimpanzees in West Africa make rockpiles for no apparent functional purpose, and hurl rocks against trees: this is construed by researchers as possible evidence of chimpanzees creating a kind of shrine and indicating sacred trees, according to the Max Planck Institute.[8] The Oubi people of West Africa refuse to kill chimpanzees, considering them to be spiritually superior to humans.[9] Gorillas build mysterious stone circles or cairns which then, after a day or so, disappear – no one knows how – an enigmatic ritual and part of the reason why researchers believe gorillas have a spiritual sensibility.[10]

Primates seem to display a sensitivity to something *beyond*, a primal spirituality in the face of the forces of nature. Maybe they are quick to the ecstatic because they live alert to the places and moments that invite a reverie or a jamboree, a meditation or a rave. Perhaps our religious texts are just doing the secretarial work of the spiritual experience, keeping the minutes of the meeting with the divine, *It Was Thus*. Perhaps animals, without our words, maintain the primal experience, the original *It Is*, and they are not taking us 'back' in evolution to our earlier selves but guiding us 'within' to our deeper and most present self, always alive and always now.

This chapter explores how many spiritual traditions welcome the animals: they may be seen as emissaries of the gods or as gods in their own right. Animals give life to the soul politic, a spiritual medicine that vitalizes the collective psyche and sacralizes the living world.

~

The worlds of the gods teem with animals. The prophet Muhammad was a lover of cats, and one of his companions, Abu Hurairah, equally devoted to them, was known as the Father of the Kittens. Animals are everywhere in Hinduism and when Lakshmi (goddess of abundance) rises from the ocean, she is seated on a lotus leaf and bathed by winged elephants pouring water from their trunks over her, a sumptuous way to be showered with blessings.

Animals, like the divine, have shades of immortality: the individual kingfisher dies, but Kingfisher lives on, at the same spot on a riverbank. While one otter sickens, Otter lives, the capitalized Idea rather than the literal fact. In this, there is a healing and a consolation, for the animals are constellar with the gods, both eternal and immortal.

When the divine throws light across the landscapes of the soul, animals cast that light as rainbows, the infinite refractions of incalculable species and each one dazzling.

Some Maori cultures considered whales and dolphins to be divine messengers whose body language, including how they leaped from the water, were foretellings of health or sickness. In Shintoism, white horses mediate between the world of humans and spirits, while particular divinities speak through specific animals, so various gods speak through fox, dove, cockerel, rat, deer, dragon, ox and white snake.

Birds have long been thought to be divine messengers, from augury to their role in myth. The blind Greek seer Tiresias could divine the will of the gods because he learned the language of the birds. Two ravens, called Memory and Thought, brought news and prophecies to the Norse god Odin.

Birdsong is a universal language of the divine, a praise-poem for the world. Delicately interpreted in traditional Persian culture, all birds sing their *zikr*, prayers to remember and invoke God. All birds have their own *zikr* but the nightingale is incomparable because his *zikr*, never repeating itself, is endlessly new, a ceaseless creation of worlds of song, always inventing new names for God.[11] For Bosnian Muslims, the humming of bees is a *zikr* calling '*Huwe, Hū*', recalling the names of the divine, invoking love, calling the Friend and bringing the beloved closer than a bee's wing.

Birds intensify and quicken the air that is their element, and we readily find spiritual ecstasy in birds, perhaps because their flight puts them beyond our physical reach and their presence is so often caught only at the edge of sight, their voices at the edge of our hearing, while their most rapturous song is at the edges of the day, dawn and dusk.

Birds represent something timeless, slipping through the immediate instant into the eternal. One of the Cantigas de Santa Maria (a collection of thirteenth-century songs commissioned by Alphonso the Wise) tells of a monk who sat in a lush garden by a flowing fountain. He asked the Virgin Mary to give him a foretaste of heaven, at which a bird began to sing, and did so with such exquisite joy and power that the monk listened, spellbound, enraptured, enparadised, for three hundred years.[12]

The song of the skylark is sung at an ever greater pitch of intensity the higher he rises, until you cannot see him any more and he seems swept up in the rising spirals of the pitches of his own voice, as if the song itself is winged. The collective noun is an ascension of larks and as he casts his voice up into the sky he ascends, ineluctably drawn to it. The song transposes my soul into a higher key, beyond what my voice can reach, further, higher, where only the wings of spirit can attend.

The bird rises helical as he sings, spiralling in an ellipsis of space until his distilled song becomes brightness, magnetized to heaven's quintessence, pinpointing god.

By tradition, on Midsummer Day, Elders of the Eveny people of Siberia would pray for success and strength and the ritual would become so intense and powerful that, according to anthropologist Piers Vitebsky, each person was said to be carried on the back of a reindeer 'towards a land of happiness and plenty near the sun. There they received a blessing, salvation, and renewal. At the highest point, the reindeer turned for a while into a crane, a bird of extreme sacredness.'[13] It is the bird of midsummer, when the day is longest, and across many cultures the crane is a symbol of light and regeneration.

They are huge. The larger cranes stand over five feet tall with a wingspan of eight feet. A crane can fly up to forty-five miles per hour and their flight is an entire spiritual teaching for although the bird is heavy-bodied, rowing the air with powerful oar-wings, these huge beats do not rock the bird's body and, from the beak through to the tail, the bird is as straight as a compass needle aligned with the stillness at the centre of movement. Nothing sways it out of true.

The sandhill crane flies a mile high and can soar far higher, to 20,000 feet and beyond, while the Eurasian demoiselle cranes can fly over the Himalayas, three miles above sea level. In doing this they disappear from human sight, which could have given rise to the legends of those birds as the messengers of highest heaven.[14]

The collective noun is a dance of cranes, and the dance of two mating cranes is a symmetry of pure, divine grace. Their *pas de deux* is a *pas de dieu*. They spiral together, the two making one image from the curve of the breast to their long, S-shaped necks, rising into the shape of life's original signature, the DNA helix, even as they dance together to engender life, a coupling spiralling down countless generations.

In Japan, the crane is holy and by legend if someone folds a thousand origami cranes, the bird will answer their prayer. In Christianity, the crane is considered an enemy of Satan and a force for good. In pre-Islamic Arabia, the three chief goddesses were called the 'three exalted cranes'. Cranes are venerated in Hinduism, Buddhism and Taoism and revered among Native Americans.

This most sacred bird in the world is, intriguingly, also the oldest. A fossil of a ten-million-year-old sandhill crane was found in Nebraska, making them the oldest known surviving bird species, but in all the generations who ascribed sacredness to the bird, not one person could have known this objectively. The bird's specialness was intuited.

In an iconic stance, the crane stands on one leg, and this has engendered a particular, and exquisite, connection in a wide variety of cultures. The bird is seen to be standing with one foot in this world and one in the otherworld, and can move between them. There is a word in Irish, *corrguinecht*,[15] that denotes the essential crane-ness of something, and the term is associated with divination and satire, conveying the stance required in their performance, standing on one foot, with one hand tucked away in a pocket and one eye closed. The diviner (an early version of the poet) stands half in the real and visible world, and half in the otherworld, which is both a spiritual concept and the other mind, or the imagination. The open eye suggests sight. The closed eye suggests insight.

Crane is profoundly associated with letters and writing and the poetic sensibility. The Roman god Mercury, inventor of letters, god of writers, and a winged messenger, was said to have created the alphabet after watching the flight of cranes, and carried a 'crane bag' made of the skin of a crane for his treasures. Such a bag was the symbolic vessel in which the Irish sea god Manannán carried his most valuable possessions: folklore and, later, the alphabet. As Irish author Manchán Magan writes, the crane could reliably carry that priceless heritage of knowledge because it held the contents 'in an entirely different dimension'.[16]

This is spiritual healing for poets, who can feel so sundered by the divide between the otherworld of imagination where they dwell well and the ordinary world which they may find hard to navigate.

Watching a murmuration of starlings is like watching a black-and-white film of the Northern Lights, as the flocks sway, held together and stretched apart as if the sky is breathing the breath of god. If this isn't holy, I don't know what is. A murmuration of starlings is co-created beauty in *how* many dimensions? They gather in my memory, my mind lost in their multitudes, ego evaporated as birds take us beyond the solo into the irrefutable unity of sky.

In the twelfth-century Persian epic *The Conference of the Birds*, a huge flock of thirty thousand birds flies as one to find the ruler of birds, called the simorgh.[17] They fly through seven valleys, each representing the seven stages of the Sufi Way. The Valley of Searching. The Valley of Love. The Valley of Wisdom. The Valley of Praise. The Valley of Contentment. The Valley of Wonderment. The seventh valley is where the seeker's individuality is lost in God, as a drop of water is lost in an ocean and only divinity remains. But the birds, having gone through many trials on their pilgrimage, are drastically reduced in number when they reach that seventh valley: only thirty birds remain, one thousandth of the number who began. And – after all this – a herald forbids them from entering the simorgh's presence. They leave, turning back demoralized and weak, but then they fly over a lake and see themselves reflected back as one being. There is more. Together, in their oneness, they form the image of the simorgh. They think and they reflect. God is in all, and all is in God.

Oneness is an essential aspect of many spiritual traditions – being inseparable from Allah, being at one with the Christian God, or at one with everything in Buddhism. Animism and paganism likewise draw people into a oneness with the natural world, and ayahuasqueros and forest shamans seek that egoless affinity with all of livingkind.

It is rare, though, to hear a scientist describe this transcendence of the self as the primatologist Barbara Smuts has done. In Kenya, Smuts devoted herself to observing baboons in the Great Rift Valley, including spending nearly two years with just one troop, joining them when they woke at dawn, and staying close as they travelled through the day until they gathered to rest at night. Her sense of subjective consciousness seemed to merge with the group-mind of the baboons, and she began to feel part of something larger, a feeling she had never had before. 'I relinquished my separate self.'

When Smuts was researching the behaviour of baboons in the Gombe Stream National Park, she was with them one evening as they were walking to their sleeping area down a stream with many small pools in it. At one point, apparently without a sign given, they stopped at one pool and each baboon sat on a stone around it. Seemingly entranced by the water, they stayed there, quiet. In this concentrated contemplation, even the youngsters were still. After about half an hour, again with no clear signal, they just as quietly left. Smuts saw this happen only twice, and to her it seemed a spiritual event like a Buddhist *sangha*, a group of people joining in a time of meditation.[18]

~

A tiny caterpillar has just fallen out of my hair on to the pencil I'm writing with. The little thing is pale yellowy green, and only as long as the letters STA on my STAEDTLER pencil. I encourage it off, on to my index finger, and it climbs up, right to the top of the nail, where it lifts its head, turning each way, north, south, east and west, before it decides downwards is the best choice, and I help it on to a plant. (After this and the mating moths, I have to wonder at this point what *else* is in my hair?)

STA ET CONSIDERA MIRACULA DEI. Stand and consider the marvels of God.

'Every creature is a word of God. If I spent enough time with the tiniest creature – even a caterpillar – I would never have to prepare a sermon. So full of God is every creature,' wrote Meister Eckhart (*c*.1260–*c*.1327), German philosopher and theologian.

Animals have long been understood as soul guides. Donkeys, translucent to goodness, are accorded a special perception of divinity. Only two animals are given a speaking role in the Bible: the snake in Eden and the donkey belonging to the prophet Balaam. Balaam has been paid to make a journey that will betray his people and, although God tells him not to go, he disobeys and sets out. Nothing stops him, not even an angel with a drawn sword blocking the path. Balaam doesn't see the angel but the donkey does, and in order to obey the angel she disobeys Balaam, who beats her three times in retaliation, displeasing the angel.

It takes a donkey to recognize the angelic. In the Qur'an too, a donkey, unlike the humans, can perceive divinity. The donkey, named Ya'fur, can answer questions posed by Allah Himself and became the Prophet's companion on journeys. Ya'fur would knock on people's doors with his muzzle, and when the door was opened, the donkey would nod to the householder and indicate the Prophet, acting as a bridge between the human world and the divine, pointing out what the householders might otherwise overlook.

'Do but ask the animals and they will teach you: the birds of the air, and they will tell you,' Job cries, deeming them moral arbiters. In a contemporary parallel, Rod Coronado, an American environmentalist, calls to fellow activists: 'Pray to the powers of earth for guidance – stealth of Cougar, night sight of Owl.'[19] A dove was the guide for Noah. A giant three-legged crow was the guide for Jimmu, the legendary first emperor of Japan, and when the bird appeared, the gods were said to be intervening in human affairs.

In the village of Somié, Cameroon, people use spider divination, known as *nggàm dù*. According to local myth, spiders used to talk and they still do communicate. People ask questions seeking guidance, and the diviners convert these words into a series of tappings: vibration is the language of spiders. The spiders shift various leaves notched with symbols, each with a symbolic meaning, and the diviners interpret these movements back to the listening community. The diviners note the importance of different ways of knowing, both human and animal, suggesting that the spiders are social medicine, healing the soul politic. '*Nggàm dù* is understood as a sort of compass or as a guide that helps understand the future and prevents various problems that threaten our society,' the diviners say. (The practice may be a subtle, kind and wise way for village elders to unobtrusively guide their communities.) 'Our intention is, above all else, to listen; to find ways to work with acute sensitivity, guided by a sense of reciprocity and justice.'[20]

Animals are often considered a moral compass, offering ethical orientation. Seven animals are guides to the Seven Sacred Laws among the Anishinaabe. Respect is the Buffalo. Love is the Eagle. Courage is the Bear. Honesty is the Sasquatch (the mythical Big Foot creature). Wisdom is the Beaver. Humility is the Wolf. Truth is the Turtle.

On the last page of a thirteenth-century Jewish Bible kept in the Ambrosian Library in Milan, there is a miniature painting. It depicts a feast for the righteous on the Last Day where the guests are invited to dine and perhaps also to judge. The righteous are not people but animals, including a cock, eagle, ox, lion, donkey, leopard and monkey. David Brooks, Australian author and professor, remarks of this: 'to see the earth as God sees it we must view it . . . through the eyes of the other creatures.'[21]

In the period of the early saints of Wales and Ireland, if animals were on your side, it showed you were walking a divine path. So a curlew saves St Beuno's book of sermons from being lost at sea, and a bird drops a feather for St Laisrén of Devenish when he decides to write a book.[22] St Ciarán, founder of the Clonmacnoise monastery, who was gentle with animals, found they blessed his ways: a pet fox carried his psalter; and a deer would accompany him, letting him rest his prayer book in their antlers.

Hildegard of Bingen (1098–1179), herbalist, healer and visionary, was abbess of Fraumünster and this abbey was said to have been founded because of an animal guide. Hildegard and her sister Bertha were walking through a forest to pray at a chapel when in the heart of the forest a deer appeared with lighted antlers, glowing in the deep green. They considered the deer to be sent by God and followed the creature to a site by a river where, they surmised, the deer was giving them a sign that this was where the abbey should be built.

The feeling of awe – a perception of the divine beyond the self – is proven to be good for the human mind.[23] In a study fresh from Harvard University, spirituality has been demonstrated to be a vital part of health and well-being, both for those who are seriously ill and for the maintenance of overall good health in those who are not sick. The study noted that for those without a specific illness, spirituality is associated with healthier lives, greater longevity, less depression and suicide and less substance use.[24] The study's definition of spirituality included meaning, purpose, connection and transcendence, found not only in religion but importantly through nature, including of course the animals.

Meanwhile, fresh from the Middle Ages, the concept of *viriditas*, or 'greening', was the key to health. *Viriditas* is the divine healing power of green, according to Hildegard of Bingen, who minted the word. The very colour of the soul was green. *Viriditas* contains, through Latin, a forest of meanings – greenness, growth, vigour, freshness and vitality – and it expresses a heaven on Earth, the life force in nature being a physical and spiritual medicine. (I think there is a bit of *vir* in *viriditas* too, a virility that rises like green shoots in springtime.)

Viriditas is as leafy as lemon balm, as fresh as chives and as medicinal as rosemary. It is, for Hildegard, the opposite of *ariditas*, the shrivelled aridity, the craquelure of the desertified soul and dried-up uncreative spirit that leads to bodily infection. *Viriditas* as a healing force is oriented towards wholeness, its power joining humans to all of creation, including animals, who are symbols of the virtues. Green is thus more than a colour: it is an attitude, a power and a direction, the joy of life and the quintessence of health.

In one of Hildegard's visions, she saw animals, including crab, deer and leopard, blowing winds on to the image of a human because humans could not live 'if they were not enlivened by the breath of these winds',[25] the animating breath of the animals making the human soul healthy and singing.

Both Harvard and Hildegard agree.

~

Animals have often been seen as spiritual guardians. Lions guard the British Museum and Trafalgar Square. The ancient Egyptians and modern Britons alike have used lions at the doors of palaces to ward off evil. There are more than ten thousand lions in London alone, including at Buckingham Palace and Chinatown, while across the country, lions safeguard the gateposts of houses and offer stone prayers for protection, even if people erect them for mere prestige.

In parts of Vietnam, villages are guarded by tiger temples. A dragon protects many churches of Wales, while in the mountain forests of Radnor the last dragon of Wales is said to be sleeping and protecting the spiritual heart of the Welsh.[26]

The Bird of the Heart, perhaps a hen, rooster, pigeon or grackle (whose appearance is a delight; whose song is not), is one of many souls that the Tzeltal Maya of Chiapas, Mexico, believe inhabit each human and protect them, keeping them alive and well.[27]

Many individuals adopt an animal talisman, feeling spirit-strengthened if they see it. Children, with their perennially prehistoric minds, do this naturally. A fox, perhaps, or a red kite or hare. Then come the objects, the hare earrings, hare paintings, hare mugs and plates.

Owl motifs were carved on vases, cups and perfume holders in ancient Athens because this was the bird of Athene. The owl symbolized wisdom, and the Greek expression 'bringing owls to Athens' means much the same as 'bringing coals to Newcastle', as Athens had so much wisdom it needed no more. My home city of Manchester takes the symbol of the bee, promoting its identity as an industrious city, community-focused, good at thinking with the hive mind. The bee is on the city's coat of arms, on people's tattoos and T-shirts, and on bollards and bins.

'We are red macaws!' was the proud cry of men from the Bororo people in Brazil, considering the macaw to be their totem animal.

'Maharajah, let me pass!' members of the Kathiota Kol tiger-clan in India would call out in greeting, *salaaming* a tiger in the jungle, using these words as a passport to safe passage. The tiger, they said, would accept the homage and would never attack clan members.[28]

Totemic animals give the collective psyche ever greater dimensions of divinity. The Mirning and Kondoledjeri of South Australia are known as the 'Whale People' and their most sacred sites on land are close to, and correspond with, the places at sea where the southern right whales come to mate, give birth and play. Elders would go to the sacred sites of the Rainbow Serpent, which included sea caves and small openings in the rocky shoreline where the sea spray would create rainbows in the mists. There, at a special clifftop site, the Elders would sing to the whales, inviting them close, and the whales would approach while the Elders paid homage to these guardians.[29]

Many cultural beliefs include gods becoming animals. European mythology tells of Zeus regularly slipping into animal form, including the swan, while the goddess Ino takes the form of a shearwater. The Buddha takes many animal incarnations and was himself fathered by a divine elephant who used his trunk to impregnate Queen Maya, while the incarnations of the Dalai Lamas include rabbit and parrot.

~

Animals may experience spirituality (the chimps at the waterfall). They may offer humans spiritual protection (from spiders to lions). They may represent the spiritual realm (the crane) and they may be messengers, associates and lovers of the gods. For many cultures the animals are creator-gods in their own right.

The hare is the first creator for Native American Algonquin people, the one who makes sun, moon and Earth.[30] The heron's cry sets time in motion in Egyptian myth.[31] Snakes, we've seen, are dazzlingly magnificent creators in origin myths from Amazonia to Indigenous Australia.

I have a special fondness for hummingbirds, so named because these tiny birds beat their wings so fast that they hum. They can fly backwards as well as forwards, and can hover as well. So swift is their flight that they seem to appear and disappear in an instant. In the lore of the Mbyá people of Paraguay, the hummingbird is the divine creator. In order to create, the bird begins with primordial nothing – and itself. While its beak, seeking nectar, suggests the probing mind, this most iridescent of birds represents wisdom, the most iridescent of qualities. In a fantastically subtle perception of creative power, Mbyá philosophy suggests that when wisdom is actualized, it unfurls the world, first conceiving the idea of things and then creating them.[32]

When the ancient Aztecs saw Spanish conquistador Hernán Cortés arriving, they allegedly considered him a god and placed red cloth on the ground for him. Is it just me who finds this a rather self-serving story on the part of the Europeans? Perhaps it was not Cortés they considered a god but rather the *horses* that he and his soldiers rode. Aztecs, who saw divinity in so many animals (including hummingbirds), had never seen a horse before and had never known an animal so large, powerful, graceful and intelligent. When they saw a creature that seemed half man and half horse, perhaps it was the horse half that they saw as a god. (The horse was the only European animal that succeeded in becoming part of the myths and stories of Indigenous people of the Americas.)[33]

God is a horse. As sensitive as she is strong, as fast as she is intuitive. She does not know things *beyond* possibility but *between* possibilities, between fear and anxiety, between confidence and pride. Northern China had a cult of Heavenly Horses. Hinduism and Buddhism have a horse deity, and she is the goddess of the corn in Europe, the White Horse of Uffington.

God is a monkey, bouncing the breath of life like a ping-pong ball from now to eternity and back in a split second, circulating *qi*. In Hinduism, Hanuman is a monkey god and monkeys may be worshipped and fed in temples, and in Daoism, monkeys were considered transcendent and immortal. Chinese deities can take the guise of monkeys, including the Monkey King, born from a stone, who has god powers, runs at the speed of meteors, leaps 34,000 miles in one somersault, can shapeshift at will and can remember every monkey that ever there was.

God is a mouse. In India some temples are dedicated to the worship of wild mice, survivors who deserve respect. God is a rat. At the Karni Mata Temple in India, there are more than twenty-five thousand sacred rats. Banksy would be in heaven.

God is a cow, the milk of intimacy and mighty benevolence flowing together from heaven. Cow is sacred in Hinduism, with myths of the divine cow-mother and a cow heaven, provisioning all the Earth's abundance in fruit and vegetables, its mangoes, pomegranates, aubergines, courgettes, bananas and cauliflowers.

God is a goat. Cunnus and cock, the rude god, horny, each sperm-jet a new guffaw, the great god Pan was full-on goat. Worshipped in Greece, Italy and Egypt, god was profligate and promiscuous.

God is a fox. A blaze of intelligence, a perfect nose for night, a

Wild Alleluia

heightened awareness and a gift for friendship. The Japanese deity of foxes presides over tea and sake, fertility, rice and household well-being.

God is crocodilian. The Egyptian god Sobek was a fierce protector against evil and took the form of a crocodile, and Sobek's main temple was in the city of Crocodilopolis.

God is a frog. For the ancient Egyptians, the frog goddess Heqet was goddess of fertility and particularly associated with both the final stages of the Nile in flood and the final part of childbirth. Frog is a divine midwife.

God is a raven. He has a beak and wings. He hops. God is a scamp with beady eyes and black feathers. God is not solemn and never goes to church, because he is easily bored. He is a fire-bringer and sun-finder for Koyukon people. (The sun was lost under a blanket in a woman's house; raven found it, rolled it to the door and then up into the sky.)[34] He lived first in bird-land, the land of spirits, but got sick of it. He carried a stone in his beak until he got tired of that too and tossed it down into the ocean, where it grew and grew, swelling and plumping up to become the land. God is a career-buffoon, an omniscient fool, power-clown, messenger, way-finder, jester, yes sir, Yes Men. A light-fingered thief, raven fingers light itself. He then gives it away in the refracted poetry of sun, moon and stars. He is a major god for Native Americans of the northwest including Haida, Tlingit, Kwakiutl and Dene peoples.[35]

God is a bear. The good brown bruin of the soil. God is all paws with a taste for berries; he enjoys a tipple and has a sweet tooth. God has a big bum and a good waddle on him to get him over rivers and mountains to his second home in the otherworld. God is a furry soul-mender, he is mighty, mysterious and a myth unto himself. A winterer, god hibernates tucking his nose between his paws for the sleep of a giant comma in the pause of the year. Bear has been worshipped widely across the world, by everyone from Finnish people and the Celts of Gaul and Britain to Ainu people and across North America.

Why *wouldn't* all these be gods?

As far back as we can know, societies have considered animals to be gods, as necessary as the air we breathe. We are, already and again, walking within the transcendent. There are gods in the woods, a wren on the flute, hedgehog on sax, bat on piccolo, stag on bassoon, with brittle stars on timpani and octopus on the violin, while whale sings the basso profundo of it all, in the wild orchestra. Animals ensoul the world, giving the collective psyche limitless dimensions of sacredness.

We could, with relief, acknowledge divinity again in the real and living world, knowing it as the truth that has so far vouchsafed humanity's time on Earth. Then the collective psyche could come to its senses and the individual soul come home to itself, letting the soul-medicine that has always surrounded us work its ordinary miracles, in the holy and reckless plurality of the animals, each one an iteration of life's deepest prayer: *let there be life.*

15

Spiderling, Chickadee, Finch and Friends

'Myths are public dreams, dreams are private myths'
— Joseph Campbell

Look! I want to cry out to everyone I have ever met and ever will.

Look at this glistening sphere, sheltering a world of dreams! Look at this: the eye of the spider!

Jumping spiders go to bed at night in little silken pouches called 'retreats', their own sleeping bags, and if you approach very quietly and gaze into the eyes of baby jumping spiders, you can see them dreaming. In the first ten days of life, the spiderling's exoskeleton has no pigmentation and you can look clean through the head, right into the eyes that, like other dreaming eyes, have flurries of rapid eye movement (REM).[1]

In another indication that they are dreaming while they are in this state, their little legs twitch into a curl and then spring out uncurled again, while their spinnerets go crazy in spinning their silk threads. Spider silk has, per weight, the tensile strength of steel and they rely on it, for although jumping spiders don't make webs they do set tiny anchors of silk so when they take a leap they always have a safety cord, like a bungee rope, tucked into the back of their trousers.

Okay, I made up the trousers.

But nothing else.

For all of us, the dreaming mind lets out skeins of silk both fine and strong that connect the inner world and the outer. Dreams are anchored to the real and yet take place in the realm of reverie as a spider spins the silk from inside herself, attaching it to something outside herself.

In Lakota stories, Iktomi is a Trickster spirit who often takes the form of a spider. Long ago, they say, when the world was young, a Lakota healer had gone to a mountain, taking a hoop made of willow decorated with feathers and beads. He was on a quest for a vision.

He saw a spider and recognized him as Iktomi. Iktomi took the man's hoop and began to spin a web. As he did so, he spoke of how life, like a spiderweb, contained many different possible turnings and of how important it was to listen to the right voices to make good decisions. Iktomi made the hoop into the first dreamcatcher, that decorative web hung above a sleeper's bed that may catch the good dreams and let nightmares float away. (In an explanation considered equally valid, dreamcatchers are also interpreted as trapping nightmares in the web, to stop them getting to the dreamer.) The fact that some spiders are themselves dreamers gives the symbol an extra layer of significance.

A couple of days ago my friend Anita Roy, writer and editor, came to stay. I told her about baby jumping spiders. She in return told me of going to spend the previous night in the woods and dreaming of an owl. Dreams were in the air. We wanted to walk, and set off for the source of the River Severn, picking our way through a forest. There was a dense autumn mist, and tiny beads of moisture had settled on a myriad of spiderwebs that were cast everywhere. Every fern, every fir-tree needle, every patch of heather, gorse and bilberry were traced with silver light.

This landscape is always filled with spiderwebs and although I've walked here many times I have never seen it spider-laced like this. On this day the landscape, decorated in every inch with that haze of silk, had a penumbra rarely seen. Only in that mist-light could this happen and as it changed the literal view, the opaque light also seemed to shift our minds to the dreamscape of the forest. Just as the webs are always there but seldom visible, so dream surrounds us all the time but is rarely present to the waking mind. The landscape was dreaming and we could see through the exoskeleton, right into its eyes.

~

This chapter explores the dreamworld where we dwell with the animals: they dream, and we dream of them. The chapter then considers how the collective psyche also dreams, through fairy tales and medicine stories. Over thousands of years, communities have created collaborative, collective dreams, catching them and spinning them into stories that help and guide the collective psyche. Fairy tales and medicine stories are cures for the individual soul and they are also remedies for the soul politic. More: these stories have animal medicine right at their heart.

Dreaming is delicate as spider silk and yet has an influence so strong we cannot argue with it. Dreaming is a subtle, diffuse dimension of life, and we're all there.

Who's *we*?

Spiders. Rats. Cats. Dogs. Zebra finches. Humans and other primates. Many animals dream.

Cats dream of hunting, of jumping, of grooming and defending, in what is called 'paradoxical sleep',[2] when the body is almost inactive but the mind has put on its seven-league boots. If I'm sleeping on my side, Otter may sleep alongside me, his back to my front, and push his paws into my palms and then if he dreams, his dreams twitch in my hands so we share his dream. Blind Otter, dreaming through my paws.

If rats are presented with mazes in the daytime, they later practise running through the mazes in their dreams, remembering or relearning them, and they see and hear in their dreams what they saw and heard in the day, re-experiencing the same emotions.[3]

Both zebrafish[4] and zebra finches dream. More than this, zebra finches dream of singing.[5] They experience the REM state and then their forebrains fire neurons in a distinct pattern, one that also takes place when they are awake and singing. It seems that their sleeping brains replicate the pattern of their singing, suggesting, say researchers, that these songbirds are moving their vocal muscles to the music of their dreams.

It is thought that octopuses may dream. They are known to have different sleep stages, including a quiet sleep stage when they stay the same colour and an active sleep stage when they change their patterns and textures and may show erratic movement, thrashing their tentacles as if they are trying to escape a predator and then inking their tanks while still asleep, a known anti-predatory response.[6]

Dogs evidently dream. Sleeping dogs may well smell other animals even at a great distance and respond in the subliminal world of dream, barking accordingly.

For the Runa people of Ecuador, human knowledge is extended along the threads of a dog's dreaming, like spiders knowing what is happening at a scale far larger than themselves, by detecting (with their feet) vibrations on their webs. Runa people pay close attention to the dreams of their dogs at night, listening for the different whimpers and tiny phrases uttered in sotto voce barks. Dogs bark differently according to what they are dreaming about, say the Runa, who interpret the barks as a foreshadowing of the future. If a dog barks 'hua hua hua' while it dreams, they believe the dog is dreaming of hunting, and the following day the dog would be out chasing animals. If, by contrast, the dog barks 'cuai' in the night, it would be a sure signal that a jaguar would kill them the following day, for this is how dogs cry out when attacked by felines.[7] Dogs do, in effect, smell the future, being able to detect things that are at some distance but on their way towards us. Like a jaguar.

Michael, the gorilla who learned sign language and painted his dog friend Apple, was a dreamer and when he had been dreaming his past sometimes slipped its moorings and washed into his present. One day he woke in terrible distress and a human he trusted went to sit with him. Michael explained in sign language that he had dreamed of the morning in the rainforest in Cameroon when he had been captured as a baby and his family murdered. Michael signed the gunshot. He signed the screams of fear and pain. The shock, the trembling and the blood, he signed. He had been orphaned from babyhood and was held in terrified isolation for months. He couldn't forget, and his dreams surrounded him in an atmosphere of grief and terror.

Knowing that so many animals dream augments our experience of the world, enriching the psyche and deepening the dreaming self. The dreams of animals open the individual to wider worlds and wilder ways of perceiving, for we are not limited to our single selves but can breathe in the dreams of the others in the common air of all.

~

Sleep is medicinal, vital for the health of the psyche, and has been called 'overnight therapy'. Sleep washes over us, rinsing the mind in mental housework, and dreams sweep up and tidy away our memories.

Animals lead us towards sleep and the dreamosphere. Stroking pets is a category of touch known as 'idle play',[8] beguiling and calming at the same time. Petting them induces gentle reverie or soft fascination, as the poet William Cowper experienced when stroking his pet hares, that state as delicate as a dream in which we are entirely present and yet inattentive to anything else.

At Lydney in Gloucestershire, there is a Roman healing temple dedicated to the Celtic god Nodens where sleep was the curative element, and the medical assistant to the god was a dog.[9] The dog's role was to guide the sick to the Land of Nod. Ancient medicine and contemporary corporations concur on how animals transport our psyches into medicinal sleep. Marketing and design departments create pyjamas with dalmatians, owls, unicorns, flying horses, sleepy kittens and snoozing bear cubs. Hot water bottles, to tuck us into dream, come in the shape of rabbits, bears, penguins, turtles and frogs.

When we fall asleep, we may dream of animals. Chuang Tzu, an ancient Taoist Chinese philosopher (c.369–286 BCE), wrote that he dreamed he had turned into a butterfly, but when he woke he had not been able to decide whether he was a man dreaming of being a butterfly, or a butterfly dreaming of being a man. Dreams such as this can transform us, radically altering our perspectives.

People look for meanings in dreams about animals. Gypsy dream-interpretation suggests that dreaming of a mosquito points to persecution, whereas in Islam a mosquito in your ear denotes blessing, status and authority. In the second century CE, Artemidorus of Ephesus collected over three thousand accounts of dreams in a book, according to which dreams of dragonflies can mean change, regeneration or flightiness; a dream of a katydid means the dreamer will miss out on opportunities due to an overly laid-back attitude, while a dream of a mantis means the dreamer is involved in a destructive relationship. Dreaming of bees means good luck for farmers but to others it is a warning of destruction by a mob.

Between 30 and 50 per cent of the dreams of children below the age of ten are about animals. After that, the frequency of animals in dreams begins to drop, so, for those aged between fourteen and sixteen, animals appear in less than 14 per cent of dreams, and after the age of eighteen, in less than 7 per cent.[10]

Intriguingly, 30 per cent of dream animals, including in the dreams of adults, include a hint of faerie, with animals talking or metamorphosing into other animals or people.[11] I had one such dream when I was beginning this book, when I dreamed of a black guide dog. Like a good dog, she could find people. Like a good doctor, she could guide them. Her kennel was a treehouse, with a wooden staircase leading up to it, and she took me and her two companion dogs up into the treehouse. There were three little pallet-beds, with small mattresses for the three dogs. I felt like Goldilocks. Her gifts were communication (language in all its forms) and, evidenced by the little pallet-beds, a bestowing of healing sleep. She was a guide-dog doctor, guiding dogs and people to sleep. It was a guiding dream for me.

The artist Rima Staines paints the world of faerie. Hers is an apothecary art, distilling that otherworld of our collective dreaming, with Baba Yaga the grandmother witch and her house built on chicken legs; clogs and pipe smoke perhaps, a kettle, a claw and a lantern; feather, heather and zither and old eyes sunk deep in knowledge. In one painting, a baby nestles tenderly into the branches of a horse-chestnut tree, looked after by an owl, while a fox, badger, mouse and hedgehog are intertwined with the tree's roots, suggesting how the animals are the source of dream and story, caring for the psyche.[12]

I dreamed once that I was driving up a very old lane in Wales. (Wales is old, in rocks, language and myth.) I had to leave my car behind to walk far and farther than far, beyond the road and into myth.

Rima Staines was there. The day was old and turning to twilight. In the deft way that dreams have of catching one detail and making it spark, my old red tartan pyjamas were there, suggesting a dream within the dream. We reached a place where there were animals carved in stone. The oldest beings were the animals, acknowledged by all those who indicate the way towards them. I woke up certain of the dream's meaning, the importance of taking the old roads to the old knowers, attending to the old stories and the animals carved into the mythic lithic psyche.

In myth and folk tales, animals take on some of the psyche's jobs that seem insuperable – and often do so in our sleep. The goddess Psyche is set impossible tasks by her horrible mother-in-law, Aphrodite, who in one version of the story mixed together wheat, barley, millet, poppy seed, chickpeas, lentils and beans into an indiscriminate heap and told Psyche to sort them into separate piles. Ants take pity on her and do the necessary work, turning what is indiscriminate into distinct categories, this ability which is crucial to thought. When Cinderella's stepmother gives her the task of picking lentils out of the ashes before she can go to the ball, she is rescued by turtle doves who do this meticulous sorting-work for her. Vasilisa, in the Russian fairy tale, is similarly given an impossible task by the terrible Baba Yaga, who demands she pick over a sack of millet, seed by seed. Vasilisa falls asleep but the animals come – the tits, pigeons and sparrows – and do the mind-sorting for her as she sleeps.

~

Fairy tales are never mere entertainment. They are cures, created by the collective psyche and for the collective psyche. The soul politic has long understood that stories are healing, with Native American cultures naming them medicine stories.

Fairy tales are indeed medicine stories, although for hundreds of years the dose has been diluted, the potions mixed with piety or misplaced politics, the power of the animals reduced, their medicine rendered meek and milky. Despite this, fairy tales and folk tales are still healing, guiding people towards healthy ways to be in the world. At the heart of all the world's medicine stories are animal healers.

The stories often begin with a fracture in the moral universe. The protagonist of folk tales may be wronged, falsely accused, subject to unwarranted ridicule, unfairly treated, socially injured and forced to seek goodness in the world beyond their family. The hero is often a victim of poisonous lies told by a scheming sibling or servant in order to steal their rightful reputation or inheritance.

Animal healers have been spiritually bowdlerized to mere 'helpers' in fairy tales. But they are still there. Where there are lies, the animals speak the truth. Where there is ridicule, they restore esteem. Where there is injustice, the animals take the side of the underdog (often represented in stories by the overlooked and mistreated youngest child). The animals support the ecocratic imperative that everyone, from king to spiderling, matters.

Crucially, the stories say, when humans harm, animals heal. They guide the protagonist out of bad situations, often through a period of loneliness which the animals heal by simply accompanying them through the darkest forest, perhaps in a nonchalant saunter (for they offer healing but seldom pity) and then leading them at a dog trot to the Good Others, the kind father or worthy princess.

In the story 'The Goose Maid', a young girl is due to be married to a prince but on the way her servant steals the badges of her identity: her gold cup, silk dress and her magical horse, Falada, who has the gift of speech. The servant wears the dress and uses the cup and poses as the bride, marrying the prince. Subject to this identity theft, the true bride is forced to be a goose maid at the palace. This is bad enough, but the false bride orders Falada to be killed. Even after death, though, the horse speaks, and tells the king what has happened. The unfailing and infallible Falada is the truth-speaker and because of him, the king restores people's rightful positions. The animals, say the stories, are dedicated to remedying the situation. They are the conscience of the collective psyche.

In fairy tales, the animals help people who show certain qualities:

being kind, generous, honest, courageous, canny, curious, alert and open-hearted. The animals represent an unimpeachable ethical dimension because they behold the moral timbre of each person. Notably, they reward those whose qualities are remedial for the soul politic, working for the good of all.

In fairy tales, the animals categorically do not offer their healing help to everyone. The greedy older brothers or sisters, those who are selfish, unkind, ungenerous or dishonest, get no help from the animals and are left to suffer their own ethical sickness, stewing in a vat of their own toxic juice.

Once upon a time, there was a miller who had three sons. He was a bit of an oaf, and when he died, he left the mill to his oldest son and his donkey to his middle son, and the youngest son got nothing except the sodding cat.

One day, a dreary day inside and out, the youngest lad was sitting on an upturned bucket outside the stable, with his head in his hands, thinking how utterly miserable his life was and would always be. But just then the undauntable cat jumped on to his lap, nudged him with her paw and said, 'Pfah! There's no water in these rivers to run the manky mill and the mule is a moping mass of mange and misery – but me! I am a cat of cats, a cat of cleverness, a cat of tricks, and I can bring you mice and tell you jokes and, what is more, I will make your fortune. For I am a cat who can *talk*.'

So begins 'Puss in Boots', where the disregarded and disinherited youngest child has been made sick by cruelty and despair. Puss, ogre-beguiler and princess-finder general, provides him with not only the symbolic riches of a good life but soul-food, encouragement, *ánimo!*

I can attest to the healing power of this story: I have returned to it over and over again in my life, and Puss empowers me when I feel weak. When I first read it as a child, I sort of fell in love with Puss. The cheek of her, this cat of pure panache! (And I wanted those boots.) Going back to the story when I was older, I could feel the pain of the wronged son, the sense of depression and his desperate need to find a way out of his situation. He needs a touch of the Trickster to turn things around, to help him be bold, someone whose imagination works like crazy-paving to cross a quagmire.

And Puss is indeed indecently trickative. She joins the illustrious clan of Trickster figures. Every society knows the Trickster, and in many stories Trickster is an animal: Coyote, Raven, Fox, Rabbit, Crow, Bluejay, Raccoon and Iktomi the Spider. The Monkey King in China. Brer Rabbit, originating in African myth. The Cat in the Hat. Wile E. Coyote. Trickster stories are medicine, bringing charisma and transformation. Many Trickster stories are also coded ways to caution us about archetypal human downfalls, warning that those who seek to entrap others and who act with greed will end up caught in their own traps, the victims of their own appetites.

The animal helpers are the relics of shamanism's powerful animal healers in cultures that have temporarily forgotten their shamanic roots. The essential animal medicine survived, but only just. From the coiled vines of trance and chants, from the huge lianas of medicine stories, down the ropes of staunch myth, still strong enough to haul a cargo of culture, the medicine survived. Reduced by misogyny and hammered by zealous anti-paganism, still the stories survived, in braided nettle roots, thin but tough, and then they were whittled down again, attenuated to a hank of wool, the old wives and the grannies of misrule still carding and carding, down through the hands of the Victorians, where the tales became a thread of cotton, the white of pure innocence, not the bright red thread of living story. And then Walt Disney.

If I asked a spider, I expect they'd be glad for Disney. Better him than no one, they'd say sensibly, better there was someone to keep something of the soul-language alive, even if it's just a tiny filament, because even the thinnest strand may still carry the spider silk of soul-language woven into webs of story.

In medicine stories, animals guide the collective imagination to position its intelligence within the wider intelligences of other creatures, like the Runa people expanding their knowledge along the filaments of their dogs' dreaming.

Animals such as Falada and Puss in Boots can talk, communicating between their worlds and ours. In the tradition of folk tales, animals (including frogs, wolves, goats, snakes and birds) often help the heroes by speaking human language, but further healing can happen when they can learn the languages of the animals.

In Greek myth, Melampus is a healer who was helped in his curing work by the animals. In one tale, he showed kindness to two orphaned baby snakes, looking after them and raising them. In thanks, the little snakes licked his ears so clean that he could understand when the animals spoke.

The German fairy tale 'The White Snake' begins with a young man at court, clear-eyed and gentle-hearted, who is falsely accused of stealing the queen's ring. He sees a snake in the woods, approaches it in friendship and smiles at it. It smiles back then glides away, leaving him with the gift of understanding the languages of the animals. Because of this, he can hear the sparrows chattering about a fat duck who swallowed the queen's ring. He gets the ring back for the queen but refuses to stay at court, not trusting those who have so wronged him. He sets out to seek his fortune. On the way, he sees salmon who can't manage to jump upstream as the river current is too strong, so he helps them. Then he helps ants whose city is being trampled and later meets three starving ravens and feeds them. The salmon, ants and ravens do not forget his kindness: remembering is a moral act and a medicinal one.

As he goes along his way, he falls in love with a princess who tests him, setting him seemingly impossible tasks. She throws a ring into the sea and orders him to fetch it or drown in the attempt. The salmon bring it to him. The princess takes ten sacks of millet seed and strews them around her orchard, telling him to gather up every grain by morning. The ants do it for him. Then she tells him she wants a golden apple from the Tree of Life. The ravens bring it to him and he shares it with his beloved (if rather demanding) princess.

These stories attest to the wisdom of showing friendship to animals. In mythic terms, to speak the languages of animals 'is to appropriate a spiritual life much richer than the merely human life of ordinary mortals', comments religious historian Mircea Eliade.[13] Attend to the way of the animals and learn their languages, is the message of the fairy tales, for when someone is aligned with the sensibility of the animals, society is well served.

~

The vision quest is a widespread tradition in Indigenous cultures, from the First Nations of America to Indigenous Australians. Coming of age, a young person sets out from home, going solo into the wilderness on a quest for a vision. They fast and pray to find a spirit, very often an animal, who teaches them medicine songs so they can call on that spirit, seeking protection throughout life.

Even in cultures which have misplaced their medicine, there are nonetheless traces of exactly this same journey in their fairy tales. They typically begin with the young person setting out alone (going solo) into a forest (the wilderness) to seek their fortune (on a quest for a vision), often hungry (fasting) and making wishes (prayers) to find an animal who teaches them the words (songs) to use to invoke the animal's help. With that protection, the young person becomes strong, resilient and able to withstand danger and hostility for life. Vision quests go by other names, including the 'dream vision' of Celtic tradition.

Young people need psyche-medicine. Adolescents need glory and enormity but they are offered a soul-pittance. Coming of age, they can learn to drive, drink alcohol and have sex legally – and then lose their virginity drunk in the back of the car. They deserve better. They deserve rites of passage and journeys of significance. They deserve to hear the ethical imperative of the animals, in an elephant's roar or a wren's song: to stay alert to what really matters, where everything is a beholding.

The soul politic, too, needs young people to have psyche-medicine: it needs the chaos of adolescence to have direction and purpose. That ferocious spiritedness may be put to beautiful use if it is harnessed by, or to, the animals.

The Lakota medicine man John Fire Lame Deer wrote of the vision quest that had a profound impact on his life as a healer. He had waited a long time for it, sitting quiet and alone. Suddenly, he felt the overwhelming presence of a huge bird, whose feathers touched his back and head. With the cry of a bird, a voice spoke: 'You are sacrificing yourself here to be a medicine man. In time you will be one . . . We are the fowl people, the winged ones, the eagles and the owls . . . You are going to understand us whenever you come to seek a vision here on this hill.'[14] Understanding the languages of animals is, again, medicine.

The animals offer the dream-seeker power, skills and wisdom, but for a price. To go into the vision state, wrote Luther Standing Bear, to go into the presence of the Great Mystery, meant sacrifice and a great solitude, what he called a 'high resolve'.[15]

Dream-seekers may have an instinct to dream that magnetizes insight, as the psyche slips from the ordinary to the extraordinary, with heightened intensity and receptivity. In dreaming, the mind, that alchemical animal, shimmers with luminescence of a wholly different order. The animals reveal medicine to people in that twilight state of mind, say the Amazonian Desana people. The anthropologist Gerardo Reichel-Dolmatoff described how 'until shortly after the Creation, only the animals knew the spells, and that human beings were quite ignorant of them . . . certain spells were revealed to people by animals, often in a dream.'[16]

From Siberia to Amazonia and the Kalahari, Indigenous cultures share a perception that when animal spirits heal illness, they first appear in human dreams or visions, diagnosing the spiritual source of the problem and giving ritual guidance as to how it can be cured.[17]

The medicine-seeker must look to the animals for knowledge, said Luther Standing Bear, and 'assuming their spiritual fineness to be of the quality of his own, he sought with them a true rapport. If the man could prove to some bird or animal that he was a worthy friend, it would share with him precious secrets and there would be formed bonds of loyalty never to be broken.'[18] His words recall the fairy tales: when the hero demonstrates friendship to the animals, they share their powers with him and offer their unbreakable loyalty, like the salmon, ants and ravens of 'The White Snake', where the salmon provide their skill of knowledge, the ants their tenacity and teamwork, and the ravens their intelligence and observation.

~

A chickadee was said to have protected the Absarokee or Crow Nation, by appearing in a dream vision to Chief Plenty-Coups, born in 1848. As a child, Plenty-Coups was eager for a medicine dream, to garner the strength of an animal and to emulate it, and he was nine years old when he set out on his vision quest. He fasted, taking no food or water for four days, and exhausted himself in a sweat lodge in order to seek an animal helper. The vision so gained, people said, would be the heart of his medicine.[19]

In his dream, the vast herds of plains buffaloes were gone and a furious storm whipped up winds from all directions at once, destroying all the trees of the forest except one. That tree was the lodge of the Chickadee. Although the littlest of the birds, Chickadee was the only bird able to withstand the storm's ferocity, like the youngest, smallest child of the fairy tale's three brothers, the only one to succeed, doing so by being sensitive and intelligent. A voice told the dreaming boy to pay attention to the Chickadee: 'He is least in strength but strongest of mind among his kind. He is willing to work for wisdom.'[20] The Chickadee-person is always listening, for 'nothing escapes his ears, which he has sharpened by constant use.' Attending well to words, he learned from the mistakes of others. Chickadee was associated with knowledge and always conveying the truth of things. Chickadee was to be his medicine.

Back in his village, Plenty-Coups told the Elders his vision and they interpreted it to mean that in the child's lifetime, all the buffalo would disappear and the Whites would destroy the Native American way of life. In the chaos of war, almost all the First Nations would lose their land, as all the birds' lodges were destroyed, except for that of Chickadee. The Absarokee or Crow Nation alone would keep their land but only by adopting the qualities of the Chickadee: listen, notice the mistakes of the other Nations, adapt to the incoming Whites rather than fighting them, learn from experience. *Be More Chickadee* was the lesson. It was taken as a guiding dream so powerful that it changed the course of his nation's destiny. Although the Absarokee lost so much in terms of culture, in being willing to make treaties with the Whites they succeeded in keeping much of their land when other nations lost theirs.

Celtic tradition credits the chickadee with giving glorious words to poets, and two of the nine sacred songbirds are chickadees, the black-capped chickadee and the boreal chickadee. (I want to say that's a very high shrike-rate for one little bird, but I won't.)

In Celtic stories, salmon, eel, sow and boar all stand for wisdom and knowledge; deer for grace and swiftness; cat for defence and fierceness; bear and badger for strength, stamina and those hibernatory skills of sleep and dream; while the otter protects and heals, representing faithfulness and single-mindedness – otter is the keeper of essential strength and inner treasures.[21]

Native American lore shows animals as exponents of virtues that heal both society and the individual. Luther Standing Bear wrote: 'By acknowledging the virtues of other beings the Lakota came to possess them for himself.'[22] He described how the fox represented reliability and alertness, and brought order, harmony and peacekeeping.[23] Swift and intelligent, the fox was cherished for kindness, gentleness and the ability to induce rest and healing sleep.[24]

Eagle medicine gave people the ability to look at things from a higher and wiser perspective, soaring far above the petty and mundane. Eagle shows you the path and perceives things with adamantine clarity, warning you of negative forces to be avoided.[25] Mouse teaches the swift changeability of life, and advises you to keep your senses twitching and aware, whisking the air.[26]

Wildcat medicine includes skills of guarding and protecting, staying alert even when sleeping.[27] Coyote, that Trickster, heals stasis, unblocks the blocked, is always ready to take the piss, trip you up, spill your beans, wazz on your bonfire, always reminding you not to take yourself too seriously.[28] His medicine is mischief.

For Ojibwe people, when the Creator sought volunteers from among the animals to transmit medicine rites, the White Otter was first to offer.²⁹ Otter medicine was crucial in curing disease, and the song for the otter medicine bag is 'I am helping you'. Otter is playful, resourceful and versatile, at ease on land and in water, acutely sensitive in hearing, smell and sight, carrying sacred knowledge and ensuring well-being, Otter is attuned to the four compass points and brings all four directions together as he is the centre of north, south, west and east. Otter is called 'he that I hear laughing', his laughter heard in a myriad of situations.³⁰

One collective noun for them is a romp of otters. Watching otters elicits a romp of pleasure and playfulness in me. I have swum with otters in a loch on the Aigas estate in Scotland and doing so I felt the most astonishing invigoration of my spirits, far beyond the normal sense of being refreshed by a lake swim. It was dawn and as I swam something curved up on my left, crescent-backed beside me, then disappeared. Then reappeared on the other side. Then appeared in front of me and then behind me. My north, my south, my west and my east. I cannot tell you if it was one otter four times, or four different otters, or two twice, but Otter it was, up from the dark water into the bright air and instilling a blessing into my soul. It was so piercing and so momentary a pleasure that (ironically) it is with me forever. I can always swim with otters because I can always shut my eyes and dip back into the pool of my memory. He that I hear laughing is still laughing inside me.

Each animal brings a different remedy to help societies think well. It is necessary, the stories suggest, to be able to distinguish the medicine, to know how to discern eagle-sight from bear-power, when to make fine and necessary discriminations of thought between otter-help and fox-gentleness and chickadee-listening.

Societies need to heal sicknesses in the soul politic, and each animal is an essential trace element, a necessary mineral, a vital vitamin. *Every* animal. In medicine stories, the animals are the conscience of the collective psyche and we need to think with them. With them all – and only with them all – can we live well, in a way that is right, living with collective conscience. That word, *conscience*, comes from the Latin verb *conscire*, where *con* means 'with' and *scire* is 'to know'. We can *know with* the animals, knowing together. To be truly well, the collective psyche needs us to think with the animals, who are the conscience of fairy tales, the moral arbiters of medicine stories. In the lore of the Amazonian Tukano people, the entire Earth can be seen as an enormous horizontal spiderweb, and the threads symbolize the paths that people must travel, not straying from the path.[31] If we unravel the silken web of the animals, we dismantle and dismay the conscience of the world.

Medicine surrounds us as we, the deer, the ant and the beaver are all part of the same one Animal, call it Life, which realizes its dreams through us all, where at the centre, which is everywhere and nowhere in the dreamosphere dreamed by the animals, is a spider on a translucent thread attached to the far side of the moon.

16

Shifting the Shape of the Mind

What three words?

Ask a shaman where their healing comes from and (if they are authentic) they will point immediately not to themselves but to the animals.

Shamanism is the world's primary healing tradition and it occurs in very similar forms across the world. Everywhere it states this implacable and simple belief: *It is the animals who heal.*

In Indigenous Australia, the Rainbow Snake is the ultimate source of a shaman's powers.[1] In many cultures, from South America to Polynesia, octopuses are believed to heal the sick.[2] One shaman of northwest Siberia in the 1930s considered that a stoat and a mouse guided him along the path of every illness.[3] John Fire Lame Deer noted how animals, including badgers, butterflies and buffalo, gave their powers to healers: his nephew had 'coyote power' and his own guides were birds, particularly the owl and the eagle.[4]

Shamanism treats physical illness, mental illness, and the injury of emotional lives – 'Divorce, depression and diarrhoea,' said a shaman to me in the Amazon, 'we treat them all.' Shamans also attend to the collective psyche, healing social rifts.

They heal by *turning*: a word both common and profound. In a community they might turn a social situation around. They may turn away the danger of an illness or injury. They can turn psychological illness to wellness. All healing is in essence about the turn, as injured flesh becomes healing tissue, or a damaged relationship begins to transform.

The turning is the thing. The shifting of the shape of illness. 'Something has shifted,' we say, of a psychological improvement.

Even with a malaise as common as a headache, you can feel the turn, the moment when it softens, maybe only a very slight recalibration of pain, but noticeable nonetheless. There has been a shift. We all know that moment when the descent ('I'm going down with something') pauses and turns to rise to wellness. This is the geometry of remedy.

In shamanic ceremony, the sense of turning is everywhere. Shamanism's practices and processes recreate that core sense of change.

The first change is in outer dress. Shamans shift into animalesque costume, identifying themselves with the motley Earth and softly summoning the animals of that locality. When a shaman, a woman aged between twenty-five and thirty-five, was buried 8,500 years ago in Saxony-Anhalt in Germany, her costume included ornaments made from the bones and teeth of bison and wild boar, while roe-deer antlers were a crown for her and she is buried with tortoise shells and a medicine bag fashioned from the leg bone of that sacred bird, the crane. When the shaman-artist Pablo Amaringo from the Peruvian Amazon depicted a shaman, he showed him in the costume of the forest, with a macaw hat, boa-skin jacket, ray-fish trousers and armadillo feet, demonstrating the shaman's ability to move freely between the realms of air, earth and water, by taking on the power of different animals.[5]

Shamanic costume often includes masks, which both cover and reveal, hiding the individual human yet showing the collective self, pregnant with other minds. A shaman of the Tlingit of Alaska may have an octopus mask, and a Haida shaman (from Canada) may use a whale mask, each of which is serious, unnerving and symbolic, and a tool of transformation first for the shaman and then for the situation they address.

There is a process of double distillation whereby the landscape is distilled into the costume, which is also the distillation of the shaman, now changed to portray themselves in the costume of their ceremonial mind.

So sweep the floor, cut the wood, light a fire, put on the costume and as darkness falls let the curtain between the worlds rise. The healing ceremony is theatrical and the stage is set. For the Lakota, one healing setting included eagles' heads and claws, bear paws and antlers as the animals were wooed and coaxed to offer their medicine.[6] A traditional shamanic healing in a sacred forest in Togo was surrounded by stuffed owls, antelope heads, shells of giant tortoises, crocodile jaws, leopard claws, dried chameleons, pink flamingos, pelicans and the lyre-shaped horns of waterbuck.[7]

The ceremonial setting quivers with a more-than-human charge. Even when animals are dead, their bones retain the essence of their presence. Also, these things have usually been gathered over a large territory, and then kept at close quarters, intensifying the atmosphere. It has the psychological effect of a medicine-concentrate containing the living force of plants, condensed to make its active ingredients more potent.

Having shifted their costume and setting, shamans shift the soundscape. Around the world, shamans use rattles, drums and songs in healing. Rattles may rattle us. They have power. They demand attention, possibly recalling a rattlesnake or the death rattle. In ceremonies they are said to rattle out the bad spirits and call in the good.

Drumming, for Ojibwe healing, can be interpreted as the essential and good heart-sound at the core of life. When the drum is beaten, it calls out to the animals to aid the healing.[8] Celtic shamans considered the drum to represent animals including bear, deer or horse,[9] and shamans' drums in Mongolia are called Wind Horses, drumming up the hooves of the horse which transports the shaman into the spirit world.

Shamans in the Amazon use healing songs called *icaros* that they say they learn from animals and plants. The songs are like nothing I have ever heard and they whistle in the highest skies of my mind. A faint whisper, a fluting breath, a smoky melody, so soft, elven and elusive, a half-cadence half sung, like a memory of a dream of a prayer. Shamans use these melodies to heal the sick and protect the vulnerable by invoking or imitating the animals.

The *icaros* contain the quintessence of the animal, so an *icaro* of the sloth (an animal regarded as clean and very careful in its eating habits) is used to cure digestive problems in children, while *icaros* of slippery animals like eels are used to aid childbirth.[10]

A traditional Yakut shamanic ceremony would begin in silence tense with presence. A drumming starts, quiet as an insect's hum. Music begins, first delicate but becoming rougher like a storm, with peals of thunder, the crowing of a falcon, the croaking of eagles, the plaintive cry of lapwings, all intended to scare away the cause of the illness.[11]

Our bodies cannot become hawk or jaguar but our voices can, and with mimetic power shamans recreate the animals in the minds of others because when it is dark our sense of hearing is activated. We cannot see that the animals are not there, but we hear them as if they are nearby, in the growl, flutter, croak, rasp and howl. Their voices amplify the energy of healing, as of a medicine cabinet of animals hooting with life.

There is a temple at Chavín de Huántar in Peru, dating back to perhaps 900 BCE, and it contains many half-human, half-jaguar sculptures. Sited at the confluence of two rivers, the temple was built with extensive ducts and channels, and it is thought that water was diverted throughout the interior, deliberately making the temple an enormous musical instrument.[12] More. The sound was specifically the purring of a gigantic feline of magnificent spiritual importance. The entire edifice would have sounded like you were inside the soul of the land, as if the temple itself had shapeshifted and become an enormous jaguar, stretching, breathing and purring.

~

Of all a shaman's transformations, in costume, setting, ceremony and soundscape, the most intense is shapeshifting: turning 'into' an animal, with altered behaviour and transformed gesture. The revelation – ancient and always new – is that healing comes through taking on the metaphoric mind of an animal.

One of the earliest images of a healer is the 'dancing shaman' in the Cave of the Trois-Frères in France. He has the ears of a wolf, the paws of a bear and the antlers of a deer, yet is inherently human, as if the figure has incorporated the gifts of different animals – the wolf's hearing, the bear's dexterity and strength and the deer's weaponry. The gift of the human is a superb one: the ability to shapeshift into animal form.

A belief in shapeshifting has been widespread in the world. In Southern Africa, the Indigenous San rock art shows paintings of shapeshifters in the form of a rhebuck or leopard, half human and half animal, an image of the shaman's mind at the moment of entering a healing trance.[13] Take on kudu mind if you want to outrun a kudu, the San hunters say. They attune themselves to the animal they seek, so, hunting an antelope, they think like an antelope, mirroring the animal's responses, fears and strategies. This inner sympathy for the animal's bodily sensations is felt in the body of the human, in corresponding places – ribs, back, face and eyes, for example – so he is lit up with the sensations of the antelope.[14] Shamans do this, hunting their quarry of sickness.

When Pawnee people wanted their scouts to be acutely sensitive, they would wear wolfskins to call up the power of the wolves. Young men in rites of passage would sing more and more wildly until someone began wolf-howling. Some of the initiates would wear wolf masks, dancing in a wolf frenzy until they had taken into themselves the power of the wolf, able to prowl, run and hear like wolves. The Pawnee said that a wolf's hearing was so sharp he could hear a cloud passing overhead.[15]

One Koyukon shaman, reported Richard Nelson, would use the spirit of the raven to scare away the sickness in a patient, 'mimicking a raven's melodious cawing, spreading his arms like wings, and bouncing on both feet as a raven would'.[16]

Plenty-Coups, Chief of the Crow Nation, described a shaman trying to heal a warrior who had been shot through the chest and was bleeding badly. As the medicine drums began, the shaman put on his costume – a whole wolf's skin. When the drumbeats became faster and softer, the healer keened like a mother wolf, trotting round the body of the wounded man, sprinkling water over him and vocalizing continuously as a wolf does to her cubs. Howling like a wolf calling for help, he led the injured man to a stream, pawed at the water and splashed it over his head, nosing the water over the bullet holes, like a wolf licking a wound.[17]

It isn't for me to interpret what happens in this kind of healing. I can only say what I feel based on my own experience of being healed by shamans. It is as if, in their deliberate creation of entirely separate ceremonial space, costume, sound and psyche, they empower not only themselves but the minds of those they try to heal. It is a shock. Nothing is familiar. It jolts the psyche like a shot of adrenaline, and the mind affects the body, rousing it to find its maximum energy to fight against whatever is endangering it. The patient knows that the shaman is not only calling on their human knowledge and skills but reaching beyond, right out to the raw potency of the animals and the essential animating principle. Charged with that ferocious power, they create the best possible opportunity for healing.

The werewolf is probably the most familiar form of shapeshifting. *Were* means 'man', from the Latin *vir*, so a werewolf is half human and half wolf. But it isn't only wolves. In the Kalahari, according to the !Kung, there were were-lions who prowled the desert, leaping in giant bounds and eclipsing the very sun by covering it with a paw.[18] There are were-jaguars in the Amazon, were-hyenas in the Arabian peninsula and parts of Africa, and traditions of were-foxes in Japan, and were-swans in Europe in the form of the Valkyries or swan maidens.

Some Indigenous cultures say certain animals may themselves be shamans. In parts of the Amazon, the anaconda is a shamanistic animal while the tapir, for example, is said to be only a little bit shamanistic.[19] As the shaman typically walks a soloist's path, so the animals that are accorded a strong shamanistic association around the world are often also solitary animals: jaguar, eagle, hare and bear. In Nagaland, India, where owls may be shamans, those in need of healing may go to an animal. Explaining their reasons, people told the anthropologist Sahil Nijhawan: 'We are seeking animal shamans – what you seek in a human healer, we seek in an animal healer.'[20]

~

Visiting Oslo once, I went to the Folk Museum and asked where I could see objects from the First Nations of Norway. The museum attendant looked saddened and awkward and I didn't understand why. He gestured to a white plywood cabinet by a wall. I was confused and went over to it. It was functional and ugly, but there was a spyhole in one of the sides. In the half-second as my eyes adjusted to the darkness, I felt excited by the hint of a mystery both secret and significant.

There was nothing there. A white block of dark absence. And that absence contained a world of reproach. I pulled back sharply and read the little typed sign on the wall beside the cabinet: *This drum was used till 1900 then hidden in a cave till 1925.* This drum? It has been returned to Sámi people, said the attendant, because that is the right thing to have done. Sámi drums were decorated with animals and were the shamans' crucial medico-musical instrument: they were never just drums but, in their designs and histories, were a codex for a shamanically intensified world, the pictures acting as symbolic codes for various medicinal rituals.

Christian missionaries had outlawed shamanism, and from the seventeenth century onwards Sámi people hid their drums with all the images and symbolism they held, often burying them for safety in remote and secret places. Shamans and their animal-healing were considered of the devil, not just in northern Scandinavia but in the Amazon and widely across the world.

Witches were the shamans of Europe. They were herbalists, midwives, psychologists and healers, and like all shamans they had their animal powers or 'familiars'. But European tradition eschewed its own wisdoms. It deliberately erased its own knowledge, claiming separateness from, superiority to and dominion over the animals. Those who knew the delicate depths of the soul implicit in shapeshifting were hunted out and killed. Misogyny (and indeed early capitalism), as well as the influence of the Christian Church, meant that the shamanism of Britain and much of Europe was demonized into something hateful and fearful. When that process was complete, it was belittled into a cartoon freak.

Language gets bent out of shape here, as though my pencil, soft and slow, is buckled by hundreds of years of cruelty, derision and stupidity. I can't write 'witchcraft' without risking the evocation of spooky turrets in moonlight, with evil-lit eyes and warty arts. I can't describe the wise hands that held healing knowledge deepening with age, without conjuring the haggard hands of comic-book witches. And if I write of flight, the crazed, crack-throated screech of witches on cartoon broomsticks will buzz your brain.

Witches shapeshifted as shamans do and for the same reasons, seeking the power of the animals and the extra perspective that another mind provides, because if you can look from more than one viewpoint your thinking becomes more skilful. Two eyes: all the better to see you with. Two ears: all the better to hear you with. Two minds: all the better to think you with. The animals provided stereoscopic thought: who thinks with hare?

Like all shamans, witches travelled not in literalism but in metaphor, shifting perception. In shapeshifting, a shaman can access her greatest awareness, forgetting herself to increase her empathy with another. Daylight-knowledge, including observation of an animal's territory, how it navigates and senses the world, helps towards this, as does dream-knowledge, but the highly charged sensitivity of the trance-state opens the mind to its best imaginings.

In various parts of the world, including old Europe, shamans fly with hallucinogens such as peyote, fly agaric mushrooms, ayahuasca and psilocybin. In its latest iteration of its antipathy to shamanism, modernity outlaws these medicines whose astonishing gift is to open up the self to the minds of others.

Shamans become birds and soar in mind-flight, seeking a bird's-eye view. In fact the ability to turn into a bird is said to be the common property of shamanism.[21] Each Yakut shaman has a mythical 'Bird-of-Prey Mother' that gives them the power to heal,[22] and they say that on their journeys they learn from cranes: in order to deal with someone's fears they must fly downwards, having turned into a hooded crane, while to fly to the upper world, the shaman has to become a white crane.[23]

Shamans fly between worlds, communicating on many levels. They are society's spiritual messengers: they discover and reveal, they are the knowers and tellers, and they find their wings with the birds.

The word for *messenger* in ancient Greek is *angelos*. This is the root of the English word *angel*, messenger and herald of the gods, necessarily winged as a bird and as necessarily human. How would you design an angel prototype without the birds for inspiration? How might you imagine the imagination without the idea of flight? I hate the idea of a world that had never known wings, where nothing had ever flown. I feel dread if I think of the psyche grounded and flightless, the mind all thumbs, numbed and halted in the dreary mundane. How would we truly know how to think if birds had not angelized the air?

'What gave me this mind/bird mind/to fly with,' wrote Nils-Aslak Valkeapää,[24] one of the few shamans I can introduce you to on the page.

~

Shamans don't tend to advertise. They are often appalling at self-promotion, holding to an austere and old-fashioned code of humility. In the Amazon, I was told: 'Generally, if you call yourself a shaman, you're not.' They often go by other names: healer, teacher, poet, artist, musician. Their work is enshadowed because its dealings are in the twilight mind, the half-light of candled allusion not the bright spotlights of self-publicity.

Nils-Aslak Valkeapää, though, left traces of his work in music and print. He was born into a reindeer-herding family in Sapmi (Sámi land) in 1943, trained as a teacher and then spent his too-short life as a singer, poet, artist, actor, dreamer and healer. He was tender and sensitive, porous to the world. His voice was soft, his words half whispered with a saddened smile, as if he was possessed of a secret so powerful it was almost unsayable, and he spoke with an intimacy and charisma that would seduce the Northern Lights.

His poetry is an incantation of his landscape, and he invoked the animals by naming them as if calling in his friends, inviting the fox, wolf, bear, otter, ermine, hare, trout, grayling and whale to a convocation – but birds were his spirit signature: 'We know each other.'

In February 1996, he was severely injured in a car accident from which he never fully recovered, and he died in 2001. 'I would like to die/ as I have lived/. . . be transformed into birdsong.'[25]

His work was societally medicinal, as he gave strength to a then-weakened culture. He turned things around for the Sámi. In part because of his work, the drums began to be taken out of hiding, drawn out of the caves where fear had hidden them. The land could, just, begin to whisper once more its lively Indigenous insights.

Across the world, when people have been attacked for shamanism and shapeshifting, they have had to hide their accoutrements and themselves. They have had to shift their own shape, transforming themselves and masking their identities. Many, like Valkeapää, have gravitated towards the arts, particularly poetry. Here they can still take the shamanic role with the particular cast of mind of the serious dreamer, mesmerized by meaning, dwellers in the ecstatic.

Poetry is short-form shamanism.

Shamans and poets alike are rhymers, sometimes literally rhyming and sometimes rhyming as a way of thinking, linking things together. Both shamans and poets operate in the sound world, and the beat of the shaman's drum is the rhythm of the poem. Like shamanic ceremonies, poems become more intense, growing towards the turn: in poetry, this is when the poem's thought lifts off, taking wing. That exact moment is called, in French, *le tourne*, and in sonnets the turn of the argument is the *volta*, meaning the 'turn' in Italian. The shapeshifting turn is the core of both the poem and the shaman's art. In both cases it is done to effect change, to transform and to heal.

Walt Whitman knew poetry as a healing art, picturing himself disguised as a shaman with his costume 'stucco'd with quadrupeds and birds all over'. Shifting into animal form was a remedy for the collective psyche, Whitman's work argues: 'The soul or spirit transmits itself into all . . . and can feel itself . . . into an animal, and feel itself a horse, a fish or bird.'[26]

Many poets have known the healing power of animals, including Christopher Smart and his cat, William Cowper and his hares, Emily Dickinson and her dog, Byron and his. At the beginning of *A Midsummer Night's Dream*, the lifeless court of Athens embodies a collective psyche that is profoundly sick. It urgently needs a tincture of animal spirits to be healed into natural vitality. Shakespeare knew exactly what he was doing by introducing the shapeshifter, Puck, who flits between being a horse, a hound, a hog and a bear, and uses shapeshifting medicine. The court comes alive, sweetened with honeysuckle and musk-rose, invigorated with wild thyme, garlic, and mustard seed.

In the last act of the play, the Duke of Athens, in wonderment at the transformation, considers how:

> as imagination bodies forth
> The forms of things unknown, the poet's pen
> Turns them to shapes.

Note the exact words: the poet turns them – shifts them – to shapes. Shapeshifting. The poet is the shaman, even if they have to be masked for the role.

~

When the mind is on its knees and in pure survival mode, the animals come. The poet Pascale Petit's story is heartbreaking. Her father raped her mother, and the poet, part French, part Indian and part Welsh, was born of this. The mother, traumatized, sick and made cruel, both neglected and punished the child, who was then abused by the father. She was abandoned in orphanages at some points of her early childhood, and her parents' rejection and their merciless abuse led to decades of agonizing depression from her teenage years.

When her psyche had been damaged to a point that seems unsurvivable, the animals healed her. Her poetry began when she met her father again, after he had been missing for thirty-five years. He was dying of emphysema in Paris, and she began visiting him regularly, although it was grievous.

She tells me in an interview that her experience of her parents was 'the overwhelming subject' of her life: 'I knew I *must* write about it.' But she couldn't. Although she felt compelled to do so, she was at first unable to meet the demand. Then, one day, she explored the Jardin des Plantes Zoo in Paris and suddenly she could see her way. 'The animals just appeared, like a miracle. They magically appeared there, the animals that I needed. They became totems to me.' Almost all those she mentions are the big cats: a black jaguar, a gold jaguar, a puma and a lion.

The fact that they were caged caused her a great deal of pain, and yet there is a rhyme here because dangerous depressions had caged her for years and the animals offered her a way out, giving her the freedom to be able to see her father and write. She began portraying her father through 'animal masks', and in one poem she wrote of her father as a giant anteater, shapeshifting him out of a human rapist and into a creature compelled by its own nature to force its way into nests.

What Petit does is shamanism on the page. In order not to be completely broken, she shapeshifts her parents. Retaining human form, they would never cease to torment her, but through the animals and insects, the poet makes poem-spells to heal herself and indeed her readers.

I feel acutely aware, as she speaks, of the innocence stolen from her as a child, and the love denied. In an extraordinary act of grace, she bestows both innocence and love on her father through the animals.

She shapeshifted herself, turning into a bird. She tells me she had felt like 'a very vulnerable little hummingbird baby' but had transposed herself, dissociating her own innocence and transferring it to these birds whose very feathers quiver with intense sensitivity. In the process of poetry her bird-self grows to strength and maturity: 'By becoming a hummingbird you become powerful, you can fly, fly sideways, backwards, hover and breathe very fast. The hummingbirds have their power and incredible beauty and shapeshifting colours, shot-silk, they are changing something for me *and* they are masters of change.'

When she began to write about her mother, she transforms her into a jaguar, 'my were-mama'. In the poem 'Jaguar Girl', we see the psychiatric damage that her mother endured, which Petit transmutes into the fierce glory of the forest. Her poem prowls and leaps, deadly accurate: each of her words a pencil-claw sharpened to its most exact meaning. In her work, she turns her mother into the Amazon rainforest and says it was 'a revelation to me. Once I'd turned her into a giant water lily, into a flower, she became something I could love. What had happened to her (I mean my father) becomes a beetle or cockroach, a harmless pollinator. It was like magic, and the moment I started writing that poem, something changed in my *heart*. I tried to look at the world through her eyes, forget the emotional abuse and terror I got, and the antipathy. In that book I found a way of loving her.'

Petit's poetry is electric, as if childhood cruelty was a fork of lightning that first burned her but then fired her with the force of forest animals whose medicine is wild and radiant. After the lightning storm, a feral rainbow. Her writing affects me profoundly, as its unflinching notation of cruelty blazing with pain is nonetheless transmuted and in the flames of furious hurt she forges gold.

The depressions she had suffered lifted. 'It did heal me. Writing about the animals, or about my abusive parents as animals, transformed the pain, metamorphosed it into healing poetry. In the poems I worked – or rather played – at being those animals, so I am no longer just a human child in pain.'[27] Jaguar medicine had worked.

~

Ted Hughes, whose work is unquestionably shamanic, told an interviewer: 'When I was feeling good, I'd have dreams full of giant pike that were perhaps also leopards . . . They'd become symbols of deep, vital life.'[28] *Perhaps also leopards.* There's a thing going on between big cats and poets. In Allen Ginsberg's poem 'The Lion for Real', a lion enters the poet's home (his psyche) and the man flees. But the lion has chosen and gives no quarter, his calling is the 'roar of the Universe'.[29] The poet, finally, accepts the call – the howl – of poetry that cannot and must not be denied. The very vocation of poet comes in the shape of big cats, according to American poet Jane Hirshfield: 'what creates an artist . . . is exposure to the tiger, for even the briefest of moments . . . a savage pursuit of truth becomes more important than kindness, than connection, than any ties.'[30]

It is a calling that obliterates normal, that turns a bathtub into a tsunami, a candle into a wildfire. It is a ferocious vocation that demands all you have and everything you are. You are avowed to it and 'the tiger nature works within', as the poet Stevie Smith wrote.[31] Surrendering to that tiger is a frequent image of a life given in service to poetry. Shamans describe their vocation similarly, for the shaman's calling must be followed and if it is refused it will wreak havoc, taking revenge on a person's mental and physical health.

'Tyger, tyger, burning bright, in the forests of the night,' wrote William Blake. What other animal provides such symmetry for this precise calling, in the human mind? What, other than tyger, known around the world as the revenge animal, could so frame the fierce anger if its demand were ignored?

The tiger is both quintessential poet-animal and quintessential shaman-animal. For the Tukano people of the north-western Amazon, the jaguar, a thunder-animal,[32] is so closely connected to shamans that the same word, *yee*, is used for both shaman and jaguar. The Tukano shaman would drink *yahé* to take on the jaguar's form, slipping into the cat's skin to speak with the Master of Animals, feline to feline: the association twisting the two together so profoundly that just as the shaman becomes a jaguar, so the Master of Animals is both a jaguar and a wise shaman.[33]

The jaguar moves between worlds and between elements, representing for many the very soul of the Amazon, the volcanic spirit flickering like living fire, the visible soul of the land, and its greatest medicine.

~

I've suffered depressions in my life that have felt immovable, as if I was mired in claggy mud that filled my mind and days until I could barely walk. I've turned to many things, and been grateful for them all. I've taken antidepressants and visited a soul-saving GP. I've seen a therapist of exquisite sensitivity, and I've turned to friends, again and gratefully again. But for preference, if I could, it is to shamans I would turn every time, because of their profound recognition that healing occurs through the animals.

In one episode of depression so devastating that I had become suicidal, I went to a newly established healing centre in the Peruvian Amazon called Mayantuyacu. There were a few huts, hot springs, a river and a handful of extraordinary people. There, I was treated by ayahuasqueros – shamans who use ayahuasca – and in one of the healing ceremonies, I could feel a sense of jaguarness, an experience so intense, so physical, so immense that it shaped my thinking, my writing and indeed my life.

Evening had fallen, the shamans had created a ceremonial space and readied themselves. They had also prepared the ayahuasca. It is an extreme medicine, known to taste foul and to induce vomiting. I'd never taken it before, and I felt anxious. But the sickness of depression was clutching me, right inside my mind-body. Words alone could not touch it. The shamans knew I was suffering, and they felt sure of their own doctoring skills.

I drank.

I have already taken the memories and given the experience words, in my book *Wild: An Elemental Journey*. Here, I want to concentrate on the exact moment when the depression began to shift: the *volta* of my soul.

I began to experience the visions that ayahuasca gives you, and a jaguar was there in my mind's eye. I didn't feel frightened but quite the reverse – I felt magnetized, as if I knew without question that I needed her. Depression is a predator, loaded with poison, dangerous and sometimes deadly. It sniffs at your life, drinking your vitality, and will prey on you until it has drunk all of your beautiful liquid spirit, until there is nothing left except a husk. Few things are stronger than depression, but a jaguar is. A jaguar is the apex predator of these forests, and tonight depression would be her quarry. This is an animal whose ferocious life force – sudden, always and now – could vanquish the slow, wan death of depression.

Drawn to it, mesmerized in my ayahuasca visions, I began to merge with the jaguar and my shape began to alter. To be precise, the shape that my psyche inhabited began to shift, like a dream or like a metaphor which was so deeply heard that my body took up the song. My psyche did not feel as if it were inhabiting a human body but the body of an animal, the jaguar that I suddenly felt myself apprenticed to. This was obviously not a literal shifting of shape, but an experience of the mind so exact that I felt I was on the very edge of understanding what a shaman might mean, saying they shifted their shape. Ayahuasca activates the mind to feel its own animal remedy, and I ingested the spirit of raw jaguar. It roared through my veins.

A terrible professional betrayal had triggered this depression. My writing hand had felt crushed. But when the jaguar within began to merge with me, she walked into my paws. I could feel the turn, the shift of shape which was also, crucially, the turning of the damage and the illness. My hands, so shaken and weak, grew huge, stretched into their rightful claws and paw-pads, strong enough to defend themselves against anything and anyone. I felt the enormous pouring potency through my paws that were also tender to the tiniest twig.

The pull of my imagination was tautened by all the aspects of the occasion – the medicine, the forest, the night and the shamans' songs – until I lost my singular self and stepped across the border in the wild, charged, ferocious tutelage of a jaguar.

I felt my whiskers. I could smell things I would never have been able to smell ordinarily. All my senses went gigantic as the medicine flowed through me and I felt this animal's archetypal vigour, ancient breath and spirit humming through me. Drink it. Eat it. Become it. I was ravenous to re-feel the strength of my own being and to know the primal power of the animal I am.

My eyes were burning to fully see with this jaguar vision, and it was a moment of acute 'crisis' in the sense of the turning. After months of illness, the animal medicine healed me in minutes. Depression didn't stand a chance against this, the hot, fierce *fuerza* that flooded through me like molten lava, burning out the sickness of depression.

And then I came back to myself. That is also part of the medicine, to return to one's own proper self, scale and senses. And in the hours and days afterwards, I realized that not only had that desolate depression been cured but a deeper transformation was taking place. I felt my oneself evaporating into the far-soul, the infinitely greater thing, a kind of world-soul so far exceeding me in importance, in scope and in meaning that the 'I' is no more than a microbe in a teaspoon of soil, a speck in the universe, an iota, the dot of one 'i' in the infinite literature of life. I am nothing, and that doesn't matter a bit. Because life does.

So I was healed by a jaguar. It worked. Was that important? My friends would have been sad if I'd committed suicide, but a world without me in it is not really much affected. No biggie, to be honest. What did matter in those ceremonies was seeing the utter and priceless sacredness of all life and the imperative of being in service to that. If what I felt was a metamorphosis, it was for the meta-soul, for the sake of the more-than-me. The most important aspect of my healing was this sense of the raw, lustrous divinity of life which has never entirely left me, and which came through a sense of identification with the knowers of the forest. In pelt and paw and breath, I could feel from within my body a radical love for the Earth as strong as the gravitational force.

~

What three words?

Mind wide open.

Be more animal.

Animals heal us.

There is, it seems, no animal which cannot lead the human mind to wellness. We are surrounded by an abundance of healing in worldwide animal transformation. If we make our raven muscles bounce in our bodies, our minds may hop like intelligent corvids. Growl with the jaws of a wolf so you can stand up to bullies. Take lessons from the chickadee.

And it breaks my heart because all that sweet healing is being poisoned. The world's soul – its animals – is being extinguished and the silent and aggrieved emptiness is a reproach that sends me staggering.

You wouldn't keep a jaguar chained in your yard, slowly bleeding to death as you slice off a piece of her body every now and then. Cruelty comes stealthily and this is its path. Step one: most of us eat beef, pork and chicken, and the eggs and dairy products they provide. Step two: those pigs, chickens and cows are very likely fed on soya. Step three: the soya is grown around the world, including in vast tracts of the Amazon – jungles and forests are destroyed for that crop. Step four: those forests are the necessary home of the original peoples of that land, home of the animals, including the jaguar. Without their home they die as slowly, as horribly and as completely as if you were keeping that jaguar for your personal consumption just outside the back door. Unless you are a cat, or other obligate carnivore, what three words? Don't eat meat.

What has happened is unhallowed. We have stormed the great green hospital of the Amazon, and we are slaughtering the doctors. The surgeons have been shot in the operating theatres. There are snipers out to shoot the ambulance drivers, and the paramedics are being starved to death.

How is the murderous malignity of this culture going to be healed? Not with statistics or diagrams or percentages, vital though these are. Facts are necessary but insufficient for the level of change required, because this transformation needs an entire shift of the shape of the collective psyche. The turn that is needed is soul-shifting.

Where might it begin? Close to the earth, the human staying humble in a suspension of that false belief that one species' mind is all there is. If we apprentice our attention to another creature, to their story, priorities, senses and needs, we may imaginatively step towards them. Paying attention to one other mind – one ant, perhaps, one mollusc or blackbird – opens a chink of light to the shiningness that is there – and here – all the time, turning up a vibrant tile in the infinite mosaic that makes up life, everlastingly and diversely proliferating.

You are no longer only you. You can become more than yourself, breathing in the glinting air of all the intelligences, electric and animal and wild. You can shift the shape of your mind.

Belonging solely to one single species seems an intolerable and dangerous limitation to me now. It would be like being limited to life within one household, both maddening and stupefying in its confinement, eschewing all the varieties of culture and knowledge beyond, losing all the grace of the diverse world.

When I was a student, I read a line by E. M. Forster that I knew I would need all my life, so I learned it, tucking it into my heart to be a part of me forever. You may know it.

'Only connect! . . . Only connect the prose and the passion, and both will be exalted.' Because the spirit holds together by connecting the real and the metaphoric, the facts and the significance. Because life holds together by connecting everything to everything, the least and the tiniest: a worm, a wasp, a wallaby, a whale and you. The parrotfish, by feeding on coral, encourages it to grow, so the coral in turn needs the parrotfish. We live because of the endlessly branching filaments of connection between everything and everything else, and not one part can be subtracted, nothing lost, because without it the whole is sundered.

Indigenous philosophy, and the shamanism that is its most profound and poetic expression, is founded on the ethic of the necessary-everything, knowing what the discipline of ecology has painstakingly retaught, that all that exists interdepends and interrelates. For our health depends on the animals, the insects and birds and fish and mammals, the all, and all the connections between them.

The animals connect us, not only outside ourselves but inside, connecting us to our truest selves. There are animals within us. The prose of common ancestry (we share common ancestry with the animals, and my bones from shoulder to fingertip are mirrored in a million animals) has its passion in shapeshifting. Because inside you is the animal you already are, always were and always will be.

Turning through eternal spirals of life, generous and regenerative, our bodies die but pass on, through an earthworm, caddisfly or mistle thrush, endlessly rebecoming as even death is healed by the animals. While the individual is mortal, the life spirit is immortal, transforming death to birth because, like the bear and all her cargo of meaning, returning with cubs in spring after the denning of winter, life itself is a shapeshifter, shapeshifting through the animating animals.

Coda

Sometimes, authors are asked if writing their books changed them, and I can say for sure that this book did. Researching it left me breathtaken, and the world feels radically different to me now, as the animals are the great transformers, lighting up a specific part of the brain, electrifying us on the inside with vitality and brilliance.

I now know I'm never further than six feet from someone who giggles and chirrups. I look at games with a double gaze now, wondering which animal gave us Tag or King of the Castle. I can never be lonely again, as I can't even walk past a tree without listening for someone (not something) singing in it. We are surrounded by animal minds that communicate with us and are demonstrably good for us.

If I want a shot of instant healing, I can find a donkey, simply to be near it. Service dogs give the world depths of skill and devotion I never knew. Now, if I learn of someone suicidal, I would not only try to get them human help but I would also try to get a dog to them as a matter of the utmost urgency, one of a zodiac of potential rescuers around us.

I now know to listen to the dogs who can detect the presence of disease and predict medical emergencies. And I also know that the dogs' call for back-up in *The Hundred and One Dalmatians* is not a piece of fiction after all.

I've learned to listen to the guiding voices of animals warning us of danger and showing us remedies. As someone who has long been frightened of death, I've been consoled by knowing that animals can willingly accompany us and when it's time, I want animals with me at the end.

When I hear bees buzzing now, I hear medicine, knowing there is healing in the animal soundscape, from a cat's purr to pondlife. Without what I've learned, I wouldn't have known how to say yes with the female treehopper, warmly humming *yes I will Yes*.

I'm humbled and astonished at learning how the animal world has ethics and kindness and that it developed them aeons before us. I will forever sense an ocean of forgiveness just as I carry whale breath in my lungs, and I am changed by both. There is fairness in the animal world that comforts me when human unfairness hurts, and the scales of justice balance in ways I'd never known before, through the minds of the animals. I have learned to salute the animals as part of the resistance, to understand them as political players, and I would vote for them in every election.

I cannot now take animals for granted in art: they emerge as the artists behind every brushstroke, the eloquence in our phrases, the key signature of our music and its original spirit. In considering spirituality, I am changed as if the grandeur of god was suddenly multiplied by all the animals, a scaled-up divinity, god refracted in everything, and everything exploding into godness.

I used to be a bit scared of spiders, but now when I see a spider I wonder what it dreamed last night. I see the world as a greater dreamscape now, because it is dreamed by a multitude of animals. This real and living dream is intuited in folk tales and medicine stories, where animals are the guides who vouchsafe the conscience of our collective psyche.

In quiet, persistent voices, the earth doctors, since the beginning of human thought, have considered the source of healing to be animals. In writing this book, the shape of my spirit has been shifted by the animals, transformed utterly. The shape of healing has been shifted. Medicine surrounds us like rainbows, different remedies shining through the prism of different animals, and in writing this book, the animals have shifted my soul.

Notes

PART ONE
How Animals Heal the Individual Psyche

1: Bouncing with Rude Health

1. S. Savage-Rumbaugh and R. Lewin, *Kanzi: The Ape at the Brink of the Human Mind* (London: Doubleday, 1994), p. 144.
2. N. S. Akimbekov and M. S. Razzaque, 'Laughter Therapy: A Humor-Induced Hormonal Intervention to Reduce Stress and Anxiety', *Current Research in Physiology*, 4 (2021), 135–8. doi: 10.1016/j.crphys.2021.04.002.
3. R. Fouts and S. T. Mills, *Next of Kin: What Chimpanzees Have Taught Me About Who We Are* (New York: William Morrow, 1997), p. 67.
4. M. Bekoff, *The Emotional Lives of Animals* (Novato, California: New World Library, 2007), p. 56.
5. Bekoff, *The Emotional Lives of Animals*, p. 56.
6. S. L. Winkler and G. A. Bryant, 'Play Vocalisations and Human Laughter: A Comparative Review', *Bioacoustics* (2021). doi: 10.1080/09524622.2021.1905065.
7. C. Blomqvist, I. Mello and M. Amundin, 'An Acoustic Play-Fight Signal in Bottlenose Dolphins (*Tursiops truncatus*) in Human Care', *Aquatic Mammals*, 31 (2005). doi: 10.1578/AM.31.2.2005.187.
8. *Guardian* (17 November 2015).
9. D. Rothenberg, *Why Birds Sing: A Journey Through the Mystery of Bird Song* (New York: Basic Books, 2005), p. 10.
10. M. Webb, *The Spring of Joy* (Adelaide: Michael Walmer, 2016), p. 39.
11. N. Park, C. Peterson and M. E. P. Seligman, 'Strengths of Character and Well-being', *Journal of Social and Clinical Psychology*, 23 (2004), 603–19.
12. Fouts and Mills, *Next of Kin*, p. 31.

13. *New Scientist* (27 March 2014).
14. J. Ackerman, *The Genius of Birds* (London: Corsair, 2016), p. 170.
15. G. Delorme, *Deer Man: Seven Years in the Forest* (London: Hachette, 2022), p. 139.
16. R. K. Nelson, *Make Prayers to the Raven* (Chicago: University of Chicago Press, 1983), pp. 77–8.
17. A. Beck and A. Katcher, *Between Pets and People* (West Lafayette, Indiana: Purdue University Press, 1996), pp. 82–3.
18. Beck and Katcher, *Between Pets and People*, p. 43.
19. J. M. Masson, *Dogs Never Lie About Love* (London: Vintage, 1997), p. 125.
20. Bekoff, *The Emotional Lives of Animals*, p. 95.
21. J. R. Jíménez, *Platero and I* (Lincoln, Nebraska: iUniverse, 2000), p. 45.
22. F. de Waal, *Mama's Last Hug: Animal Emotions and What They Teach Us About Ourselves* (London: Granta, 2020), p. 74.
23. G. M. Burghardt, 'The Comparative Reach of Play and Brain Perspective, Evidence, and Implications', *American Journal of Play*, 2:3 (2015).
24. S. Eisenbeiser, E. Serbe-Kamp, G. Gage and T. Marzullo, 'Gills Just Want to Have Fun: Can Fish Play Games, Just Like Us?', *Animals*, 12:13 (2022), 1684. doi:10.3390/ani12131684.
25. Burghardt, 'The Comparative Reach of Play and Brain Perspective'.
26. Eisenbeiser et al., 'Gills Just Want to Have Fun'.
27. Burghardt, 'The Comparative Reach of Play and Brain Perspective'.
28. C. Moss, *Elephant Memories* (Chicago: University of Chicago Press, 2000), p. 161.
29. Eisenbeiser et al., 'Gills Just Want to Have Fun'.
30. Burghardt, 'The Comparative Reach of Play and Brain Perspective'.
31. E. H. Radinger, *The Wisdom of Wolves: How They Think, Plan and Look After Each Other – Amazing Facts about the Animal That Is More Like Man Than Any Other* (London: Penguin, 2019), pp. 139–40.
32. B. Lopez, *Of Wolves and Men* (New York: Scribner, 2004), p. 4.
33. Radinger, *The Wisdom of Wolves*, pp. 139–40.
34. M. Bekoff, *Minding Animals: Awareness, Emotions, and Heart* (New York: Oxford University Press, 2003), p. 16.
35. https://www.wilddolphinproject.org/plastic-is-bad-real-bad/.
36. T. Mass and D. Sipperly, *Freedive!* (Ventura, California: Blue Water Freedivers, 1998), pp. 120–22.
37. R. Payne, *Among Whales* (New York: Scribner, 1995), p. 119.
38. S. L. Swartz, *Lagoon Time* (Washington DC: The Ocean Foundation, 2014), p. 84.
39. Swartz, *Lagoon Time*, p. 128.

40. B. J. King, *How Animals Grieve* (Chicago: University of Chicago Press, 2013), p. 100.
41. Ackerman, *The Genius of Birds*, pp. 107–8.
42. S. Wensley, *Through a Vet's Eyes* (London: Hachette, 2022), pp. 126–33.
43. Burghardt, 'The Comparative Reach of Play and Brain Perspective'.
44. D. Everett, *Don't Sleep, There are Snakes: Life and Language in the Amazonian Jungle* (London: Profile Books, 2008), p. 12.
45. Fouts and Mills, *Next of Kin*, p. 157.
46. Savage-Rumbaugh and Lewin, *Kanzi*, p. 277.
47. C. Henderson, *A Book of Noises: Notes on the Auraculous* (London: Granta, 2023), p. 91.
48. Joyce Poole, quoted in L. Watson, *Elephantoms* (New York: W. W. Norton, 2003), p. 63.
49. Katy Payne and the Elephantlisteningproject.org.
50. B. Sax, *Avian Illuminations: A Cultural History of Birds* (London: Reaktion Books, 2021), pp. 132–3.
51. E. Yong, *An Immense World: How Animal Senses Reveal the Hidden Realms Around Us* (London: The Bodley Head, 2022), pp. 196 and 187.
52. Caitlin O'Connell, quoted in Yong, *An Immense World*, p. 202.
53. B. Krause, *The Great Animal Orchestra* (New York: Hachette, 2013), p. 62.
54. A. Horowitz, *Inside of a Dog* (New York: Scribner, 2012), p. 99.
55. 'Six Surprising Benefits of Curiosity', *Greater Good* magazine, Berkeley University (24 September 2015), https://greatergood.berkeley.edu/article/item/six_surprising_benefits_of_curiosity.
56. T. B. Kashdan, P. E. McKnight, F. D. Fincham and P. Rose, 'When Curiosity Breeds Intimacy: Taking Advantage of Intimacy Opportunities and Transforming Boring Conversations, *Journal of Personality*, 76:6 (2011), 1369–402. doi: 10.1111/j.1467-6494.2010.00697.x. Erratum in *Journal of Personality*, 80:1 (2012), 254. PMID: 22092143; PMCID: PMC3356784.
57. M. Sakaki, A. Yagi and K. Murayama, 'Curiosity in Old Age: A Possible Key to Achieving Adaptive Aging', *Neuroscience & Biobehavioral Reviews*, 88 (2018), 106–16.
58. Jaak Panksepp, quoted in T. Grandin and C. Johnson, *Animals in Translation* (London: Bloomsbury, 2006), p. 94.
59. Yong, *An Immense World*, p. 66.
60. BBC documentary *Spy in the Pod* (2014), produced by zoologist Robert Pilley.
61. https://www.smithsonianmag.com/smart-news/what-wild-animals-were-really-doing-during-covid-19-lockdowns-180982351/.
62. Yong, *An Immense World*, p. 277.

63. F. Mormann, J. Dubois, S. Kornblith, M. Milosavljevic, M. Cerf et al., 'A Category-Specific Response to Animals in the Right Human Amygdala', *Nature Neuroscience*, 14:10 (2011), 1247–9. doi: 10.1038/nn.2899.

2: A Remedy for the Lonely

1. *The Lancet* (24 June 2024).
2. S. C. Tiwari, 'Loneliness: A Disease?', *Indian Journal of Psychiatry*, 55:4 (October 2013), 320–22. doi: 10.4103/0019-5545.120536.
3. J. Lynch, *The Broken Heart: The Medical Consequences of Loneliness* (New York: Basic Books, 1977), p. 26.
4. J. Serpell, *In the Company of Animals: A Study of Human–Animal Relationships* (Oxford: Basil Blackwell, 1986), p. 91.
5. 'How a Dutch Tragedy Made People Take Loneliness Seriously', BBC Online (17 December 2023), https://www.bbc.co.uk/news/world-europe-67714026.
6. T. Fischer, L. C. Cory, K. Carr and S. Kwi, *Animal Music: Sound and Song in the Natural World*, ed. G. Kreens (London: Strange Attractor Press, 2015), p. 79.
7. C. Safina, *Beyond Words: What Animals Think and Feel* (London: Souvenir Press, 2016), p. 202.
8. K. Guo, K. Meints, C. Hall, S. Hall et al., 'Left Gaze Bias in Humans, Rhesus Monkeys and Domestic Dogs', *Animal Cognition*, 12: 3 (May 2009), 409–18. doi: 10.1007/s10071-008-0199-3.
9. Tatiana Safonova and István Sántha, in M. Brightman, V. E. Grotti and O. Ulturgasheva (eds), *Animism in Rainforest and Tundra: Personhood, Animals, Plants and Things in Contemporary Amazonia and Siberia* (New York: Berghahn Books, 2014), p. 84.
10. I. Robinson (ed.), *The Waltham Book of Human–Animal Interaction: Benefits and Responsibilities of Pet Ownership* (Oxford: Pergamon Press, 1995), p. 24.
11. A. Beck and A. Katcher, *Between Pets and People* (West Lafayette, Indiana: Purdue University Press, 1996), p. 14.
12. M. Becker and D. Morton, *The Healing Power of Pets* (New York: Hyperion, 2001), pp. 30 and 37.
13. PDSA Animal Wellbeing (PAW) Report, 2020.
14. D. Prince, 'Cultural Commentary: The Silence Between: An Autoethnographic Examination of the Language Prejudice and Its Impact on the Assessment of Autistic and Animal Intelligence', *Disability Studies Quarterly*, 30:1 (2010).
15. E. A. Cartmill and R. W. Byrne, 'Orangutans Modify Their Gestural Signaling According to Their Audience's Comprehension', *Current Biology*, 17:15 (August 2007), 1345–8. doi: 10.1016/j.cub.2007.06.069.

16. S. Hurn, *Humans and Other Animals: Cross-Cultural Perspectives on Human–Animal Interactions* (London: Pluto Press, 2012), pp. 33–4.
17. L. M. Silko, *Ceremony* (New York: Penguin, 1986), p. 95.
18. W. Lyon, *Black Elk: The Sacred Ways of a Lakota* (New York: HarperCollins, 1991), p. 33.
19. L. J. Wood, B. Giles-Corti, M. K. Bulsara and D. A. Bosch, 'More Than a Furry Companion: The Ripple Effect of Companion Animals on Neighborhood Interactions and Sense of Community', *Society and Animals*, 15 (2007), 43–56.
20. Becker and Morton, *The Healing Power of Pets*, p. 75.
21. L. A. Hart in J. Serpell (ed.), *The Domestic Dog: Its Evolution, Behaviour and Interactions with People* (Cambridge: Cambridge University Press, 1995) and A. Rennie, 'The Therapeutic Relationship Between Animals and Humans', *Society for Companion Animal Studies Journal*, 9:4 (1997), 1–4.
22. Interview on Hearing Dogs for Deaf People website.
23. Interview on Hearing Dogs for Deaf People website.
24. T. Grandin and C. Johnson, *Making Animals Happy* (London: Bloomsbury, 2009), p. 77.
25. N. Nemquimo and M. Anderson, *We Will Not Be Saved* (London: Wildfire, 2024), pp. 5, 23, 30 and 72.
26. M. Magan, *Thirty-Two Words for Field* (Dublin: Gill Books, 2020), p. 307.
27. M. Oliver, *Upstream: Selected Essays* (New York: Penguin Press, 2016), p. 16.
28. Serpell, *In the Company of Animals*, p. 51.
29. Serpell, *In the Company of Animals*, p. 48.
30. Serpell, *In the Company of Animals*, p. 50.
31. J. Briggs, *Never in Anger: Portrait of an Eskimo Family* (Cambridge, Massachusetts: Harvard University Press, 1970), p. 70.
32. Serpell, *In the Company of Animals*, p. 65.
33. A. L. Podberscek, E. S. Paul and J. A. Serpell (eds), *Companion Animals and Us: Exploring the Relationships Between People and Pets* (Cambridge: Cambridge University Press, 2005), p. 176.
34. G. Delorme, *Deer Man: Seven Years in the Forest* (London: Hachette, 2022), p. 173.
35. K. Murata, M. Nagasawa, T. Onaka, N. Kanemaki et al., 'Increase of Tear Volume in Dogs After Reunion with Owners is Mediated by Oxytocin', *Current Biology*, 32:16 (August 2022), R869–R870. doi: 10.1016/j.cub.2022.07.031.
36. 'How a Dutch Tragedy Made People Take Loneliness Seriously', BBC Online.

37. L. Dossey, 'The Healing Power of Pets: A Look at Animal-Assisted Therapy', *Alternative Therapies in Health and Medicine*, 3:4 (July 1997), 8–16. PMID: 9210769.
38. P. Tedeschi and M. A. Jenkins (eds), *Transforming Trauma: Resilience and Healing Through Our Connections with Animals* (West Lafayette, Indiana: Purdue University Press, 2019), p. 101.
39. Beck and Katcher, *Between Pets and People*, pp. 73–4.
40. Wood, Giles-Corti, Bulsara and Bosch, 'More Than a Furry Companion'.
41. Beck and Katcher, *Between Pets and People*, pp. 73–4.
42. Podberscek, Paul and Serpell, *Companion Animals and Us*, pp. 169–70.
43. N. N. Ladygina-Kohts, *Infant Chimpanzee and Human Child: A Classic 1935 Comparative Study of Ape Emotions and Intelligence*, ed. F. B. M. de Waal (New York: Oxford University Press, 2001).
44. Tedeschi and Jenkins, *Transforming Trauma*, p. 59.
45. F. B. M. de Waal, 'The Antiquity of Empathy', *Science*, 336:6083 (2012), 874–6.
46. J. Bräuer, K. Schönefeld and J. Call, 'When Do Dogs Help Humans?', *Applied Animal Behaviour Science*, 148 (September 2013), 138–49.
47. Stanford University's Center for Compassion and Altruism Research and Education, reported in E. Kinsey, 'What Humpback Whales Can Teach Us About Compassion', *Smithsonian Magazine* (August 2017), first published in *Hakai Magazine*.
48. R. Fouts and S. T. Mills, *Next of Kin: What Chimpanzees Have Taught Me About Who We Are* (New York: William Morrow, 1997), p. 291.
49. Fouts and Mills, *Next of Kin*, p. 15.
50. B. J. King, *How Animals Grieve* (Chicago: University of Chicago Press, 2013), pp. 78 and 79.
51. R. Stone, 'My Friend Koko', *Evening Standard* (13 April 2012).
52. D. Prince-Hughes, *Songs of the Gorilla Nation: My Journey Through Autism* (New York: Three Rivers Press, 2004), p. 112.
53. Prince-Hughes, *Songs of the Gorilla Nation*, pp. 129–31.
54. Tedeschi and Jenkins, *Transforming Trauma*, p. 222.
55. M. Bekoff, *The Emotional Lives of Animals* (Novato, California: New World Library, 2007), p. 20.
56. Podberscek, Paul and Serpell, *Companion Animals and Us*, pp. 168–9.
57. Serpell, *In the Company of Animals*, p. 29.
58. H. J. Jerison, 'The Perceptual World of Dolphins', in R. J. Schusterman, J. A. Thomas and F. G. Wood (eds), *Dolphin Cognition and Behavior: A Comparative View* (Hillsdale, New Jersey: Lawrence Erlbaum Associates, 1986), pp. 158–60.

59. D. Rothenberg, *Thousand Mile Song: Whale Music in a Sea of Sound* (New York: Basic Books, 2008), pp. 159–61.
60. F. de Waal, *Mama's Last Hug: Animal Emotions and What They Teach Us About Ourselves* (London: Granta, 2020), p. 96.
61. Safina, *Beyond Words*, p. 182.
62. L. Morino and C. M. Colvin, 'Thinking Pigs: A Comparative Review of Cognition, Emotion, and Personality in *Sus domesticus*', *International Journal of Comparative Psychology*, 28:1 (2015), ISSN 0889-3675, https://escholarship.org/uc/item/8sx4s79c Journal.
63. P. Broly and J.-L. Denueubourg, 'Behavioural Contagion Explains Group Cohesion in a Social Crustacean', *PLOS Computational Biology*, 11:6 (2015).
64. Safina, *Beyond Words*, p. 19.

3: Untangling the Psyche

1. M. Becker and D. Morton, *The Healing Power of Pets* (New York: Hyperion, 2002), p. 55.
2. Becker and Morton, *The Healing Power of Pets*, p. 55.
3. G. Gaffney, *Half Broke* (New York: W. W. Norton, 2020), pp. 65 and 68.
4. L. J. Keeling, L. Jonare and L. Lanneborn, 'Investigating Horse–Human Interactions: The Effect of a Nervous Human', *Veterinary Journal*, 181:1 (2009), 70–71. doi: 10.1016/j.tvjl.2009.03.013.
5. C. Wilson, 'Sirona Therapeutic Horsemanship Evaluation Impact Report 2020', Hartpury University, https://sironatherapeutichorsemanship.files.wordpress.com/2020/11/hartpury-report-2020-rev-5-23.11.20.pdf.
6. H. L. Burgon, 'Horses, Mindfulness and the Natural Environment: Observations from a Qualitative Study with At-Risk Young People Participating in Therapeutic Horsemanship', *International Journal of Psychosocial Rehabilitation*, 17:2 (2013), 51–67.
7. A. Liefooghe, *Equine-Assisted Psychotherapy and Coaching* (Oxon: Routledge, 2020), p. 125.
8. A. Beck and A. Katcher, *Between Pets and People* (West Lafayette, Indiana: Purdue University Press, 1996), pp. 102–3.
9. J. R. Nurenberg, S. J. Schleifer, T. M. Shaffer, M. Yellin et al., 'Animal-Assisted Therapy with Chronic Psychiatric Inpatients: Equine-Assisted Psychotherapy and Aggressive Behavior', *Psychiatric Services*, 66:1 (2014). doi: 10.1176/appi.ps.201300524; S. B. Barker and K. S. Dawson, 'The Effects of Animal-Assisted Therapy on Anxiety Ratings of Hospitalized Psychiatric Patients', *Psychiatric Services*, 49:6 (1998), 797–801; P. Nepps, C. Stewart

and S. Bruckno, 'Animal-Assisted Therapy: Effects on Stress, Mood, and Pain', *Journal of Lancaster General Hospital*, 6:2 (2011), 56–9; J. Serpell, *In the Company of Animals: A Study of Human–Animal Relationships* (Oxford: Basil Blackwell, 1986), p. 81.
10. P. Tedeschi and M. A. Jenkins (eds), *Transforming Trauma: Resilience and Healing Through Our Connections with Animals* (West Lafayette, Indiana: Purdue University Press, 2019), p. 101.
11. Liefooghe, *Equine-Assisted Psychotherapy and Coaching*, p. 97.
12. Tedeschi and Jenkins, *Transforming Trauma*, p. 309.
13. Becker and Morton, *The Healing Power of Pets*, p. 55.
14. Serpell, *In the Company of Animals*, pp. 76–8.
15. Tedeschi and Jenkins (eds), *Transforming Trauma*, p. 101.
16. Serpell, *In the Company of Animals*, p. 78.
17. D. Wells, 'The Value of Pets for Human Health', *Psychologist* (11 March 2011).
18. B. M. Levinson, 'Pets and Personality Development', *Psychological Reports*, 42 (1978), 1031–8.
19. Beck and Katcher, *Between Pets and People*, pp. 142–7.
20. J. Wittenauer and M. Ascher, ' "Prescribing" Companion Animals for Patients with Mental Illness', *Clinical Psychiatry News* (10 May 2013).
21. Andreas Liefooghe, pers. comm. (9 January 2023).
22. Wells, 'The Value of Pets for Human Health'.
23. Levinson, 'Pets and Personality Development'.
24. Wells, 'The Value of Pets for Human Health'.
25. Tedeschi and Jenkins, *Transforming Trauma*, p. 101.
26. M. A. Rivera, *On Dogs and Dying* (West Lafayette, Indiana: Purdue University Press, 2010), p. 5.
27. K. Kruger, S. Trachtenberg and J. Serpell, 'Can Animals Help Humans Heal? Animal-Assisted Interventions in Adolescent Mental Health' (2004), conference paper.
28. Liefooghe, *Equine-Assisted Psychotherapy and Coaching*, p. 2.
29. Kruger, Trachtenberg and Serpell, 'Can Animals Help Humans Heal?'.
30. Kruger, Trachtenberg and Serpell, 'Can Animals Help Humans Heal?'; N. Bardill and S. Hutchinson, 'Animal-Assisted Therapy with Hospitalized Adolescents', *Journal of Child and Adolescent Psychiatric Nursing*, 10:1 (1997), 17–24.
31. Nurenberg, Schleifer, Shaffer, Yellin et al., 'Animal-Assisted Therapy with Chronic Psychiatric Inpatients'.
32. Kruger, Trachtenberg and Serpell, 'Can Animals Help Humans Heal?'

33. Kruger, Trachtenberg and Serpell, 'Can Animals Help Humans Heal?'; Nurenberg, Schleifer, Shaffer, Yellin et al., 'Animal-Assisted Therapy with Chronic Psychiatric Inpatients'.
34. Serpell, *In the Company of Animals*, p. 77.
35. Wittenauer and Ascher, '"Prescribing" Companion Animals for Patients with Mental Illness'.
36. V. V. Vidovic, V. V. Stetic and D. Brathko, 'Pet Ownership, Type of Pet, and Socio-Emotional Development of School Children', *Anthrozoos*, 12:4 (1999).
37. P. Shepard, *The Others: How Animals Made Us Human* (Washington DC: Island Press, 1996), p. 148.
38. P. N. Schultz, G. A. Remick-Barlow and L. Robbins, 'Equine-Assisted Psychotherapy: A Mental Health Promotion/Intervention Modality for Children Who Have Experienced Intra-Family Violence', *Health & Social Care Community*, 15:13 (May 2007), 265–71. doi: 10.1111/j.1365-2524.2006.00684.x.
39. Liefooghe, *Equine-Assisted Psychotherapy and Coaching*, p. 89.
40. N. Kawamura, M. Niiyama and H. Niiyama, 'Long-Term Evaluation of Animal-Assisted Therapy for Institutionalized Elderly People', *Psychogeriatrics*, 7 (2007), 8–13.
41. Tedeschi and Jenkins, *Transforming Trauma*, p. 101; S. M. Arduini, 'Evaluation of an Experimental Program Designed to Have a Positive Effect on Adjudicated, Violent, Incarcerated Male Juveniles Age 12–25 in the State of Oregon', unpublished doctoral dissertation, Pepperdine University, California, 2000.
42. Liefooghe, *Equine-Assisted Psychotherapy and Coaching*, p. 89.
43. Beck and Katcher, *Between Pets and People*, pp. 125–7.
44. Serpell, *In the Company of Animals*, p. 78.
45. D. Preece-Kelly, *Unleashing the Healing Power of Animals* (Dorchester: Veloce, 2017), p. 75.
46. Kruger, Trachtenberg and Serpell, 'Can Animals Help Humans Heal?'
47. T. Henley, *Rediscovery: Ancient Pathways, New Directions* (Edmonton, Canada: Lone Pine, 1996), pp. 96–9.
48. D. Hunter and C. Sawyer, 'Blending Native American Spirituality with Individual Psychology in Work with Children', *Journal of Individual Psychology*, 62:3 (2006).
49. PBS News, 'Meet the "Courtroom Dogs" Who Help Child Crime Victims Tell Their Stories' (27 May 2016), https://www.pbs.org/newshour/show/meet-the-courtroom-dogs-who-help-child-crime-victims-tell-their-stories; Tedeschi and Jenkins, *Transforming Trauma*, p. 18.

50. M. Bekoff, *The Emotional Lives of Animals* (Novato, California: New World Library, 2007), p. 20.
51. Burgon, 'Horses, Mindfulness and the Natural Environment'.
52. Beck and Katcher, *Between Pets and People*, p. 7.
53. Serpell, *In the Company of Animals*, p. 77.
54. V. Hearne, *Adam's Task: Calling Animals by Name* (1986; New York: Skyhorse, 2007), p. 188.
55. M. J. Sams, E. V. Fortney and S. Willenbring, 'Occupational Therapy Incorporating Animals for Children with Autism: A Pilot Investigation', *American Journal of Occupational Therapy*, 60:3 (May–June 2006), 268–74. doi: 10.5014/ajot.60.3.268.
56. *Illustrated London News* (24 and 31 March 1860).
57. Wells, 'The Value of Pets for Human Health'.
58. G. E. Evans and D. Thomson, *The Leaping Hare* (London: Faber & Faber, 2017), pp. 243–4.
59. Tedeschi and Jenkins, *Transforming Trauma*, pp. 429, 437 and 451.
60. Tedeschi and Jenkins, *Transforming Trauma*, p. 21.
61. Becker and Morton, *The Healing Power of Pets*, p. 160.
62. A. Parton and S. Parton, *Endal: How One Extraordinary Dog Brought a Family Back from the Brink* (London: HarperTrue, 2009).
63. Becker and Morton, *The Healing Power of Pets*, p. 149.
64. J. Froling, 'Service Dog Tasks for Psychiatric Disabilities', Sterling Service Dogs, Michigan, 1998; ADA, Assistance Dogs of America, https://assistancedogregistry.com/law_information/.
65. Paws for Life USA, https://animalsdeservebetter.org/.
66. NBC Philadelphia, 'Service Dog Saves Blind Owner's Life During House Fire' (6 August 2015).
67. Froling, 'Service Dog Tasks for Psychiatric Disabilities'.
68. Tedeschi and Jenkins, *Transforming Trauma*.

4: Oh God, Get That Young Woman a Dog

1. Ken Baldwin, reported in 'Jumpers' by T. Friend, *New Yorker* (5 October 2003).
2. '"Amazing" Therapy Dog Helps Woman on Motorway Bridge', BBC News (16 June 2021).
3. A. Beck and A. Katcher, *Between Pets and People* (West Lafayette, Indiana: Purdue University Press, 1996), p. 200.

4. P. Tedeschi and M. A. Jenkins (eds), *Transforming Trauma: Resilience and Healing Through Our Connections with Animals* (West Lafayette, Indiana: Purdue University Press, 2019), pp. 379–80.
5. F. Bua, (2023): 'A Qualitative Investigation into Dogs Serving on Animal-Assisted Crisis Response (AACR) Teams: Advances in Crisis Counselling', thesis, La Trobe, 2023. doi: 10.26181/21844344.v1.
6. M. Becker and D. Morton, *The Healing Power of Pets* (New York: Hyperion, 2002), p. 49.
7. M. E. Rogers, 'Disaster Mental Health Field Work Enhanced by Animal-Assisted Crisis Response', HOPE Animal-Assisted Crisis Response (4 April 2014), www.hopeacr.org.
8. J. Rogers, L. A. Hart and R. P. Bolt, 'The Role of Pet Dogs in Casual Conversations of Elderly Adults', *Journal of Social Psychology*, 133:3 (June 1993), 265–77. doi: 10.1080/00224545.1993.9712145.
9. M. Bearzi, *Dolphin Confidential: Confessions of a Field Biologist* (Chicago: Chicago University Press, 2012), pp. 87–8.
10. H. A. Love, 'Best Friends Come in All Breeds: The Role of Pets in Suicidality', *Anthrozoös*, 34:2 (2021), 1–12. doi: 10.1080/08927936.2021.1885144.
11. A. M. Barcelos, N. Kargas, C. Packham and D. S. Mills, 'Understanding the Impact of Dog Ownership on Autistic Adults: Implications for Mental Health and Suicide Prevention', *Scientific Reports*, 11:23655 (2021).
12. 'Paws for Thought' report (2019), Simon Community Scotland, working with Dogs Trust, to support homeless people and their pets.
13. L. Scanlon, P. Hobson-West, K. Cobb, A. McBride et al., 'Homeless People and Their Dogs: Exploring the Nature and Impact of the Human–Companion Animal Bond', *Anthrozoös*, 34:1 (2021), 1–16. doi: 10.1080/08927936.2021.1878683.
14. 'Paws for Thought' report.

PART TWO

How Animals Heal the Individual Body

5: Emergency Services

1. 'Animal Heroes: Lulu the Pig', BBC Online (17 April 2015).
2. M. Bekoff, 'Pigs are Intelligent, Emotional, and Cognitively Complex', *Psychology Today* (12 June 2015).
3. '10 Fun Facts About Pigs', British Columbia Society for the Prevention of Cruelty to Animals website, https://spca.bc.ca/news/fun-facts-about-pigs/.

4. 'Parrot Saved Toddler's Life with Warning', *Telegraph* (25 March 2009).
5. A. Franklin, *Animals and Modern Cultures: A Sociology of Human–Animal Relations in Modernity* (London: Sage Publications, 1999), p. 87.
6. C. Safina, *Beyond Words: What Animals Think and Feel* (London: Souvenir Press, 2016), p. 61.
7. Safina, *Beyond Words*, p. 61.
8. Nan Hauser, interviewed for BBC Earth, 'A Whale Saved My Life', *Close Encounters* (broadcast 7 September 2021).
9. R. L. Pitman, V. B. Deecke, C. M. Gabriele, M. Srinivasan et al., 'Humpback Whales Interfering When Mammal-Eating Killer Whales Attack Other Species: Mobbing Behavior and Interspecific Altruism?', *Marine Mammal Science*, 33:1 (2017), 7–58.
10. 'Dolphins Shield Swimmers', news24 (23 November 2004), https://www.news24.com/news24/dolphins-shield-swimmers-20041123.
11. Safina, *Beyond Words*, pp. 351–2.
12. Safina, *Beyond Words*, pp. 351–3.
13. P. Tedeschi and M. A. Jenkins (eds), *Transforming Trauma: Resilience and Healing Through Our Connections with Animals* (West Lafayette, Indiana: Purdue University Press, 2019), p. 331.
14. S. Coren, 'Dogs Learn by Modeling the Behavior of Other Dogs', *Pyschology Today* (23 January 2013).
15. '5 Tales of Amazing Dog Heroics', CNN (9 December 2013).
16. 'Most Humans Rescued by a Dog in 24 Hours', Guinness World Records website, https://www.guinnessworldrecords.com/world-records/382221-most-humans-rescued-by-a-dog-in-24-hours.
17. R. Fouts and S. T. Mills, *Next of Kin: What Chimpanzees Have Taught Me About Who We Are* (New York: William Morrow, 1997), pp. 5–6.
18. H. Waddell, *Beasts and Saints* (London: Constable, 1934), p. 60.
19. P. Newman, *Tracking the Weretiger: Supernatural Man-Eaters of India, China and Southeast Asia* (Jefferson, North Carolina: McFarland, 2012), p. 32.
20. M. Brightman, V. E. Grotti and O. Ulturgasheva (eds), *Animism in Rainforest and Tundra: Personhood, Animals, Plants and Things in Contemporary Amazonia and Siberia* (New York: Berghahn Books, 2014), p. 54.
21. Brightman, Grotti and Ulturgasheva, *Animism in Rainforest and Tundra*, pp. 52–3.
22. M. Pomedli, *Living with Animals: Ojibwe Spirit Powers* (Toronto: University of Toronto Press, 2014), p. 156.
23. Pomedli, *Living with Animals*, p. 102.

24. D. Thomson, *The People of the Sea* (Edinburgh: Canongate Books, 1996), pp. 58–9.
25. M. Newton, *Savage Girls and Wild Boys: A History of Feral Children* (London: Faber & Faber, 2002), p. 6.
26. R. Louv, *Our Wild Calling* (Chapel Hill, North Carolina: Algonquin Books, 2019), pp. 106–7.
27. 'Abandoned Boy Said to Have Been Raised by a Dog', *New Zealand Herald* (4 August 2004).
28. 'Siberian Boy, 7, Raised by Dogs After Parents Abandoned Him', *Independent* (4 August 2004).
29. 'Chile's "Dog Boy" Flees Care Center', Reuters (14 November 2001), https://rense.com/general16/chiliDogBoy.htm.
30. M. Margaritoff, 'Ivan Mishukov: The Boy Who Was Saved by Dogs', All That's Interesting website (17 December 2001), https://allthatsinteresting.com/feral-children/7; M. Newton, *Savage Girls and Wild Boys: A History of Feral Children* (London: Faber, 2003), pp. 1 and 2.

6: Dog Doctors

1. 'Study Shows Dogs Can Accurately Sniff Out Cancer in Blood', *Science Daily* (8 April 2019).
2. A. Bowman, F. J. Dowell and N. P. Evans, 'The Effect of Different Genres of Music on the Stress Levels of Kennelled Dogs', *Physiology and Behavior*, 171 (2017), pp. 207–15.
3. C. Guest, *Daisy's Gift* (London: Virgin Books, 2017), pp. 117–19.
4. I. Tucker, 'Diseases That Dogs Can Detect', *Guardian* (4 November 2018).
5. M. Becker and D. Morton, *The Healing Power of Pets* (New York: Hyperion, 2002), p. 92.
6. 'Study Shows Dogs Can Accurately Sniff Out Cancer in Blood', *Science Daily*.
7. Guest, *Daisy's Gift*, p. 267.
8. Tucker, 'Diseases That Dogs Can Detect'.
9. Guest, *Daisy's Gift*, p. 253.
10. Guest, *Daisy's Gift*, pp. 207–10.
11. Becker and Morton, *The Healing Power of Pets*, p. 155.
12. Becker and Morton, *The Healing Power of Pets*, pp. 60–76.
13. 'Making Perfect Scents of PoTs', *The Sniff*, 21 (May/June 2022), Medication Detection Dogs magazine, ed. G. Butlin.
14. 'Making Perfect Scents of PoTs', *The Sniff*.
15. Author interview with Claire Guest (15 July and 13 October 2022).

16. Guest, *Daisy's Gift*, pp. 197–9.
17. Becker and Morton, *The Healing Power of Pets*, p. 93.

7: The Animal Apothecaries

1. J. Serpell, *In the Company of Animals: A Study of Human–Animal Relationships* (Oxford: Basil Blackwell, 1986), p. 74.
2. M. Pomedli, *Living with Animals: Ojibwe Spirit Powers* (Toronto: University of Toronto Press, 2014), p. 176.
3. A. Albert, 'Care Homes Use Snake Massage to Reduce Anxiety in Elderly', Home Care (17 October 2019), https://www.homecare.co.uk/news/article.cfm/id/1616410/Snake-therapist-charms-elderly
4. H. Bennett, 'Why Protecting Your Vagus Nerve is Key to Optimal Mental Health', BBC Science Focus (31 May 2024), https://www.sciencefocus.com/the-human-body/vagus-nerve.
5. 'This Nerve Influences Nearly Every Internal Organ: Can It Improve Our Mental State Too?', *The New York Times* (2 June 2022).
6. Serpell, *In the Company of Animals*, p. 75.
7. I. Robinson (ed.), *The Waltham Book of Human–Animal Interaction: Benefits and Responsibilities of Pet Ownership* (Oxford: Pergamon Press, 1995), p. 55.
8. A. Horowitz, *Inside of a Dog* (New York: Scribner, 2012), p. 312.
9. S. Ouanes and J. Popp, 'High Cortisol and the Risk of Dementia and Alzheimer's Disease: A Review of the Literature', *Frontiers in Aging Neuroscience*, 11 (2019).
10. Horowitz, *Inside of a Dog*, p. 312.
11. Rebecca Johnson, Research Center for Human/Animal Interaction at the University of Missouri College of Veterinary Medicine, quoted on NPR, 'Pet Therapy: How Animals and Humans Heal Each Other' (5 March 2012).
12. P. Tedeschi and M. A. Jenkins (eds), *Transforming Trauma: Resilience and Healing Through Our Connections with Animals* (West Lafayette, Indiana: Purdue University Press, 2019), p. 311.
13. Tedeschi and Jenkins, *Transforming Trauma*, p. 101.
14. A. L. Podberscek, E. S. Paul and J. A. Serpell (eds), *Companion Animals and Us: Exploring the Relationships Between People and Pets* (Cambridge: Cambridge University Press, 2005), pp. 125–40.
15. M. Bekoff, *The Emotional Lives of Animals* (Novato, California: New World Library, 2007), p. 16.
16. Tedeschi and Jenkins, *Transforming Trauma*, p. 26.

17. T. Nagasawa, Y. Kimura, K. Masuda and H. Uchiyama, 'Effects of Interactions with Cats in Domestic Environment on the Psychological and Physiological State of Their Owners: Associations among Cortisol, Oxytocin, Heart Rate Variability, and Emotions, *Animals*, 13:13 (2023), 2116. doi: 10.3390/ani13132116.
18. Tedeschi and Jenkins, *Transforming Trauma*, p. 302.
19. A. Beck and A. Katcher, *Between Pets and People* (West Lafayette, Indiana: Purdue University Press, 1996), p. 7.
20. Podberscek, Paul and Serpell, *Companion Animals and Us*, pp. 125–40.
21. R. Isaacson, *The Horse Boy* (London: Penguin, 2010), p. 53.
22. Beck and Katcher, *Between Pets and People*, p. 149.
23. Beck and Katcher, *Between Pets and People*, pp. 57–8.
24. Beck and Katcher, *Between Pets and People*, p. 7.
25. Podberscek, Paul and Serpell, *Companion Animals and Us*, pp. 125–40.
26. Pomedli, *Living with Animals*, pp. 105 and 113.
27. S. Hurn, *Humans and Other Animals: Cross-Cultural Perspectives on Human–Animal Interactions* (London: Pluto Press, 2012), p. 158.
28. Pomedli, *Living with Animals*, p. 141.
29. J. Lame Deer and R. Erdoes, *Lame Deer, Seeker of Visions: The Life of a Sioux Medicine Man* (New York: Touchstone, 1973), pp. 163–4.
30. Hurn, *Humans and Other Animals*, pp. 157–8.
31. M. A. Huffman, 'Current Evidence for Self-Medication in Primates: A Multidisciplinary Perspective', *Yearbook of Physical Anthropology*, 40 (1997), 171–200.
32. T. Grandin and C. Johnson, *Making Animals Happy.* (London: Bloomsbury, 2009), p. 241.
33. N. Klein, F. Fröhlich and S. Krief, 'Geophagy: Soil Consumption Enhances the Bioactivities of Plants Eaten by Chimpanzees', *Naturwissenschaften*, 95:4 (2008), 325–31.
34. 'Peculiar Potions' episode of BBC series *Weird Nature* (2002).
35. N. Miller, 'The Animals That Detect Disasters' (15 February 2022), BBC Future Planet, https://www.bbc.com/future/article/20220211-the-animals-that-predict-disasters.
36. *New Scientist* (7 March 2007), 'Letter: For the Record', https://www.newscientist.com/letter/mg19325941-000-for-the-record/.
37. L. Hogan, *The Radiant Lives of Animals* (Boston: Beacon Press, 2020), p. 89.
38. H. Witt, Polynesian navigation historian, 'The Soft, Warm, Wet Technology of Native Oceania', *Whole Earth Review* (Fall, 1991).

39. R. Sheldrake, *Dogs That Know When Their Owners are Coming Home* (London: Arrow Books, 2000), p. 216.
40. B. Sax, *Avian Illuminations: A Cultural History of Birds* (London: Reaktion Books, 2021), p. 72.
41. *Totem Latamat* (2021), dir. Michael Walling, commissioned by Border Crossings, https://www.youtube.com/watch?v=gebkkrKQyoI.
42. E. O. Wilson, 'My Wish: Build the Encyclopedia of Life', TED 2007 (March 2007), https://www.ted.com/talks/e_o_wilson_my_wish_build_the_encyclopedia_of_life?
43. 'Meta-Analysis Reveals Declines in Terrestrial but Increases in Freshwater Insect Abundances', *Science*, 368:6489 (24 April 2020), https://www.science.org/doi/10.1126/science.aax9931; 'Plummeting Insect Numbers Threaten Collapse of Nature', *Guardian* (10 February 2019).

8: Midwives for the Dying

1. M. Pomedli, *Living with Animals: Ojibwe Spirit Powers* (Toronto: University of Toronto Press, 2014), pp. 44–5.
2. L. Standing Bear, *Land of the Spotted Eagle* (Lincoln, Nebraska: University of Nebraska Press, 1978), pp. 211–12.
3. Pomedli, *Living with Animals*, pp. 109–10.
4. E. Doolittle, 'Crickets in the Concert Hall: A History of Animals in Western Music', *Transcultural Music Review*, 12 (2008).
5. Doolittle, 'Crickets in the Concert Hall'.
6. C. Safina, *Beyond Words: What Animals Think and Feel* (London: Souvenir Press, 2016), p. 364.
7. J. M. Lockhart, *Raptor: A Journey Through Birds* (London: Fourth Estate, 2016), p. 25.
8. R. Jeffers, 'Vulture', in *The Beginning and the End* (New York: Random House, 1963).
9. J. Marzluff and T. Angell, *Gifts of the Crow: How Perception, Emotion, and Thought Allow Smart Birds to Behave Like Humans* (New York: Simon & Schuster, 2012), pp. 137–46.
10. M. Bekoff, 'Animal Emotions, Wild Justice and Why They Matter: Grieving Magpies, a Pissy Baboon, and Empathic Elephants', *Emotion, Space and Society*, 2:2 (2009), 82–5.
11. B. J. King, *How Animals Grieve* (Chicago: University of Chicago Press, 2013), p. 47.

12. M. Bekoff, *The Emotional Lives of Animals* (Novato, California: New World Library, 2007), pp. 63–8.
13. B. Krause, *The Great Animal Orchestra* (New York: Hachette, 2013), p. 114.
14. Krause, *The Great Animal Orchestra*, pp. 117–18.
15. C. Moss, *Elephant Memories* (Chicago: University of Chicago Press, 2000), p. 270.
16. M. Ryan and P. Thornycroft, 'Jumbos Mourn Black Rhino Killed by Poachers', IOL (Independent Online), South Africa (18 November 2007).
17. E. von Muggenthaler, 'The Felid Purr: A Healing Mechanism', *Journal of the Acoustical Society of America*, 110:5 (2001), 2666.
18. Dr Stephanie Hodgkinson, pseudonym by request, pers. comm. (25 October 2022).
19. D. Dosa, *Making Rounds with Oscar: The Extraordinary Gift of an Ordinary Cat* (New York: Hyperion, 2010).
20. J. Lempin, ' "Doctor Peyo": The Horse Comforting Cancer Patients in Calais – in Pictures', *Guardian* (12 March 2021).
21. Safina, *Beyond Words*, p 71.
22. R. K. Nelson, *Make Prayers to the Raven* (Chicago: University of Chicago Press, 1983), p. 192.
23. M. A. Rivera, *On Dogs and Dying* (West Lafayette, Indiana: Purdue University Press, 2010), pp. 11–16.
24. Rivera, *On Dogs and Dying*, pp. 27–8.
25. J. Goddard, 'Faithful Tip's 105-Day Vigil Next to His Fallen Master Touched the Hearts of a Nation', Derbyshire Live (21 February 2018).
26. King, *How Animals Grieve*, p. 21.
27. BBC News, 'Greyfriars Bobby Tale is Wrong Claims Cardiff Historian' (5 August 2011), https://www.bbc.co.uk/news/uk-wales-14424513.
28. J. Cressey, 'Making a Splash in the Pacific: Dolphin and Whale Myths and Legends of Oceania', *Rapa Nui Journal*, 12:3 (September 1998), pp. 75–84.
29. M. Brightman, V. E. Grotti and O. Ulturgasheva (eds), *Animism in Rainforest and Tundra: Personhood, Animals, Plants and Things in Contemporary Amazonia and Siberia* (New York: Berghahn Books, 2014), p. 6.
30. B. Sax, *Avian Illuminations: A Cultural History of Birds* (London: Reaktion Books, 2021), pp. 302–3.
31. Sax, *Avian Illuminations*, p. 72.
32. L. Jensen, *Your Wild and Precious Life: On Grief, Hope and Rebellion* (Edinburgh: Canongate, 2024), p. 131.
33. Liz Jensen, pers. comm. (30 November 2023).

34. Liz Jensen, pers. comm. (30 November 2023).
35. Jensen, *Your Wild and Precious Life*, p. 205.
36. Liz Jensen, pers. comm. (30 November 2023).
37. R. L. Spaniol, M. D. S. Mendonça, S. M. Hartz et al., 'Discolouring the Amazon Rainforest: How Deforestation is Affecting Butterfly Coloration', *Biodiversity and Conservation*, 29:11 (August 2020). doi: 10.1007/s10531-020-01999-3.
38. J. G. Neihardt, *Black Elk Speaks* (Lincoln, Nebraska: University of Nebraska Press, 1988), p. 184.

PART THREE
How Animals Heal the Body Politic
9: Key Signatures for a Sound World

1. 'The Assessment Report of the Intergovernmental Science-Policy Platform on Biodiversity and Ecosystem Services on Pollinators, Pollination and Food Production', ed. S. G. Potts, V. L. Imperatriz-Fonseca and H. T. Ngo, IPBES (2016). doi: 10.5281/zenodo.3402856.
2. Walter Kaiser, quoted in 'Do Honeybees Sleep?', British Beekeepers Association website, https://www.bbka.org.uk/do-honeybees-sleep?
3. L. Jašarević, 'Can Honeybees Teach Us How to Live?', *Sapiens* (13 December 2018), https://www.sapiens.org/culture/apiaries-beekeeping-bosnia/.
4. M. Pomedli, *Living with Animals: Ojibwe Spirit Powers* (Toronto: University of Toronto Press, 2014), p. xxxi.
5. K. Cohen, *Honoring the Medicine* (New York: Ballantine Books, 2006), p. 307.
6. Cohen, *Honoring the Medicine*, p. 2.
7. R. Katz, *Boiling Energy: Community Healing Among the Kalahari !Kung* (Cambridge, Massachusetts: Harvard University Press, 1982), p. 33.
8. J. Blancou, B. B. Chomel, A. Belotto and F. X. Meslin, 'Emerging or Re-emerging Bacterial Zoonoses: Factors of Emergence, Surveillance and Control', *Veterinary Research*, 36 (2005), 507–22.
9. J. Coulehan, 'Navajo Indian Medicine: Implications for Healing', *Journal of Family Practice*, 10:1 (1980), 55–61.
10. L. Jašarević, *Beekeeping in the End Times* (Bloomington: Indiana University Press, 2024), p. 6; Jašarević, 'Can Honeybees Teach Us How to Live?'.
11. M. Magan, *Thirty-Two Words for Field* (Dublin: Gill Books, 2020), pp. 195–8.
12. L. Herbowski, 'The Maze of the Cerebrospinal Fluid Discovery', *Anatomy Research International* (December 2013). doi: 10.1155/2013/596027.

13. M. Zoldas, 'The Therapeutic Sound of Slovenian Bees', BBC Reel (21 July 2020).
14. Jašarević, *Beekeeping in the End Times*, p. 170; Jašarević, 'Can Honeybees Teach Us How to Live?'.
15. E. von Muggenthaler, 'The Felid Purr: A Healing Mechanism?', *Journal of the Acoustical Society of America*, 110:5 (2001), 2666.
16. A. Cochrane and K. Callen, *Dolphins and Their Power to Heal* (London: Bloomsbury, 1992), p. 15.
17. G. Reichel-Dolmatoff, *The Forest Within: The World-View of the Tukano Amazonian Indians* (Totnes: Themis Books, 1996), pp. 149 and 182.
18. Cohen, *Honoring the Medicine*, p. 40.
19. David Dunn in D. Rothenberg and M. Ulvaeus (eds), *The Book of Music and Nature* (Middletown, Connecticut: Wesleyan University Press, 2000), p. 106.
20. Pomedli, *Living with Animals*, p. 106.
21. Pomedli, *Living with Animals*, p. 103.
22. Cymin Samawatie, quoted in D. Rothenberg, *Nightingales in Berlin: Searching for the Perfect Sound* (Chicago: University of Chicago Press, 2019), p. 142.
23. E. Stobbe, J. Sundermann, L. Ascone and S. Kühn, 'Birdsongs Alleviate Anxiety and Paranoia in Healthy Participants', *Scientific Reports*, 12 (2022), 16414. doi:10.1038/s41598-022-20841-0.
24. R. Hammoud, S. Tognin, L. Burgess, N. Bergou et al., 'Smartphone-Based Ecological Momentary Assessment Reveals Mental Health Benefits of Birdlife', *Scientific Reports*, 12 (2022), 17589. doi: 10.1038/s41598-022-20207-6.
25. R. T. Buxton, A. L. Pearson, H.-Y. Lin, J. C. Sanciangco et al., 'Exploring the Relationship Between Bird Diversity and Anxiety and Mood Disorder Hospitalisation Rates', *Geo: Geography and Environment*, 10 (2023), e127.
26. J. Methorst, A. Bonn, M. Marselle, K. Böhning-Gaese et al., 'Species Richness is Positively Related to Mental Health: A Study for Germany', *Landscape and Urban Planning*, 211 (2021), 104084.
27. R. S. Johnson, *Messiaen* (Berkeley, California: University of California Press, 1975), p. 117.
28. D. Rothenberg, *Why Birds Sing: A Journey Through the Mystery of Bird Song* (New York: Basic Books, 2005), p. 194.
29. D. Rothenberg, *Secret Sounds of Ponds* (New York: Roof Books, 2023), p. 28.
30. E. Doolittle, 'Crickets in the Concert Hall: A History of Animals in Western Music', *Transcultural Music Review*, 12 (2008).
31. B. Krause, 'How Can Natural Soundscapes Provide a Refuge from Our Hyper-Stimulated World?', *Literary Hub* (28 September 2021).
32. B. Krause, *The Great Animal Orchestra* (New York: Hachette, 2013), p. 87.

33. Krause, *The Great Animal Orchestra*, p. 84.
34. P. Shepard, *The Others: How Animals Made Us Human* (Washington DC: Island Press, 1996), p. 154.
35. Krause, *The Great Animal Orchestra*, p. 92.
36. J. Lewis, 'A Cross-Cultural Perspective on the Significance of Music and Dance on Culture and Society, with Insight from BaYaka Pygmies', in M. Arbib (ed.), *Language, Music and the Brain: A Mysterious Relationship* (Cambridge, Massachusetts: MIT Press, 2012).
37. Krause, 'How Can Natural Soundscapes Provide a Refuge?'
38. Jašarević, *Beekeeping in the End Times*, pp. 1 and 177; Jašarević, 'Can Honeybees Teach Us How to Live?'.

10: Wolves at the Core of Ethics

1. T. Grandin and C. Johnson, *Animals in Translation* (London: Bloomsbury, 2006), p. 304.
2. B. Hare and V. Woods, *Survival of the Friendliest: Understanding Our Origins and Rediscovering Our Common Humanity* (London: Oneworld, 2020).
3. Grandin and Johnson, *Animals in Translation*, pp. 304–6.
4. Wolfgang M. Schleidt, retired director of the Konrad Lorenz Institute of Ethology in Vienna.
5. R. McIntyre, *The Reign of Wolf 21* (Vancouver: Greystone Books, 2022), pp. 138–9.
6. B. Lopez, *Of Wolves and Men* (New York: Scribner, 2004), pp. 103–5.
7. Lopez, *Of Wolves and Men*, pp. 128–9.
8. Lopez, *Of Wolves and Men*, p. 121.
9. M. Bekoff, 'Animals Can be Ambassadors for Forgiveness, Generosity, Peace, Trust, and Hope', *Psychology Today* (8 July 2009).
10. D. Prince-Hughes, *Songs of the Gorilla Nation: My Journey Through Autism* (New York: Three Rivers Press, 2004), p. 218.
11. Prince-Hughes, *Songs of the Gorilla Nation*, p. 142.
12. G. Reichel-Dolmatoff, *The Forest Within: The World-View of the Tukano Amazonian Indians* (Totnes: Themis Books, 1996), p. 150.
13. A. McGinnis, A. T. Kincaid, M. J. Barrett, C. Ham et al., 'Strengthening Animal–Human Relationships as a Doorway to Indigenous Holistic Wellness', *Ecopsychology* (September 2019), 162–73.
14. R. W. Kimmerer, *Braiding Sweetgrass* (London: Penguin, 2020), p. 9.
15. M. Bekoff and J. Pierce, *Wild Justice* (Chicago: University of Chicago Press, 2009), p. 19.

16. M. Pomedli, *Living with Animals: Ojibwe Spirit Powers* (Toronto: University of Toronto Press, 2014), p. 101.
17. Tim Ingold in A. Manning and J. Serpell (eds), *Animals and Human Society* (London: Routledge, 1994), p. 9.
18. D. Rothenberg and M. Ulvaeus (eds), *The Book of Music and Nature* (Middletown, Connecticut: Wesleyan University Press, 2000), p. 181.
19. M. Bekoff, *Minding Animals: Awareness, Emotions, and Heart* (New York: Oxford University Press, 2003), p. 123.
20. Bekoff, *Minding Animals*, p. 123.
21. B. Keenan, *An Evil Cradling* (London: Vintage, 1993), p. 288.
22. E. T. Frank, M. Wehrhahn and K. E. Linsenmair, 'Wound Treatment and Selective Help in a Termite-Hunting Ant', *Proceedings of the Royal Society B*, 285:1872 (14 February 2018). doi: 10.1098/rspb.2017.2457.
23. McIntyre, *The Reign of Wolf 21*, p. 90.
24. McIntyre, *The Reign of Wolf 21*, pp. 232–5.
25. M. Becker and D. Morton, *The Healing Power of Pets* (New York: Hyperion, 2002), p. 57.
26. R. Fouts and S. T. Mills, *Next of Kin: What Chimpanzees Have Taught Me About Who We Are* (New York: William Morrow, 1997), p. 289.
27. Fouts and Mills, *Next of Kin*, p. 111.
28. J. Kluger, 'What Makes Us Moral', *Time* magazine (21 November 2007).
29. *Naturebang*, BBC Radio 4 (21 January 2022).
30. Bekoff, *Minding Animals*, p. x.
31. F. de Waal, *Mama's Last Hug: Animal Emotions and What They Teach Us About Ourselves* (London: Granta, 2020), p. 151.
32. F. Patterson, 'Conversations with a Gorilla', *National Geographic* (October 1976).
33. Fouts and Mills, *Next of Kin*, p. 271.
34. J. E. Sprinkle, 'Animals, Empathy, and Violence: Can Animals be Used to Convey Principles of Prosocial Behavior to Children?', *Youth Violence and Juvenile Justice*, 6:1 (2008), 47–58.
35. McIntyre, *The Reign of Wolf 21*, pp. xiv–xv.
36. V. Hearne, *Adam's Task: Calling Animals by Name* (1986; New York: Skyhorse, 2007), p. 207.
37. 'Indisputable with Dr Rashad Richey', https://www.youtube.com/watch?v=JTm1kjDeAqU.
38. Pomedli, *Living with Animals*, p. 152.
39. J. Serpell, *In the Company of Animals* (Oxford: Basil Blackwell, 1986), p. 144.

40. R. K. Nelson, *Make Prayers to the Raven* (Chicago: University of Chicago Press, 1983), p. 21.
41. M. Brightman, V. E. Grotti and O. Ulturgasheva (eds), *Animism in Rainforest and Tundra: Personhood, Animals, Plants and Things in Contemporary Amazonia and Siberia* (New York: Berghahn Books, 2014), p. 39.
42. Reichel-Dolmatoff, *The Forest Within*, p. 85.
43. *Feminine Power* exhibition at the British Museum (May 2022).

11: The Fair Play of Justice

1. K. Sewall, 'The Girl Who Gets Gifts from Birds', BBC News (25 February 2015).
2. J. Ackerman, *The Genius of Birds* (London: Corsair, 2016), p. 121.
3. D. Prince-Hughes, *Songs of the Gorilla Nation: My Journey Through Autism* (New York: Three Rivers Press, 2004), p. 36.
4. J. H. Leuba, 'Morality Among the Animals', *Harper's Monthly*, 937 (1928), 97–103.
5. 'Animal Minds', *Radiolab* podcast (3 December 2021).
6. F. Range, K. Leitner and Z. Virányi, 'The Influence of the Relationship and Motivation on Inequity Aversion in Dogs', *Social Justice Research*, 25:2 (2012), 170–94. doi: 10.1007/ s11211-012-0155-x.
7. C. A. F. Wascher and T. Bugnyar, 'Behavioral Responses to Inequity in Reward Distribution and Working Effort in Crows and Ravens', *PLoS ONE*, 8:2 (2013), e56885, https://doi.org/10.1371/journal.pone.0056885.
8. F. de Waal, *Are We Smart Enough to Know How Smart Animals Are?* (London: Granta, 2016), p. 197.
9. de Waal, *Are We Smart Enough*, p. 198.
10. F. de Waal, *Mama's Last Hug: Animal Emotions and What They Teach Us About Ourselves* (London: Granta, 2020), p. 215.
11. Ackerman, *The Genius of Birds*, pp. 120–21.
12. T. Grandin and C. Johnson, *Animals in Translation* (London: Bloomsbury, 2006), p. 282.
13. Richard Wilkinson, 'Unhealthy Societies: The Afflictions of Inequality', in M. Bekoff and J. Pierce, *Wild Justice* (Chicago: University of Chicago Press, 2009), p. 130.
14. B. Jackson, L. Kubzansky and R. Wright, 'Linking Perceived Unfairness to Physical Health: The Perceived Unfairness Model', *Review of General Psychology*, 10 (2006), 21–40. doi: 10.1037/1089-2680.10.1.21.
15. Bekoff and Pierce, *Wild Justice*, p. 130.

16. C. Leineweber, C. Eib, P. Peristera and C. Bernhard-Oettel, 'The Influence of and Change in Procedural Justice on Self-Rated Health Trajectories: Swedish Longitudinal Occupational Survey of Health Results', *Scandinavian Journal of Work, Environment & Health*, 42:4 (1 July 2016), 320–28. doi: 10.5271/sjweh.3565.
17. M. Bekoff, *The Emotional Lives of Animals* (Novato, California: New World Library, 2007), pp. 89–91.
18. Bekoff, *The Emotional Lives of Animals*, p. 89.
19. Bekoff, *The Emotional Lives of Animals*, p. 98.
20. Bekoff, *The Emotional Lives of Animals*, p. 102.
21. Bekoff, *The Emotional Lives of Animals*, pp. 89 and 91.
22. Bekoff, *The Emotional Lives of Animals*, p. 109.
23. de Waal, *Mama's Last Hug*, p. 214.
24. de Waal, *Mama's Last Hug*, p. 215.
25. J. R. Anderson, B. Bucher, H. Chijiiwa and H. Kuroshima et al., 'Third-Party Social Evaluations of Humans by Monkeys and Dogs', *Neuroscience and Biobehavioral Reviews*, 82 (2017), 95–109.
26. C. Moss, *Elephant Memories* (Chicago: University of Chicago Press, 2000), pp. 186–7.
27. de Waal, *Mama's Last Hug*, p. 98.
28. Marc Bekoff, 'The Animal Manifesto: Six Reasons for Expanding our Compassion Footprint', quoted in S. Colling, *Animal Resistance in the Global Capitalist Era* (East Lansing: Michigan State University Press, 2021), pp. 41–2.
29. J. Marzluff and T. Angell, *In the Company of Crows and Ravens* (New Haven, Connecticut: Yale University Press, 2005), p. 24.
30. E. Westermarck, *The Origin and Development of Moral Ideas* (London: Macmillan, 1912).
31. L. Watson, *Elephantoms* (New York: W. W. Norton, 2003), pp. 113–19.
32. C. Williams, 'Elephants on the Edge Fight Back', *New Scientist* (15 February 2006).
33. M. Bekoff, *Minding Animals: Awareness, Emotions, and Heart* (New York: Oxford University Press, 2003), p. 6.
34. R. Fouts and S. T. Mills, *Next of Kin: What Chimpanzees Have Taught Me About Who We Are* (New York: William Morrow, 1997), p. 142.
35. 'Baboons Ambush Motorist', News24 (2 December 2000), https://www.news24.com/news24/baboons-ambush-motorist-20001202.
36. J. Hribal, *Fear of the Animal Planet: The Hidden History of Animal Resistance* (Petrolia, California: CounterPunch, 2010), pp. 21 and 24.
37. Sahil Nijhawan, pers. comm. (23 September 2022).

38. J. Vaillant, *The Tiger: A True Story of Vengeance and Survival* (London: Sceptre, 2010), p. 153.
39. Vaillant, *The Tiger*, p. 14.
40. Vaillant, *The Tiger*, p. 319.
41. Colling, *Animal Resistance in the Global Capitalist Era*, p. 66.
42. S. L. Swartz, *Lagoon Time* (Washington: The Ocean Foundation, 2014), p. 83.
43. R. Kessler, 'Hugs Follow a 3-Second Rule', *Science* (28 January 2011), https://www.science.org/content/article/hugs-follow-3-second-rule.
44. Swartz, *Lagoon Time*, p. 36.
45. S. Nightingale, *Touched: Revelations at San Ignacio Lagoon* (Reno, Nevada: Samara Press, forthcoming), p. 4.
46. Swartz, *Lagoon Time*, pp. 107–9.
47. Swartz, *Lagoon Time*, p. 60.
48. C. Siebert, 'Watching Whales Watching Us', *The New York Times* (8 July 2009).
49. R. Payne, *Among Whales* (New York: Scribner, 1995), p. 345.
50. Payne, *Among Whales*, p. 220.
51. Siebert, 'Watching Whales Watching Us'.
52. de Waal, *Mama's Last Hug*, pp. 134–5.
53. de Waal, *Mama's Last Hug*, p. 125.
54. Nightingale, *Touched*, p. 14.

12: Political Animals

1. O. Hogstad, 'Nest Defence Strategies in the Fieldfare *Turdus Pilaris*: The Responses on an Avian and a Mammalian Predator', *Ardea*, 92 (2004).
2. *Turdus* is Latin for 'thrush', whose family fieldfares belong to.
3. M. Beckman, 'Farting Fish Keep in Touch', *Science* (7 November 2003), https://www.science.org/content/article/farting-fish-keep-touch.
4. L. Conradt and T. J. Roper, 'Group Decision-Making in Animals', *Nature* 421:6919 (2003), 155–8.
5. Conradt and Roper, 'Group Decision-Making in Animals'.
6. D. R. Farine, 'Collective Behaviour: Jackdaws Vote to Leave with Their Voice', *Current Biology*, 32:10 (2022), R467–R469.
7. T. Seeley, *Honeybee Democracy* (Princeton: Princeton University Press, 2010), p. 226.
8. G. B. Shaw, *Man and Superman* (1903).
9. J. Bridle, *Ways of Being* (London: Allen Lane, 2022), pp. 259–61.
10. Bridle, *Ways of Being*, p. 145.

11. J. Cressey, 'Making a Splash in the Pacific: Dolphin and Whale Myths and Legends of Oceania', *Rapa Nui Journal*, 12:3 (September 1998), 75–84.
12. R. K. Nelson, *Make Prayers to the Raven* (Chicago: University of Chicago Press, 1983), p. 83.
13. P. Kropotkin, *Mutual Aid: A Factor of Evolution* (New York: Dover, 2006), p. 9.
14. M. A. Elgar, 'House Sparrows Establish Foraging Flocks by Giving Chirrup Calls if the Resources are Divisible', *Animal Behaviour*, 34:1 (1986), 169–74.
15. G. Delorme, *Deer Man: Seven Years in the Forest* (London: Hachette, 2022), pp. 118–24.
16. L. E. Steckermeier, 'The Value of Autonomy for the Good Life: An Empirical Investigation of Autonomy and Life Satisfaction in Europe', *Social Indicators Research*, 154 (2021), 693–723; D. Cosme and E. T. Berkman, 'Autonomy Can Support Affect Regulation During Illness and in Health', *Journal of Health Psychology*, 25:1 (2020); A. Kukita, J. Nakamura and M. Csikszentmihalyi, 'How Experiencing Autonomy Contributes to a Good Life', *Journal of Positive Psychology*, 17:1 (2022).
17. 'Will No Cage Hold Him? Monkey Again Escapes Zoo', *The New York Times* (15 August 2007).
18. R. Fouts and S. T. Mills, *Next of Kin: What Chimpanzees Have Taught Me About Who We Are* (New York: William Morrow, 1997), p. 151.
19. J. Hribal, *Fear of the Animal Planet: The Hidden History of Animal Resistance* (Petrolia, California: CounterPunch, 2010), p. 96.
20. Hribal, *Fear of the Animal Planet: The Hidden History of Animal Resistance*, p. 109.
21. 'Escaped Goat, Rumored to Have Freed Others from Slaughter, Has Been Captured', *Huffington Post* (30 August 2018).
22. 'Elephant Sets Antelopes Free', IOL (Independent Online), South Africa (8 April 2003).
23. 'Wild Horses of Newbury', https://www.facebook.com/filmsforaction/videos/wild-horses-of-newbury/10153379308455983/.
24. G. Monbiot, *Regenesis* (London: Penguin, 2022), p. 136.
25. G. Cajete, *Look to the Mountain: An Ecology of Indigenous Education* (Durango, Colorado: Kivaki Press, 1994), p. 88.
26. L. Standing Bear, *Land of the Spotted Eagle* (Lincoln, Nebraska: University of Nebraska Press, 1978), p. 193.
27. J. Goodall and D. Peterson, *Visions of Caliban: On Chimpanzees and People* (Athens, Georgia: University of Georgia Press, 1993), p. 145.
28. 'Elephant was Beaten 4 Days, Wild Animal Park Worker Says', *Los Angeles Times* (4 June 1988).

29. Hribal, *Fear of the Animal Planet*, p. 151.
30. Hribal, *Fear of the Animal Planet*, pp. 144 and 150.
31. M. Magan, *Thirty-Two Words for Field* (Dublin: Gill Books, 2020), p. 335.
32. S. Hattenstone, *Guardian* (6 January 2022).
33. 'Chimpanzees "Addicted" to Mobile Phones', *Global Times* (23 March 2023); 'Why the Toronto Zoo Wants You to Stop Showing Its Gorillas Videos from Your Phones', CTV News Toronto (7 July 2023); 'US Zoo Fears Teen Gorilla's Exposure to Phones is Behind Anti-Social Behavior', *Guardian* (6 April 2022).
34. 'Why the Toronto Zoo Wants You to Stop Showing Its Gorillas Videos', CTV News Toronto.
35. Hollie Ross, behavioural husbandry supervisor at Toronto Zoo, in an interview with Canadian broadcaster CP24; *Toronto Star* (7 July 2023).

PART FOUR
How Animals Heal the Soul Politic

13: Pink Pink Stink Nice Drink

1. B. Sax, *Avian Illuminations: A Cultural History of Birds* (London: Reaktion Books, 2021), pp. 164–5.
2. R. K. Nelson, *Make Prayers to the Raven* (Chicago: University of Chicago Press, 1983), p. 104.
3. J. Serpell, *In the Company of Animals: A Study of Human–Animal Relationships* (Oxford: Basil Blackwell, 1986), p. 61.
4. J. Hribal, *Fear of the Animal Planet: The Hidden History of Animal Resistance* (Petrolia, California: CounterPunch, 2010), p. 5.
5. S. Hurn, *Humans and Other Animals: Cross-Cultural Perspectives on Human–Animal Interactions* (London: Pluto Press, 2012), p. 100.
6. Hurn, *Humans and Other Animals*, p. 104.
7. 'Banksy Creates New "Working from Home" Artwork', *Bristol 24/7* (15 April 2020).
8. A. Franklin, *Animals and Modern Cultures: A Sociology of Human–Animal Relations in Modernity* (London: Sage Publications, 1999), p. 99.
9. G. Reichel-Dolmatoff, *Rainforest Shamans: Essays on the Tukano Indians of the Northwest Amazon* (Totnes: Themis Books, 1997), pp. 221–2.
10. K. Cohen, *Honoring the Medicine* (New York: Ballantine Books, 2006), p. 29.
11. Sax, *Avian Illuminations*, p. 118.
12. S. Pike, *For the Wild: Ritual and Commitment in Radical Eco-Activism* (Oakland, California: University of California Press, 2017), p. 117.

13. L. Standing Bear, *Land of the Spotted Eagle* (Lincoln, Nebraska: University of Nebraska Press, 1978), p. 207.
14. J. G. Neihardt, *Black Elk Speaks* (Lincoln, Nebraska: University of Nebraska Press, 1988), p. 26.
15. F. B. Linderman, *Plenty-Coups: Chief of the Crows* (Lincoln, Nebraska: University of Nebraska Press, 1962), p. 6.
16. T. Hughes, 'The Thought-Fox', in *The Hawk in the Rain* (London: Faber, 1957).
17. BBC Radio 4, *Today* (8 February 2024).
18. C. Safina, *Beyond Words: What Animals Think and Feel* (London: Souvenir Press, 2016), p. 350.
19. G. Mackay Brown, 'A Country Boy Goes to School', in *The Collected Poems of George Mackay Brown*, ed. A. Bevan and B. Murray (London: John Murray, 2005).
20. Stroke Association, stroke.org.uk.
21. Interview by Dr Luz Mar González-Arias, 'Fox Talks: Species Intersections and Healing in "A Quarter of an Hour"', *The Polyphony* (4 April 2022), https://thepolyphony.org/2022/04/04/fox-talks-species-intersections-and-healing-in-a-quarter-of-an-hour/.
22. Sax, *Avian Illuminations*, p. 51.
23. A.-S. Tribot, N. Blanc, T. Brassac, F. Guilhaumon et al., 'What Makes a Teddy Bear Comforting? A Participatory Study Reveals the Prevalence of Sensory Characteristics and Emotional Bonds in the Perception of Comforting Teddy Bears', *Journal of Positive Psychology*, 19 (2023), 1–14. doi: 10.1080/17439760.2023.2170273.
24. L. Hogan, *The Radiant Lives of Animals* (Boston, Massachusetts: Beacon Press, 2020), p. 10.
25. J. Cressey, 'Making a Splash in the Pacific: Dolphin and Whale Myths and Legends of Oceania', *Rapa Nui Journal*, 12:3 (September 1998), 75–84.
26. Etymonline.com.
27. B. Krause, *The Great Animal Orchestra* (New York: Hachette, 2013), p. 66.
28. Siyabona Africa, 'San', www.krugerpark.co.za/africa_bushmen.html.
29. M. Pomedli, *Living with Animals: Ojibwe Spirit Powers* (Toronto: University of Toronto Press, 2014), p. 31.
30. M. Robinson, 'Animals of the Serranía de la Lindosa: Exploring Representation and Categorisation in the Rock Art and Zooarchaeological Remains of the Colombian Amazon', *Journal of Anthropological Archaeology*, 75 (September 2024).
31. E. Wilmer, 'Of a Word', in *Tourist in Hell* (Chicago: University of Chicago Press, 2010), p. 94.

14: Wild Alleluia

1. J. Goodall, 'Primate Spirituality', in *The Encyclopedia of Religion and Nature*, ed. B. Taylor (New York: Thoemmes Continuum, 2005), pp. 1303–6.
2. B. Wallauer, 'Exploring Evolution and Spirituality in Chimpanzees and Humans' (6 June 2017), Jane Goodall Institute website, https://janegoodall.org/.
3. Wallauer, 'Exploring Evolution and Spirituality in Chimpanzees and Humans'.
4. M. Bekoff, 'Great Apes', *Psychology Today* (16 March 2023).
5. J. Harrod, 'The Case for Chimpanzee Religion', *Journal for the Study of Religion, Nature and Culture*, 8 (2014), 8–45. doi: 10.1558/jsrnc.v8i1.8.
6. J. Pruetz and T. LaDuke, 'Brief Communication: Reaction to Fire by Savanna Chimpanzees (*Pan troglodytes verus*) at Fongoli, Senegal: Conceptualization of "Fire Behavior" and the Case for a Chimpanzee Model', *American Journal of Physical Anthropology*, 141:4 (2010).
7. C. Safina, *Beyond Words: What Animals Think and Feel* (London: Souvenir Press, 2016), p. 55.
8. H. Kühl, A. Kalan, M. Arandjelovic, F. Aubert et al., 'Chimpanzee Accumulative Stone Throwing', *Scientific Reports*, 6: 22219 (2016). doi: 10.1038/srep22219.
9. R. Fouts and S. T. Mills, *Next of Kin: What Chimpanzees Have Taught Me About Who We Are* (New York: William Morrow, 1997), p. 48.
10. D. Prince-Hughes, *Songs of the Gorilla Nation: My Journey Through Autism* (New York: Three Rivers Press, 2004), p. 98.
11. D. Rothenberg, *Why Birds Sing: A Journey Through the Mystery of Bird Song* (New York: Basic Books, 2005), p. 133.
12. S. Nightingale, *Granada: The Light of Andalucia* (Boston, Massachusetts: Nicholas Brealey Publishing, 2015), p. 168.
13. P. Vitebsky, *Reindeer People: Living with Animals and Spirits in Siberia* (London: Harper Perennial, 2005), p. 11.
14. P. Matthiessen, *The Birds of Heaven: Travels with Cranes* (London: Vintage, 2003).
15. M. Magan, *Thirty-Two Words for Field* (Dublin: Gill Books, 2020), p. 306.
16. Magan, *Thirty-Two Words for Field*, p. 308.
17. Farid ud-Din Attar, *The Conference of Birds* (originally published 1177).
18. B. Smuts, 'Encounters with Animal Minds', *Journal of Consciousness Studies*, 8:5–7 (January 2001), 293–309.
19. S. Pike, *For the Wild: Ritual and Commitment in Radical Eco-Activism* (Oakland, California: University of California Press, 2017), p. 210.

20. 'Meet the Diviners', Nggam Dù website, https://nggamdu.org/; Tomás Saraceno in Collaboration: *Web(s) of Life*, Serpentine Gallery, London (2023).
21. D. Brooks, *Animal Dreams* (Sydney: Sydney University Press, 2021), p. 253.
22. T. Bullough, *Sarn Helen: A Journey Through Wales, Past, Present and Future* (London: Granta, 2023), pp. 224–5.
23. V. E. Sturm, S. Datta, A. R. K. Roy, I. J. Sible et al., 'Big Smile, Small Self: Awe Walks Promote Prosocial Positive Emotions in Older Adults', *Emotion*, 22:5 (2020), 1044–58. doi: 10.1037/emo0000876.
24. T. A. Balboni, T. J. VanderWeele, S. D. Doan-Soares, K. N. G. Long et al., 'Spirituality in Serious Illness and Health', *JAMA*, 328:2 (12 July 2022), 184–97.
25. Hildegard von Bingen, *Liber Divinorum Operum*, https://sufipathoflove.files.wordpress.com/2019/12/liber-divinorum-operum-.pdf.
26. T. Hughes, *Wales's Best One Hundred Churches* (Bridgend: Seren, 2007), p. 136.
27. B. Sax, *Avian Illuminations: A Cultural History of Birds* (London: Reaktion Books, 2021), p. 93.
28. P. Newman, *Tracking the Weretiger: Supernatural Man-Eaters of India, China and Southeast Asia* (Jefferson, North Carolina: McFarland, 2012), p. 31.
29. J. Cressey, 'Making a Splash in the Pacific: Dolphin and Whale Myths and Legends of Oceania', *Rapa Nui Journal*, 12:3 (September 1998), 75–84.
30. G. E. Evans and D. Thomson, *The Leaping Hare* (London: Faber & Faber, 2017), p. 130.
31. Sax, *Avian Illuminations*, p. 88.
32. J. D. Forbes, *Columbus and Other Cannibals*, revised edn (New York: Seven Stories Press, 2008), pp. 2–4.
33. L. Hogan, *The Radiant Lives of Animals* (Boston, Massachusetts: Beacon Press, 2020), p. 33.
34. R. K. Nelson, *Make Prayers to the Raven* (Chicago: University of Chicago Press, 1983), p. 17.
35. Sax, *Avian Illuminations*, p. 122.

15: Spiderling, Chickadee, Finch and Friends

1. D. Rößler, 'Regularly Occurring Bouts of Retinal Movements Suggest an REM Sleep-like State in Jumping Spiders', *Proceedings of the National Academy of Science*, 199:33 (8 August 2022). doi: 10.1073/pnas.2204754119.
2. B. Handwerk, 'Animals Dream Too', *National Geographic* (2 November 2022).
3. Handwerk, 'Animals Dream Too'.
4. Handwerk, 'Animals Dream Too'.

5. K. J. Wu, 'Zebra Finches Dream a Little of Melody', *Smithsonian* (1 August 2018).
6. R. Kemeny, 'Do Octopuses Dream?', *National Geographic* (24 May 2023).
7. E. Kohn, 'How Dogs Dream: Amazonian Natures and the Politics of Trans-species Engagement', *American Ethnologist*, 34:1 (2007), 3–24.
8. A. Beck and A. Katcher, *Between Pets and People* (West Lafayette, Indiana: Purdue University Press, 1996), pp. 87–8.
9. J. Matthews, *The Celtic Shaman* (Shaftesbury: Element Books, 1991), p. 146.
10. Beck and Katcher, *Between Pets and People*, p. 72.
11. M. Schredl and M. Blagrove, 'Animals in Dreams of Children, Adolescents, and Adults: The UK Library Study', *Imagination, Cognition and Personality*, 41:1 (2021), 87–104. doi: 10.1177/0276236620960634.
12. Rima Staines, *Anja in the Horse Chestnut*, watercolour on paper (2010), www.rimastaines.com.
13. M. Eliade, *Myths, Dreams and Mysteries* (New York: Harper and Row, 1960), p. 61.
14. J. Lame Deer and R. Erdoes, *Lame Deer, Seeker of Visions: The Life of a Sioux Medicine Man* (New York: Touchstone, 1973), pp. 12–15.
15. L. Standing Bear, *Land of the Spotted Eagle* (Lincoln, Nebraska: University of Nebraska Press, 1978), pp. 203–5.
16. G. Reichel-Dolmatoff, *Rainforest Shamans: Essays on the Tukano Indians of the Northwest Amazon* (Totnes: Themis Books, 1997), p. 169.
17. A. L. Podberscek, E. S. Paul and J. A. Serpell (eds), *Companion Animals and Us: Exploring the Relationships Between People and Pets* (Cambridge: Cambridge University Press, 2005), pp. 113–14.
18. Standing Bear, *Land of the Spotted Eagle*, pp. 203–5.
19. F. B. Linderman, *Plenty-Coups: Chief of the Crows* (Lincoln, Nebraska: University of Nebraska Press, 1962), p. 28.
20. Linderman, *Plenty-Coups*, p. 66.
21. Matthews, *The Celtic Shaman*, pp. 59–63.
22. Standing Bear, *Land of the Spotted Eagle*, pp. 203–5.
23. Standing Bear, *Land of the Spotted Eagle*, pp. 143–4.
24. Standing Bear, *Land of the Spotted Eagle*, pp. 218–19.
25. K. Cohen, *Honoring the Medicine* (New York: Ballantine Books, 2006), p. 54.
26. Cohen, *Honoring the Medicine*, p. 57.
27. M. Pomedli, *Living with Animals: Ojibwe Spirit Powers* (Toronto: University of Toronto Press, 2014), p. 175.
28. Cohen, *Honoring the Medicine*, p. 60.
29. Pomedli, *Living with Animals*, p. 13.

30. Pomedli, *Living with Animals*, pp. 89–91.
31. G. Reichel-Dolmatoff, *The Forest Within: The World-View of the Tukano Amazonian Indians* (Totnes: Themis Books, 1996), p. 42.

16: Shifting the Shape of the Mind

1. A. P. Elkin, 'The Rainbow-Serpent Myth in North-West Australia', *Oceania*, 1:3 (1930), 349–52, http://www.jstor.org/stable/40327333.
2. H. Toner, 'Octopus Legends and Urban Myths', PBS website (1 October 2019).
3. P. Vitebsky, *Shamanism* (Norman, Oklahoma City: University of Oklahoma Press, 2001), p. 58.
4. J. Lame Deer and R. Erdoes, *Lame Deer, Seeker of Visions: The Life of a Sioux Medicine Man* (New York: Touchstone, 1973), p. 165.
5. Vitebsky, *Shamanism*, p. 92.
6. Lame Deer and Erdoes, *Lame Deer, Seeker of Visions*, p. 192.
7. T. Kpomassie, *Michel the Giant* (Dublin: Penguin Classics, 2022), pp. 31–2.
8. M. Pomedli, *Living with Animals: Ojibwe Spirit Powers* (Toronto: University of Toronto Press, 2014), p. 7.
9. J. Matthews, *The Celtic Shaman* (Shaftesbury: Element Books, 1991), p. 117.
10. T. Fischer, L. C. Cory, K. Carr and S. Kwi, *Animal Music: Sound and Song in the Natural World*, ed. G. Kreens (London: Strange Attractor Press, 2015), p. 9.
11. M. Eliade, *Shamanism: Archaic Techniques of Ecstasy* (London: Arkana, 1989), p. 230.
12. C. Solomon, 'The Sound of History: Mescaline, Music, and Terror', *Pacific Standard* (24 July 2012).
13. G. Anderson, *Bushman Rock Art* (Cape Town: Art Publishers, 1990), p. 23.
14. M. Guenther, 'Animals in Bushman Thought, Myth and Art', in *Hunters and Gatherers 2: Property, Power and Ideology*, ed. T. Ingold, D. Riches and J. Woodburn (Oxford: Berg, 1988), pp. 192–202.
15. B. Lopez, *Of Wolves and Men* (New York: Scribner, 2004), pp. 111–12.
16. R. K. Nelson, *Make Prayers to the Raven* (Chicago: University of Chicago Press, 1983), p. 29.
17. F. B. Linderman, *Plenty-Coup: Chief of the Crows* (Lincoln, Nebraska: University of Nebraska Press, 1962), pp. 258–65.
18. J. Vaillant, *The Tiger: A True Story of Vengeance and Survival* (London: Sceptre, 2010), p. 131.
19. Vitebsky, *Shamanism*, p. 23.
20. Sahil Nijhawan, pers. comm. (23 September 2022).

21. Eliade, *Shamanism*, p. 8.
22. J. M. Lockhart, *Raptor: A Journey Through Birds* (London: Fourth Estate, 2016), p. 26.
23. P. Matthiessen, *The Birds of Heaven: Travels with Cranes* (London: Vintage, 2003), p. 17.
24. N.-A. Valkeapää, *The Sun, My Father*, 2nd edn (Guovdageaidnu/Kautokeino, Samiland: DAT, 2003), poem 119.
25. N.-A. Valkeapää, *Trekways of the Wind* (Guovdageaidnu, Norway: DAT, 1994), p. 147.
26. E. Holloway (ed.), *The Uncollected Poetry and Prose of Walt Whitman* (New York: Doubleday, 1921), pp. 11 and 64–5.
27. Pascale Petit, pers. comm. (15 December 2022).
28. Ted Hughes interviewed by T. Pero, 'Poet, Pike and a Pitiful Grouse', *Guardian* (8 January 1999).
29. A. Ginsberg, 'The Lion for Real', in *Howl and Other Poems* (San Francisco: City Lights Books, 1958).
30. J. Hirshfield, *Nine Gates: Entering the Mind of Poetry* (New York: HarperCollins, 1997), pp. 156–7.
31. S. Smith, 'The Photograph', in *A Good Time Was Had by All* (London: Jonathan Cape, 1937).
32. G. Reichel-Dolmatoff, *Rainforest Shamans: Essays on the Tukano Indians of the Northwest Amazon* (Totnes: Themis Books, 1997), p. 177.
33. Reichel-Dolmatoff, *Rainforest Shamans*, p. 48.

Select Bibliography

Abram, D., *Becoming Animal* (New York: Pantheon, 2010).
Ackerman, J., *The Genius of Birds* (London: Corsair, 2016).
Anderson, G., *Bushman Rock Art* (Cape Town: Art Publishers, 1990).
Arbib, M. (ed.), *Language, Music and the Brain: A Mysterious Relationship* (Cambridge, Massachusetts: MIT Press, 2012).
Bachelard, G., *The Poetics of Space* (Paris: Presses universitaires de France, 1958).
Bachelard, G., *Air and Dreams: An Essay on the Imagination of Movement* (Dallas: Dallas Institute Publications, 1988).
Bearzi, M., *Dolphin Confidential: Confessions of a Field Biologist* (Chicago: Chicago University Press, 2012).
Beck, A., and Katcher, A., *Between Pets and People* (West Lafayette, Indiana: Purdue University Press, 1996).
Becker, M., and Morton, D., *The Healing Power of Pets* (New York: Hyperion, 2002).
Bekoff, M., *Minding Animals: Awareness, Emotions, and Heart* (New York: Oxford University Press, 2003).
Bekoff, M., *The Emotional Lives of Animals* (Novato, California: New World Library, 2007).
Bekoff, M., 'Animal Emotions, Wild Justice and Why They Matter: Grieving Magpies, a Pissy Baboon, and Empathic Elephants', *Emotion, Space and Society*, 2:2 (2009), 82–5.
Bekoff, M., and Pierce, J., *Wild Justice* (Chicago: University of Chicago Press, 2009).
Blancou, J., Chomel, B. B., Belotto, A., and Meslin, F. X., 'Emerging or Re-emerging Bacterial Zoonoses: Factors of Emergence, Surveillance and Control', *Veterinary Research*, 36 (2005), 507–22.

Select Bibliography

Bledsoe, B., 'The Significance of the Bear Ritual Among the Sami and Other Northern Cultures', University of Texas, https://www.laits.utexas.edu/sami/diehtu/siida/religion/bear.htm (accessed 14 October 2024).

Bridle, J., *Ways of Being* (London: Allen Lane, 2022).

Briggs, J., *Never in Anger: Portrait of an Eskimo Family* (Cambridge, Massachusetts: Harvard University Press, 1970).

Brightman, M., Grotti, V. E., and Ulturgasheva, O. (eds), *Animism in Rainforest and Tundra: Personhood, Animals, Plants and Things in Contemporary Amazonia and Siberia* (New York: Berghahn Books, 2014).

Brooks, D., *Animal Dreams* (Sydney: Sydney University Press, 2021).

Brum, E., *Banzerio Òkòtó: The Amazon as the Centre of the World* (London: The Indigo Press, 2023).

Bullough, T., *Sarn Helen: A Journey Through Wales, Past, Present and Future* (London: Granta, 2023).

Burkert, W., *Creation of the Sacred* (Cambridge, Massachusetts: Harvard University Press, 1998).

Burnside, J., *Aurochs and Auks* (Bedminster: Little Toller Books, 2021).

Butlin, G. (ed.), *The Sniff*, 21 (May/June 2022), Medical Detection Dogs magazine.

Cajete, G., *Look to the Mountain: An Ecology of Indigenous Education* (Durango, Colorado: Kivaki Press, 1994).

Caras, R. A., *A Dog is Listening* (New York: Galahad Books, 1998).

Clark, J. D., *Beastly Folklore* (Metuchen, New Jersey: Scarecrow Press, 1968).

Clark, K., *Animals and Men: Their Relationships as Reflected in Western Art from Prehistory to Present Day* (New York: William Morrow, 1977).

Coates, M., *Journey to the Lower World: A Shamanic Performance by Marcus Coates After a Traditional Siberian Yakut Ritual for the Residents of Sheil Park, Liverpool, in January 2003*, ed. A. Finlay (Newcastle-upon-Tyne: Platform Projects and Morning Star, 2005).

Cochrane, A., and Callen, K., *Dolphins and Their Power to Heal* (London: Bloomsbury, 1992).

Cohen, K., *Honoring the Medicine* (New York: Ballantine Books, 2006).

Coleman, L., *The Puma Years* (New York: Little A, 2011).

Colling, S., *Animal Resistance in the Global Capitalist Era* (East Lansing: Michigan State University Press, 2021).

Coulehan, J., 'Navajo Indian Medicine: Implications for Healing', *Journal of Family Practice*, 10:1 (1980), 55–61.

Cox, L., *Swimming to Antarctica* (New York: Knopf, 2004).

Cressey, J., 'Making a Splash in the Pacific: Dolphin and Whale Myths and Legends of Oceania', *Rapa Nui Journal*, 12:3 (September 1998), 75–84.

Select Bibliography

Cunningham, D., *Soundings* (London: Virago Press, 2022).

Davis, W., *The Wayfinders: Why Ancient Wisdom Matters in the Modern World* (Toronto: House of Anansi Press, 2009).

De Waal, F., *The Age of Empathy: Nature's Lessons for a Kinder Society* (London: Souvenir Press, 2011).

De Waal, F., *Are We Smart Enough to Know How Smart Animals Are?* (London: Granta, 2016).

De Waal, F., *Mama's Last Hug: Animal Emotions and What They Teach Us About Ourselves* (London: Granta, 2020).

Delorme, G., *Deer Man: Seven Years in the Forest* (London: Hachette, 2022).

Derrida, J., *The Animal That Therefore I Am*, ed. M. Mallet (New York: Fordham University Press, 2008).

Dillard, A., *Pilgrim at Tinker Creek* (Norwich: Canterbury Press, 2011).

Dobbs, H., *Journey into Dolphin Dreamtime* (London: Jonathan Cape, 1992).

Dobbs, H., *Dolphin Healing* (London: Judy Piatkus, 2000).

Donaldson, S., and Kymlicka, W., *Zoopolis: A Political Theory of Animal Rights* (Oxford: Oxford University Press, 2013).

Doolittle, E., 'Crickets in the Concert Hall: A History of Animals in Western Music', *Transcultural Music Review*, 12 (2008).

Dosa, D., *Making Rounds with Oscar: The Extraordinary Gift of an Ordinary Cat* (New York: Hyperion, 2010).

Dyer, A., *Seeing Animals* (Cambridge: The Lutterworth Press, 2019).

Eliade, M., *Shamanism: Archaic Techniques of Ecstasy* (London: Arkana, 1989).

Erdrich, L., *The Night Watchman* (New York: Hachette, 2020).

Evans, G. E., and Thomson, D., *The Leaping Hare* (London: Faber & Faber, 2017).

Everett, D., *Don't Sleep, There are Snakes: Life and Language in the Amazonian Jungle* (London: Profile Books, 2008).

Federici, S., *Caliban and the Witch: Women, the Body and Primitive Accumulation* (Brooklyn: Autonomedia, 2004).

Fischer, T., Cory, L. C., Carr, K., and Kwi, S., *Animal Music: Sound and Song in the Natural World*, ed. G. Kreens (London: Strange Attractor Press, 2015).

Forbes, J. D., *Columbus and Other Cannibals*, revised edn (New York: Seven Stories Press, 2008).

Fouts, R., and Mills, S. T., *Next of Kin: What Chimpanzees Have Taught Me About Who We Are* (New York: William Morrow, 1997).

Franklin, A., *Animals and Modern Cultures: A Sociology of Human–Animal Relations in Modernity* (London: Sage Publications, 1999).

Froling, J., 'Service Dog Tasks for Psychiatric Disabilities', Sterling Service Dogs, Michigan, (1998).

Select Bibliography

Fuller, A., *Fi* (London: Jonathan Cape, 2024).
Gaffney, G., *Half Broke* (New York: W. W. Norton, 2020).
Giddens, A., *Modernity and Self-Identity* (Cambridge: Polity, 1991).
Giggs, R., *Fathoms: The World in the Whale* (London: Scribe UK, 2020).
Gilbert, W., and Warner, S. L., *The Portrait of a Tortoise* (London: Virago Press, 1981).
Goodall, J., and Peterson, D., *Visions of Caliban: On Chimpanzees and People* (Athens, Georgia: University of Georgia Press, 1993).
Grandin, T., 'Do Animals and People with Autism Have True Consciousness?', *Evolution and Cognition*, 8 (2002), 241–8.
Grandin, T., and Johnson, C., *Animals in Translation* (London: Bloomsbury, 2006).
Grandin, T., and Johnson, C., *Making Animals Happy* (London: Bloomsbury, 2009).
Graves, R., *The White Goddess*, 2nd edn (London: Faber & Faber, 1961).
Guest, C., *Daisy's Gift* (London: Virgin Books, 2017).
Gumbs, A. P., *Undrowned: Black Feminist Lessons from Marine Mammals* (Oakland, California: AK Press, 2020).
Haraway, D., *The Companion Species Manifesto: Dogs, People, and Significant Otherness* (Chicago: Prickly Paradigm Press, 2003).
Hare, B., and Woods, V., *Survival of the Friendliest: Understanding Our Origins and Rediscovering Our Common Humanity* (London: Oneworld, 2020).
Harrell, S., and Yongxiang, L., 'The History of the History of the Yi, Part II', *Modern China*, 29:3 (2003), 362–96.
Hearne, V., *Adam's Task: Calling Animals by Name* (New York: Skyhorse Publishing, 2007).
Henderson, C., *The Book of Barely Imagined Beings* (London: Granta, 2012).
Henderson, C., *A Book of Noises: Notes on the Auraculous* (London: Granta, 2023).
Henley, T., *Rediscovery: Ancient Pathways, New Directions* (Edmonton, Canada: Lone Pine Publishing, 1996).
Hirshfield, J., *Nine Gates: Entering the Mind of Poetry* (New York: HarperCollins, 1997).
Hogan, L., *Dwellings* (New York: W. W. Norton, 2007).
Hogan, L., *The Radiant Lives of Animals* (Boston: Beacon Press, 2020).
Holloway, E. (ed.), *The Uncollected Poetry and Prose of Walt Whitman* (New York: Doubleday, 1921).
Horowitz, A., *Inside of a Dog* (New York: Scribner, 2012).
Hosey, G., and Melfi, V. (eds), *Anthrozoology: Human–Animal Interactions in Domesticated and Wild Animals* (Oxford: Oxford University Press, 2019).

Select Bibliography

Howell-Jones, G., *Do Not Call the Tortoise* (Hay-on-Wye: The Cyrus Press, 2022).
Hribal, J., *Fear of the Animal Planet: The Hidden History of Animal Resistance* (Petrolia, California: CounterPunch, 2010).
Hughes, T., *Wales's Best One Hundred Churches* (Bridgend: Seren, 2007).
Hunter, D., and Sawyer, C., 'Blending Native American Spirituality with Individual Psychology in Work with Children', *Journal of Individual Psychology*, 62 (2006).
Hurn, S., *Humans and Other Animals: Cross-Cultural Perspectives on Human–Animal Interactions* (London: Pluto Press, 2012).
Isaacson, R., *The Healing Land* (London: Fourth Estate, 2002).
Isaacson, R., *The Horse Boy* (London: Penguin, 2010).
Isaacson, R., *The Long Ride Home* (London: Penguin, 2014).
Jašarević. L., *Beekeeping in the End Times* (Bloomington: Indiana University Press, 2024).
Jayne, W. A., *The Healing Gods of Ancient Civilizations* (New York: University Books, 1962).
Jensen, L., *Your Wild and Precious Life: On Grief, Hope and Rebellion* (Edinburgh: Canongate, 2024).
Jíménez, J. R., *Platero and I* (Lincoln, Nebraska: iUniverse.com, 2000).
Johnson, R. S., *Messiaen* (Berkeley, California: University of California Press, 1975).
Karsh, E. B., and Turner, D. C., 'The Human–Cat Relationship', in *The Domestic Cat: The Biology of Its Behaviour*, ed. D. C. Turner and P. Bateson (Cambridge: Cambridge University Press, 1988).
Kast, V., *Through Emotions to Maturity: Psychological Readings of Fairytales* (New York: Fromm International, 1993).
Katz, R., *Boiling Energy: Community Healing Among the Kalahari !Kung* (Cambridge, Massachusetts: Harvard University Press, 1982).
Keenan, B., *An Evil Cradling* (London: Vintage, 1993).
Kimmerer, R. W., *Braiding Sweetgrass* (London: Penguin, 2020).
King, B. J., *How Animals Grieve* (Chicago: University of Chicago Press, 2013).
Kpomassie, T., *Michel the Giant* (Dublin: Penguin Classics, 2022).
Krause, B., *The Great Animal Orchestra* (New York: Hachette, 2013).
Krause, B., *The Power of Tranquility in a Very Noisy World* (New York: Hachette, 2021).
Kropotkin, P., *Mutual Aid: A Factor of Evolution* (New York: Dover, 2006).
Kruger, K., Trachtenberg, S., and Serpell, J., 'Can Animals Help Humans Heal? Animal-Assisted Interventions in Adolescent Mental Health' (2004), (conference paper).

Select Bibliography

Lame Deer, J., and Erdoes, R., *Lame Deer, Seeker of Visions: The Life of a Sioux Medicine Man* (New York: Touchstone, 1973).

Le Guin, U. K., *Buffalo Gals* (New York: Plume, New American Library, 1987).

LeMaster, J., and Kummings, D. (eds), *Walt Whitman: An Encyclopedia* (New York: Garland Publishing, 1998).

Levinson, B. M., 'Pets and Personality Development', *Psychological Reports*, 42 (1978), 1031–38.

Leyda, J., *The Years and Hours of Emily Dickinson*, Vol. II (New Haven, Connecticut: Yale University Press, 1960).

Liefooghe, A., *Equine-Assisted Psychotherapy and Coaching* (Oxon: Routledge, 2020).

Linderman, F. B., *Plenty-Coups: Chief of the Crows* (Lincoln, Nebraska: University of Nebraska Press, 1962).

Lockhart, J. M., *Raptor: A Journey Through Birds* (London: Fourth Estate, 2016).

London, J., *The Call of the Wild and Selected Stories* (East Rutherford, New Jersey: Signet Classics, 1960).

London, J., *White Fang* (London: William Collins, 2014).

Lopez, B., *Of Wolves and Men* (New York: Scribner, 2004).

Lopez, B., *Horizon* (New York: Knopf, 2019).

Louv, R., *Our Wild Calling* (Chapel Hill, North Carolina: Algonquin Books, 2019).

Lynch, J., *The Broken Heart: The Medical Consequences of Loneliness* (New York: Basic Books, 1978).

Lyon, W., *Black Elk: The Sacred Ways of a Lakota* (New York: HarperCollins, 1991).

McIntyre, R., *The Reign of Wolf 21* (Vancouver: Greystone Books, 2022).

McGinnis, A., Kincaid, A. T., Barrett, M. J., Ham, C., et al., 'Strengthening Animal–Human Relationships as a Doorway to Indigenous Holistic Wellness', *Ecopsychology* (September 2019), 162-73.

Magan, M., *Thirty-Two Words for Field* (Dublin: Gill Books, 2020).

Maitland, S., *Gossip from the Forest* (London: Granta, 2013).

Manning, A., and Serpell, J. (eds), *Animals and Human Society* (London: Routledge, 1994).

Marzluff, J., and Angell, T., *In the Company of Crows and Ravens* (New Haven, Connecticut: Yale University Press, 2005).

Marzluff, J., and Angell, T., *Gifts of the Crow: How Perception, Emotion, and Thought Allow Smart Birds to Behave Like Humans* (New York: Simon & Schuster, 2012).

Masson, J. M., *Dogs Never Lie About Love* (London: Vintage, 1997).

Masson, J. M., *The Pig Who Sang to the Moon* (London: Vintage, 2005).

Select Bibliography

Masson, J. M., and McCarthy, S., *When Elephants Weep* (London: Vintage, 1996).

Masud, N., *A Flat Place* (London: Penguin, 2024).

Matthews, J., *The Celtic Shaman* (Shaftesbury: Element Books, 1991).

Matthiessen, P., *The Birds of Heaven: Travels with Cranes* (London: Vintage, 2003).

Meijer, E., *Animal Languages* (London: John Murray, 2019).

Melson, G. F., *Why the Wild Things Are* (Cambridge, Massachusetts: Harvard University Press, 2001).

Merrifield, A., *The Wisdom of Donkeys* (New York: Bloomsbury, 2010).

Methorst, J., Bonn, A., Marselle, M., Böhning-Gaese, K., et al., 'Species Richness is Positively Related to Mental Health: A Study for Germany', *Landscape and Urban Planning*, 211 (2021), 104084.

Midgley, M., *Animals and Why They Matter* (Harmondsworth, Middlesex: Penguin, 1983).

Monbiot, G., *Regenesis* (London: Penguin, 2022).

Moquin, W., and Van Doren, C., *Great Documents in American Indian History* (New York: Da Capo Press, 1995).

Mort, H., *Never Leave the Dog Behind* (Sheffield: Vertebrate Publishing, 2020).

Moss, C., *Elephant Memories* (Chicago: University of Chicago Press, 2000).

Muggenthaler, E. von, 'The Felid Purr: A Healing Mechanism?', *Journal of the Acoustical Society of America*, 110:5 (2001), 2666.

Mustill, T., *How to Speak Whale: A Voyage into the Future of Animal Communication* (London: HarperCollins, 2022).

Narby, J., and Huxley, F. (eds), *Shamans Through Time* (New York: Jeremy P. Tarcher/Putnam, 2001).

Natterson-Horowitz, B., and Bowers, K., *Zoobiquity* (New York: Vintage, 2013).

Neihardt, J. G., *Black Elk Speaks* (Lincoln, Nebraska: University of Nebraska Press, 1988).

Nelson, R. K., *Make Prayers to the Raven* (Chicago: University of Chicago Press, 1983).

Nelson, R. K., *The Island Within* (New York: Vintage, 1991).

Newman, P., *Tracking the Weretiger: Supernatural Man-Eaters of India, China and Southeast Asia* (Jefferson, North Carolina: McFarland, 2012).

Newton, M., *Savage Girls and Wild Boys: A History of Feral Children* (London: Faber & Faber, 2002).

Nightingale, S., *Granada: The Light of Andalucia* (Boston, Massachusetts: Nicholas Brealey Publishing, 2015).

Nightingale, S., *Touched: Revelations at San Ignacio Lagoon* (Reno, Nevada: Samara Press, forthcoming).

Orwell, G., *Animal Farm* (London: William Collins, 2021).

Select Bibliography

Payne, R., *Among Whales* (New York: Scribner, 1995).

Parton, A., and Parton, S., *Endal: How One Extraordinary Dog Brought a Family Back from the Brink* (London: HarperTrue, 2009).

Petit, P., *Mama Amazonica* (Hexham, Northumberland: Bloodaxe Books, 2017).

Petit, P., *Tiger Girl* (Hexham, Northumberland: Bloodaxe Books, 2020).

Pike, S., *For the Wild: Ritual and Commitment in Radical Eco-Activism* (Oakland, California: University of California Press, 2017).

Podberscek, A. L., Paul, E. S., and Serpell, J. A. (eds), *Companion Animals and Us: Exploring the Relationships Between People and Pets* (Cambridge: Cambridge University Press, 2005).

Pomedli, M., *Living with Animals: Ojibwe Spirit Powers* (Toronto: University of Toronto Press, 2014).

Preece-Kelly, D., *Unleashing the Healing Power of Animals* (Dorchester: Veloce Publishing, 2017).

Prince-Hughes, D., *Songs of the Gorilla Nation: My Journey Through Autism* (New York: Three Rivers Press, 2004).

Radinger, E. H., *The Wisdom of Wolves: How They Think, Plan and Look After Each Other – Amazing Facts About the Animal That is More Like Man Than Any Other* (London: Penguin, 2019).

Reichel-Dolmatoff, G., *The Forest Within: The World-View of the Tukano Amazonian Indians* (Totnes: Themis Books, 1996).

Reichel-Dolmatoff, G., *Rainforest Shamans: Essays on the Tukano Indians of the Northwest Amazon* (Totnes: Themis Books, 1997).

Rivera, M. A., *On Dogs and Dying* (West Lafayette, Indiana: Purdue University Press, 2010).

Robinson, I. (ed.), *The Waltham Book of Human–Animal Interaction: Benefits and Responsibilities of Pet Ownership* (Oxford: Pergamon Press, 1995).

Rockwell, D., *Giving Voice to Bear: North American Indian Rituals, Myths, and Images of the Bear* (Toronto: Roberts Rinehart, 1991).

Rothenberg, D., *Why Birds Sing: A Journey Through the Mystery of Bird Song* (New York: Basic Books, 2005).

Rothenberg, D., *Thousand Mile Song: Whale Music in a Sea of Sound* (New York: Basic Books, 2008).

Rothenberg, D., *Bug Music: How Insects Gave Us Rhythm and Noise* (New York: St Martin's Press, 2013).

Rothenberg, D., *Nightingales in Berlin: Searching for the Perfect Sound* (Chicago: University of Chicago Press, 2019).

Rothenberg, D., *Secret Sounds of Ponds* (New York: Roof Books, 2023).

Select Bibliography

Rothenberg, D., and Ulvaeus, M. (eds), *The Book of Music and Nature* (Middletown, Connecticut: Wesleyan University Press, 2000).

Safina, C., *Beyond Words: What Animals Think and Feel* (London: Souvenir Press, 2016).

Sattin, A., *Nomads: The Wanderers Who Shaped Our World* (London: John Murray, 2022).

Savage-Rumbaugh, S., and Lewin, R., *Kanzi: The Ape at the Brink of the Human Mind* (London: Doubleday, 1994).

Sax, B., *Avian Illuminations: A Cultural History of Birds* (London: Reaktion Books, 2021).

Seeley, T., *Honeybee Democracy* (Princeton: Princeton University Press, 2010).

Serpell, J., *In the Company of Animals: A Study of Human–Animal Relationships* (Oxford: Basil Blackwell, 1986).

Sheldrake, R., *Dogs That Know When Their Owners Are Coming Home* (London: Arrow Books, 2000).

Shepard, P., *The Others: How Animals Made Us Human* (Washington DC: Island Press, 1996).

Silko, L. M., *Ceremony* (New York: Penguin, 1986).

Simard, S., *Finding the Mother Tree* (New York: Knopf, 2021).

Solomon, R., *A Passion for Justice: Emotions and the Origins of the Social Contract* (Boston, Massachusetts: Addison-Wesley, 1990).

Standing Bear, L., *Land of the Spotted Eagle* (Lincoln, Nebraska: University of Nebraska Press, 1978).

Stowe, H., *Move Like Water* (London: Granta, 2023).

Swartz, S. L., *Lagoon Time* (Washington DC: The Ocean Foundation, 2014).

Tedeschi, P., and Jenkins, M. A. (eds), *Transforming Trauma: Resilience and Healing Through Our Connections with Animals* (West Lafayette, Indiana: Purdue University Press, 2019).

Thomson, D., *The People of the Sea* (Edinburgh: Canongate Books, 1996).

Thoreau, H., *On Walden Pond* (1854; Ware: Wordsworth Editions, 1995).

Trommer, R. W., *All The Honey* (Reno, Nevada: Samara Press, 2023).

Vaillant, J., *The Tiger* (London: Sceptre, 2010).

Valkeapää, N., *Trekways of the Wind* (Guovdageaidnu, Norway: DAT, 1994).

Valkeapää, N., *The Sun, My Father*, 2nd edn (Guovdageaidnu/Kautokeino, Samiland: DAT, 2003).

Vitebsky, P., *Shamanism* (Norman, Oklahoma City: University of Oklahoma Press, 2001).

Vitebsky, P., *Reindeer People: Living with Animals and Spirits in Siberia* (London: Harper Perennial, 2005).

Select Bibliography

Waddell, H., *Beasts and Saints* (London: Constable, 1934).
Waterbury, F., 'Bird-Deities in China', *Artibus Asiae*, Supplementum, 10:2 (1952).
Watson, L., *Elephantoms* (New York: W. W. Norton, 2003).
Webb, M., *The Spring of Joy* (Adelaide: Michael Walmer, 2016).
Westermarck, E., *The Origin and Development of Moral Ideas* (London: Macmillan, 1912).
White, T. I., *In Defence of Dolphins: The New Moral Frontier* (Oxford: Blackwell, 2007).
Whitney, J. D., *All My Relations* (Kalispell, Montana: Many Voices Press, 2010).
Wolf, A. H., *A Good Medicine Collection* (Summertown, Tennessee: Book Publishing Company, 1991).
Wynne, W. A., *Yorkie Doodle Dandy, A Memoir* (Denver, Colorado: Top Dog Enterprises, 2012).
Yong, E., *An Immense World: How Animal Senses Reveal the Hidden Realms Around Us* (London: The Bodley Head, 2022).
Young, R., *The Secret Life of Cows: Animal Sentience at Work* (Preston: Farming Books and Videos, 2003).

Index

abandonment 43, 101, 102–4, 124, 151, 193, 194, 255, 306
abuse 49, 50, 54, 55, 208, 306–8
acknowledgement and recognition 36, 37, 38, 75, 76, 90, 120, 165, 278
Addison's disease 112
adoption by animals 101–4, 193, 194
advertising and marketing 247, 283
alerting and giving a Tell 58–61, 94, 95, 108, 111–22, 126, 136–8, 141, 154, 206
alertness 19, 51, 264, 287, 290, 293
alleluia 174, 262
altruism 89, 90
animacy 22, 23, 241, 255, 263
animal helpers 285–90
animal spirits 5, 19, 22, 24, 25, 247, 250, 251, 253, 263, 291, 306
animal trials 243
animal yoga-instructors 130
anti-corruption 219, 220
anxiety and stress 6, 19, 42, 46, 48, 50, 54, 60, 61, 68, 76, 117, 128, 130, 131, 138, 154, 170, 174, 176, 200, 202, 276
apology 191, 192
apothecary animals 124–41
art 241–61; made by animals 251–3
artifice 220, 237, 238

assistance dogs 112–20
autonomy 50, 227, 228
awe 138, 260, 264, 272
ayahuasca 135, 303, 310, 311

balance 130, 132, 133, 198, 204
beauty 99, 159, 160, 172, 177, 178, 204, 226
bees 16, 17, 101, 140, 163–6, 168–70, 177, 179, 180; ordering a death from 142–4; *see also* hive mind
bereavement 32, 144, 149–51, 158, 160, 236, 237
between, the 47–8, 253, 254, 265
beyond, the 264, 265
bipolar 59–60, 65
bird-feather-worthy 184–5
birdsong 18, 138, 139, 171–5, 185, 242, 258, 266, 281, 305
body language 28, 29, 47, 190
bodyguard *see* guardianship
brain injury 253
bullying 50, 184, 207, 208, 209

calling for back-up 115
calmness 29, 46, 48, 50, 52, 60, 138, 283
cancer 105–1, 121, 122, 132, 153

Index

capitalism *see* Götterdämmerung capitalism
care 40, 41, 69, 101, 102, 103, 104, 183
cartoons 248
cave art 258–60, 299
ceremonies of healing 297–9, 310
ceremonies of increase 140
cheating 204, 206, 286, 287
childlessness 35
children's literature 41, 254–5
chivalry 181
Christian tradition 35, 97, 98, 129, 169, 270–72, 273
circadian rhythm *see* rhythms
civilized behaviour 193
closeness 27
Cloud Cuckoo Land 246
coastguard *see* guardianship
collaboration 222–6
collective action 221, 222
collective sickness 250
comedy 5, 7, 8–9, 16, 28, 29, 277
comfort 6, 12, 31, 37, 38, 39, 40, 41, 52, 54, 57, 74, 77, 129, 131, 145, 146, 151, 152, 153, 154, 157, 158, 159, 172, 183, 187, 238, 255, 256, 261, 265, 318
coming of age 290
communication 5, 9, 27–32, 50, 64, 65, 70, 71, 79, 87, 92, 94, 122, 123, 136, 137, 142, 143, 189, 202, 217, 221, 222, 232, 251, 260, 271, 284, 286–9, 304, 317; in writing 254, 268
compassion 40, 41
connections 32, 37, 52, 63, 64, 65, 69, 70, 79, 136, 138, 165, 166, 168, 273, 314
conscience of the world, animals as the 169, 185, 186, 195–7, 203, 286, 287, 294, 295, 318
consensus decision-making 221–4

consent 189, 190
constancy of being 238
constraint 227, 228
contagious wellness 168
coronary heart disease 116, 131, 132
courage 96, 105, 231, 271, 287
courtesy 189–91
cruelty 73, 78, 184, 207, 208, 210, 211, 229, 231–7, 287, 303, 308, 313
cuddling *see* hugging, nuzzling, cuddling and stroking
curiosity 8, 19, 20, 45, 54, 105, 126, 149, 216, 249, 250, 258, 287

daemon-animal 245
dance 262, 263, 264, 265, 267; rain dance 263; waterfall dance 262; *see also* waggle dancing
dead taking animal form 146, 157–60
death-eaters 148, 149
dementia and Alzheimer's disease 130
democracy 219–23, 234
depression 6, 7, 32, 46, 50, 56, 57, 58, 63–79, 96, 128, 132, 149, 174, 227, 272, 287, 296, 306–12
diabetes 2, 111, 112, 113, 128, 167
diagnosis 107, 109, 111, 121, 123, 167, 291
disease detection 105–11, 120–23
dissent 223
diversity 172, 174, 223, 261, 313, 314
divination 268, 271
divinity 22, 126, 127, 129, 168, 169, 224, 242, 265–78
doctoring 60, 62, 105–39, 153, 155, 242, 284, 310, 313, 318
dreams 19, 125, 134, 135, 178, 184, 196, 259, 279–85, 290–95, 303–5, 308, 318
Dreamtime, the 257, 258

362

Index

dying 1, 2, 34, 36, 51, 64, 66, 74, 77, 99, 100, 127, 141–60, 164, 173, 186, 188, 196, 208, 211, 213, 230, 250, 261, 286, 306, 313, 315, 317

edges 26, 27, 28, 35–7, 266
electricity 22–5, 230, 308
emergency 58–61, 83–104
empathy 38, 39, 40, 41, 42, 43, 44, 48, 50, 75, 85–6, 87, 88, 192, 193, 303, 313
End Times 169, 180
enskyment 149
ensoulment 278
enthusiasm 8, 105, 223, 263
epilepsy 2, 113, 128
escape 208, 219, 228–30
ethics. 169, 181–97, 202, 203, 206, 209, 271, 272, 286, 287, 289, 290, 314, 318
etiquette 191
etymology 24, 25, 126, 166, 204, 207
everything 19, 155, 166–8, 170, 216, 273, 294, 312, 314
expertise 223
exuberance 212, 213, 262

fair play 202, 203
fairness and unfairness 200–206
fairy tales and folk tales 9, 10, 101, 281, 285–95, 318
faithfulness 97, 98, 155–7, 242
fertility 125, 126, 172, 241, 247, 257, 258, 277
forest music as medicine 177–9
forgiveness 184, 217, 218
freedom 56, 57, 116, 175, 219, 228–31, 307, 313
friendship 30, 31, 50, 63, 77, 79, 91–3, 150, 182, 183, 189, 190, 198, 199, 206, 214, 217, 218, 226, 228, 254, 277, 289, 291, 304, 305

generosity 54, 184, 185, 186, 195, 205, 215, 226, 228, 230, 287, 314
gentleness 46, 89, 138, 293, 294
gift-giving 198–200
glee 20
gods 265–71, 275–8
good vibes 17, 18
Götterdämmerung capitalism 233, 247, 248, 302
grace 14, 158, 182, 215, 217, 218, 267, 293, 307
gratitude 199, 200, 217
greenness 273
greetings *see* welcome and greetings
guardianship 57, 84, 88–90, 96–103, 111–19, 194–7, 255, 256; bodyguard 83, 84, 87–9; coastguard 89, 90, 96; lifeguard 90, 91; spiritual guardians 147, 148, 273–5
guiding 54, 57, 59, 60, 62, 91–3, 125–7, 134, 136, 137–9, 141–8, 153, 157, 185, 186, 224, 225, 258, 270–72, 281, 283, 284, 286, 288, 291, 293, 296; guides between the living and the dead 142–8, 151–8; ocean guide 91–3; soul guide 143, 144–8, 270–74

happiness 5, 8, 9, 10, 46, 51, 52, 90, 220, 251, 264, 267
harmony 30, 124, 133, 134, 167–70, 180, 204, 293
headaches 58, 117, 130, 131, 132, 297
help, and willingness to 83–104, 224, 225, 230, 286–90, 294
heraldry 243, 244, 246

363

Index

hive mind 222–4
holiness 180, 268, 269, 278
homelessness 76–9
honesty 46, 47, 50, 202, 203, 204, 272, 286, 287
honey scribes 165, 179, 180
hugging, nuzzling, cuddling and stroking 1, 22, 27, 31, 33, 38, 43, 45, 46, 47, 49, 53, 60, 70, 74, 85, 89, 103, 130, 131, 154, 181, 189, 212, 215, 220, 251, 255, 283
humility 185, 272, 304, 313
humour 8, 9

ideas 241, 260
imagination 15, 115, 159, 241, 242, 243, 245, 248, 257, 258, 260, 261, 268, 288, 304, 306, 311
immortality 261, 265, 276, 315
imprisonment 10, 49, 92, 174, 175, 208, 211, 228–31, 237, 238, 282
independence 51, 114, 223
Indigenous understandings 31, 32, 53, 54, 101, 127, 133, 134, 139, 140, 145, 146, 148, 157, 160, 166–8, 170, 173, 175, 183, 185, 186, 195, 209, 225, 234, 257–9, 275, 276, 290–305, 310–12, 314
inequality 202, 219, 220, 286
initiative 58, 95
insect angels 139–41
insight 59, 126, 241, 268, 291, 305
intelligence 24, 25, 58, 59, 86, 94, 95, 107, 120, 149, 182, 197, 224, 235, 253, 260, 288, 292, 293, 312–14
intelligent disobedience 59, 116, 118, 120, 121, 270
interdependence 166, 168, 223, 314, 227
Islamic ecology and the bees 164, 169

jaguar medicine 23, 135, 209, 282, 299, 301, 307–13
jeopardy 96–8
joy 7, 9, 10, 11, 251
judgement 205
justice 198–218, 271, 272, 286, 287; and medicine 205, 286

kindness 41, 46, 89, 90, 101, 102, 103, 111, 184, 187, 193, 204, 255, 287, 289, 293, 309, 318
kissing 33, 125, 198, 215, 216

language 8, 23, 28, 29, 31, 32, 44, 55, 87, 99, 126, 127, 139, 164, 183, 228, 253, 254, 256, 266, 271, 284, 288–91; of the divine 266
laughter 5–8, 294
life 278, 294, 312, 313, 315
life force 8, 23, 24, 148, 172, 173, 247, 273, 301, 308, 309, 310–12
life-saving 63–79, 136, 137, 106–9, 120, 121
lifeguard *see* guardianship
listening 7, 16, 18, 42, 55, 56, 92, 93, 105–9, 118, 121–3, 127, 137, 138, 141, 158, 171–3, 175, 176, 178, 186, 223, 224, 266, 271, 280, 282, 292, 294, 317
literature 253, 254, 261
loneliness 26–44, 51, 63, 77, 78, 237, 286
love 10, 36, 43, 44, 48, 77, 86, 103, 111, 113, 157, 165, 215, 251, 255, 256, 307, 312
loyalty 36, 43, 85, 86, 94, 156, 291
lupification of humanity 182, 183

malaria 111, 135
marvellous, the 49, 112–115, 216, 270

Index

mast cell activation syndrome 117, 118, 119
Master of Animals 195–7, 309
meanness 186, 205, 287
medicine songs 186, 290, 298, 299
medicine stories 281, 285, 286, 288, 290–95
mercy 104, 148, 199, 205, 206
message 18, 60, 61, 75, 93, 99, 108, 115, 118, 141, 143, 158, 202, 220, 225, 246, 289, 290
messengers 120, 139, 146, 158, 224, 243, 246, 253, 265, 266, 267, 268, 284, 286, 304
metaphor 261, 299, 303, 311, 314
midwives for the dying 151–5
mind-body 48, 125, 126, 129, 130, 131, 310
minor ailments 132
moral compass 271, 272
morality dictionary 242
mothering 114
music 8, 99, 100, 106, 122, 138, 146, 170–80, 216, 242, 251, 258, 281, 298, 299, 302, 304; *see also* rhythms
mythic thinking 48, 99, 257, 279, 285

name-giving 249
narcissism 166, 167, 248
natural democracy 234
nature medicine 124, 166–8
needing to be needed 132
neurodiversity 31, 34, 48, 49, 50, 55, 74
non-judgemental interaction 52, 53
nursery rhymes 254
nuzzling *see* hugging, nuzzling, cuddling and stroking

old knowing 285
oneness 269, 270

otherworld 268, 277, 284

Paddington, spirit of 145
panache 246, 287
paramedic service 75, 95, 96, 104, 139, 313
Parkinson's disease 111
peer-review process 223
perseverance 85, 86
pet-keeping 5, 13, 14, 27–35, 37, 44, 66, 67, 68, 71–9, 130, 131, 132, 133, 137, 144, 145, 147, 154–7, 189, 199, 281
pity 84, 101–4, 193, 285, 286
play and playfulness 5, 7, 8, 11–15, 19, 85, 135, 146, 181, 184, 212, 213, 215, 216, 294; wordplay 14–15
poetry 22, 41, 56, 149, 165, 174, 211, 224, 245, 253, 260, 268, 293, 304–9
policing 195–7, 209; policing the police 194, 195
political medicine 219–38
postural tachycardia syndrome 112, 117, 118, 119
prayer 128, 139, 183, 266, 267, 271–3, 278, 290, 298
prescriptions 32, 51, 53, 127, 128
pretending 9, 15, 61, 62
pride 107, 227, 250, 274, 276
prosthetic minds 62
protection 61, 62, 74, 77, 84, 88–92, 97, 98, 100, 102–4, 115, 120, 124, 154, 156, 159, 181, 183–5, 194, 196, 219, 229, 234, 255, 256, 273–5, 277, 290, 292, 293, 298
public health 126, 137, 141
purring 18, 27, 151, 171, 212, 299, 318

qualities, skills and virtues of animals 29, 53, 54, 105, 111, 151–6, 169, 193, 203, 223, 228, 229, 242, 245, 246, 251, 271–3, 275, 291–5, 300

rapid rapport 70, 71
regularity 133
remorse 97, 98, 192
resistance 221, 229, 235–7
revenge 199, 206–11, 217, 233, 309
rhythms: circadian and seasonal 133–4; musical 175, 176–8, 298, 305; of nature 133–4, 176–8, 263
ritual 140, 149, 196, 251, 263, 264, 267, 291, 302
role models 183, 184, 220, 233, 242, 244

sacrifice 96, 97, 100
safety 62, 111–19, 136–8
sanctuary 45, 46, 125, 184
screening 106, 110, 111
search and rescue, emotional and physical 71, 94, 95
seizures 81, 111, 113, 114, 115
self-medication in animals 134, 135
senses 16, 17, 18, 19, 60, 95, 112, 120, 137, 293, 303, 311, 313
sensitivity 16, 40, 46, 47, 48, 70, 71, 106, 119, 125, 126, 127, 136, 159, 196, 203, 261, 264, 276, 292, 295, 303, 304, 307, 310
service, dogs in 38, 57–62, 116
shamanism 127, 184, 186, 196, 197, 247, 248, 250, 259, 269, 288, 296–315
shapeshifting 21, 160, 170, 183, 247, 254, 259, 276, 299–308, 312, 314, 315
sharing 198, 199
shit, taking a synchronized 221
skills of animals *see* qualities, skills and virtues of animals
sky maps 257
slaughter 209, 213, 214, 217, 218, 229, 230, 313

sleep 27, 28, 58, 59, 95, 96, 112, 113, 117, 119, 125, 132, 133, 145, 146, 153, 164, 170, 171, 244, 255, 274, 277, 279–85, 293
sleeplessness 32, 58, 111, 112, 117
smelling 16, 18, 19, 45, 46, 62, 94, 105–11, 115, 116, 120, 129, 137, 150, 170, 210, 282, 311
snake remedies 125, 127, 128
social interaction 37, 38, 51, 79
socializing us 216, 217
soft fascination 56, 283
songlessness 141, 175
Songlines 258
sounds 6, 7, 16–18, 29, 32, 122, 138, 150, 160, 163, 165, 166, 168–80, 206, 212, 216, 218, 224, 225, 242, 262, 298, 299–301, 305; *see also* rhythms
soundscape healing 175, 176
speech and silence 54–6, 286
spirit 145–7, 159, 242
spiritual guardians *see* guardianship
spirituality 262–78, 289, 291
stroking *see* hugging, nuzzling, cuddling and stroking
substitute children 34, 35
substitute siblings 35
Sufi lore 169
suicide 50, 58, 63–79, 114, 272, 310, 312
symbolism of animals 9, 31, 126, 128, 146, 159, 160, 187, 193, 219, 231, 241–6, 251, 267, 268, 271, 273, 274, 280, 293, 295, 297, 302, 308
sympathetic magic 247

talisman 256, 274
teddy bears 114, 145, 146, 255, 256
telling the bees 144
tenderness 88, 89, 100, 181, 182, 187

Index

therapy with animals 45–62
thinking, good 260
thresholds 26, 36, 37, 60
totalitarianism 237
touch 27, 28
tickling 6
time 10, 19, 21, 22, 69, 71, 78, 79, 145, 213, 257, 258, 263–5, 294
totem animal 139, 140, 149, 253, 274, 307
transcendence 269, 273, 278
transformation 23, 32, 67, 77, 141, 160, 172, 173, 179, 183, 184, 247, 259, 260, 283, 288, 296–9, 305–8, 312–15
trauma 50, 54, 58, 61, 68, 69, 70, 83, 97, 128, 170, 184, 235, 251, 306–8
Trickster 249, 251, 280, 287, 288, 293
truth 60, 85, 98, 99, 102, 141, 173, 185, 186, 193, 222, 223, 227, 243, 245, 247, 261, 272, 278, 286, 287, 292, 309
turning, by shamans and poets 296–7, 305–6, 310
twats, total bunch of 226–7, 233
twilight barking 115

ugliness 204, 286, 287
Umwelt 17
understanding 30, 143, 289, 291

unforgetting 99, 188, 282, 289
unwashedness 45
Ur-Imagination 259, 261

vigil 150, 155–7
virtues of animals *see* qualities, skills and virtues of animals
vision quest 290–92
vitality 5–25, 173, 241, 248, 249, 250, 273, 306, 310
vocation 153, 308, 309

waggle dancing 222, 223
warmth and coldness 27, 101, 133, 199
ways of knowing 99, 126, 127, 271, 303, 304
welcome and greetings 26, 36, 37, 75, 182, 264, 274
welfare state 182
werewolves 184, 250, 301
wholeness 44, 166–8, 178, 273, 314
wingedness 49, 157, 266, 268, 303, 304
wisdom 35, 54, 99, 126, 141, 185, 197, 224, 242, 246, 260, 269, 272, 274, 275, 289, 291–3, 302
what three words? 312
without what? 139
wordplay *see* play and playfulness

In Thanks

For their buoyant enthusiasm and faith in this book and for their wise guidance, my deep thanks to my editor, Simon Prosser, and my agent, Jessica Woollard. For their judicious, graceful intelligence in editing and copy-editing, my gratitude to Ruby Fatimilehin and Caroline Pretty. For comments both gentle and incisive, I would like to thank Jan Parker and Mike Parker, this book's early readers, who gave it their exquisite attention.

I have sought permission from DAT publishers, Guovdageaidnu/Kautokeino, Samiland, to quote from Nils-Aslak Valkeapää's *Trekways of the Wind* (1994) and *The Sun, My Father* (2003). For funding help, I am so grateful to the Royal Literary Fund, the Society of Authors and the Authors' Foundation.

For sublimely idiosyncratic generosity, I would like to thank John Lister-Kaye and Rory MacLean. For the invitation of a lifetime – to visit the whales – I thank Steven Nightingale and Elizabeth Dilly.

For the bees: I would like to pay tribute to the memory of Daphne Shelton and John Burnside.

To Giuliana Becciu, Fran Blockley, Tom Bullough, Laurence Cranmer, Euan Crockett, Moya Crockett, Jules Date, Brian Eno, Gareth Evans, Charles Foster, Celeste Goschen, Jenny, Jonathan, David and Timothy Griffiths, Niall Griffiths, Rachel Hembery, Anna Jenkins, John and Jan Jewkes, Deborah Jones, Suzie Kobrin, Nicoletta Laude, Mel McCree, George Marshall, Thoby Miller, Mariam Motamedi Fraser, Marg Munyard, Ed O'Brien, Clare Patey, Philip Robinson, Anita Roy, Naomi Saville, Hannah Scrase, Gracie Stanley, Buz Thomas, Jen and David Tomkinson, Peredur Tomos, Michael Walling and George Williams, my heartfelt thanks for surrounding me with a kindness carved of solid oak. Your gift of deep listening was the light towards which my thoughts could grow.